Periodontology
at a Glance

Periodontology
at a Glance

Second Edition

Valerie Clerehugh
Emeritus Professor of Periodontology
School of Dentistry
University of Leeds, UK

Aradhna Tugnait
Associate Professor in Restorative Dentistry
School of Dentistry
University of Leeds, UK

Michael R. Milward
Professor of Periodontology
Birmingham Dental School
University of Birmingham, UK

Iain L. C. Chapple
Professor of Periodontology
Birmingham Dental School
University of Birmingham, UK

WILEY Blackwell

This second edition first published 2024
© 2024 John Wiley & Sons Ltd

Edition History
1e, © 2009 Valerie Clerehugh, Aradhna Tugnait and Robert Genco

The right of Valerie Clerehugh, Aradhna Tugnait, Michael R. Milward and Iain L. C. Chapple to be identified as the authors of this work has been asserted in accordance with law.

Registered Offices
John Wiley & Sons, Inc., 111 River Street, Hoboken, NJ 07030, USA
John Wiley & Sons Ltd, The Atrium, Southern Gate, Chichester, West Sussex, PO19 8SQ, UK

For details of our global editorial offices, customer services, and more information about Wiley products visit us at www.wiley.com.

Wiley also publishes its books in a variety of electronic formats and by print-on-demand. Some content that appears in standard print versions of this book may not be available in other formats.

Library of Congress Cataloging-in-Publication Data
Names: Clerehugh, Valerie, author. | Tugnait, Aradhna, author. | Milward,
    Michael R., author. | Chapple, Iain L. C. (Iain Leslie), author.
Title: Periodontology at a glance / Valerie Clerehugh, Aradhna Tugnait,
    Michael R. Milward, Iain L. C. Chapple.
Other titles: At a glance series (Oxford, England)
Description: Second edition. | Hoboken : Wiley-Blackwell, 2024. | Series:
    At a glance series | Includes bibliographical references and index.
Identifiers: LCCN 2023049868 (print) | LCCN 2023049869 (ebook) | ISBN
    9781118988428 (paperback) | ISBN 9781118988466 (adobe pdf) | ISBN
    9781118988459 (epub)
Subjects: MESH: Periodontal Diseases | Handbook
Classification: LCC RK450.P4 (print) | LCC RK450.P4 (ebook) | NLM WU 49 |
    DDC 617.6/32–dc23/eng/20231214
LC record available at https://lccn.loc.gov/2023049868
LC ebook record available at https://lccn.loc.gov/2023049869

Cover Design: Wiley
Cover Image: Courtesy of Valerie Clerehugh

Set in 9.5/11.5pt MinionPro by Straive, Pondicherry, India

Printed and bound in Great Britain by Bell & Bain Ltd, Glasgow

Contents

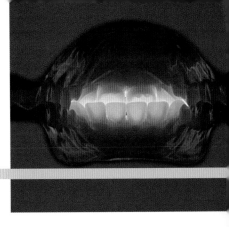

Part 6 Periodontal diseases and periodontal management 117

Preface to the second edition

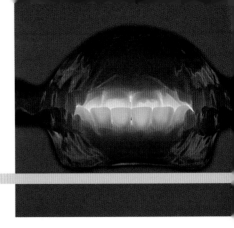

Periodontology, as the specialty of dentistry concerned with diseases of the supporting tissues of the teeth, is an exciting and constantly developing field. Periodontal diseases are widespread. From 1990 to 2019, there was an 8.44% increase in the prevalence rate of severe periodontitis worldwide. In 2022, the World Health Organisation estimated the prevalence of severe periodontitis globally was 19%, with 1.1 billion people affected. As such, any practitioner of dentistry or dental hygiene and therapy will be confronted with patients presenting with periodontal problems on a daily basis. Current research suggests that periodontal diseases are also linked to other general health problems including diabetes mellitus, atherosclerotic cardiovascular diseases, stroke, rheumatoid arthritis, chronic kidney disease, nosocomial respiratory infections, adverse pregnancy outcomes, Alzheimer disease and certain cancers. Thus, periodontal diseases and their management may have effects beyond that of the oral cavity.

In the UK and US, as in other countries, periodontal care is delivered in general dental practice, specialist periodontal practice and the dental hospital setting. Perhaps more than any other area of dentistry at the time of writing, the management of periodontal patients is often achieved by an integrated dental team. The continuing development of the roles of professions complementary to dentistry can only enhance the scope for delivery of effective patient care.

Periodontology at a Glance, 2nd edition, is the latest title in the widely known and popular 'At a Glance' series. After the success of the first edition, we were thrilled and honoured to be approached by Wiley to write this second edition. It is designed to provide a concise and current review of the field of periodontology and peri-implant diseases and conditions and includes the underpinning principles of these subjects and their clinical periodontal applications. It is designed as a study aid and revision guide for students of dentistry, hygiene and therapy. It is also a useful tool for dental practitioners, hygienists and therapists to update their knowledge of this continually developing subject.

While preparing this second edition, we were deeply saddened by the untimely death of our dear friend, colleague and co-editor Professor Robert Genco who was a true inspiration and an international icon in the field of periodontology. However, it is with huge pleasure and delight that we welcome Professor Iain Chapple and Professor Michael Milward as co-editors of this second edition alongside Professor Valerie Clerehugh and Dr Aradhna Tugnait.

In the typical visual 'At a Glance' style, this book uses a two page spread/short chapter format for each topic. Salient information has been distilled from the literature and presented in easy-to-read notes, tables, diagrams and figures. Where teeth are referred to in the text and figures, the following notation is used: UR, upper right quadrant; UL, upper left quadrant; LR, lower right quadrant; and LL, lower left quadrant. The permanent teeth are referred to as '1' (indicating central incisor) to '8' (indicating third molar), to give UR1 as the upper right permanent central incisor and UR8 as the upper right permanent third molar.

The chapters are self-contained and can therefore be read in any order. Cross-referencing will direct the reader to additional relevant chapters in the book. Each chapter ends with a box of key points to present the reader with the essential take-home messages for a particular topic. References and further reading for each chapter are provided in Appendix 5 at the end of the book.

Periodontology at a Glance has been thoroughly updated since the first edition and incorporates the latest 2018 classification findings following the 2017 World Workshop on the Classification of Periodontal and Peri-implant Diseases and Conditions, which was convened jointly by the European Federation of Periodontology (EFP) and the American Academy of Periodontology (AAP) to align and update the classification with current understanding of periodontal and peri-implant diseases and conditions. The book also includes the EFP S3-level treatment guideline and the British Society of Periodontology and Implant Dentistry (BSP) implementation of this for Stages I–III periodontitis.

We have divided our second edition into six parts, each starting with a short overview of content and with its own unique colour code, designed to enhance the visual appeal of the book and facilitate the reader's journey through the different topics: Part 1 provides the core *Foundations*; Part 2 covers *Risk and periodontal diseases* – the four chapters on risk originally authored by Bob Genco have kindly been further updated for this edition by Iain Chapple while retaining the essence of Bob's original texts, for which our heartfelt thanks; Part 3 addresses the steps in *Reaching a periodontal diagnosis and treatment plan*; Part 4 focuses on the *Fundamentals of periodontal patient care* relevant to all patients; Part 5 features *Advanced periodontal patient care: periodontal surgery; dental implants; periodontal-orthodontic interface*; and finally, Part 6 includes a diverse range of pertinent periodontal clinical topics covering *Periodontal diseases and periodontal management*.

We have loved writing the second edition of *Periodontology at a Glance* and we truly hope you enjoy using this book.

From the Editors: Professor Valerie Clerehugh, Dr Aradhna Tugnait, Professor Michael R. Milward and Professor Iain L. C. Chapple.

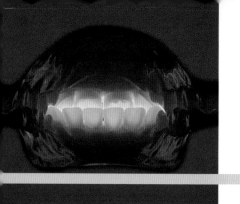

Acknowledgements

We acknowledge the many colleagues who provided figures for *Periodontology at a Glance*:

- Dr Asmaa Al-Taie: Figs 28.7 and 28.8.
- Professor Iain Chapple: Figs 7.2, 7.3a, 7.3b, 7.4, 8.1, 9.4, 32.4, 32.5, 32.6, 32.7, 32.8, 36.2, 39.6 and 41.9.
- Mr James Chesterman: Figs 29.7, 34.6 and 33.8.
- Mr Paul Gregory: Fig. 38.7.
- Mr Paul Franklin: Figs 14.9 and 33.2.
- Dr Margaret Kellett: Fig. 42.3.
- Dr Susan Kindelan: Figs 41.7 and 41.8.
- Professor Phil Marsh: Fig. 4.3.
- Professor Mike Milward: Figs 7.1 and 7.5.
- Mr Peter Nixon: Figs 25.4c, 26.5, 27.3, 28.3, 29.2 and 33.6.
- Mr Jaymit Patel: Fig. 29.3.
- Dr Bob Turner: Fig. 5.1.
- Dr Pip White: Fig 7.3b.
- Dr Simon Wood: Fig. 4.4.
- Ms Victoria Yorke: Fig. 18.6.

We extend our thanks to the Photography Department at Leeds Dental Institute for their expertise. We thank Quintessence for permission to publish the following images in *Periodontology at a Glance*: Fig. 32.2b, Fig. 32.3, Fig. 32.4, Fig. 32.6, Fig. 32.7, Fig. 32.8 and Fig. 38.6b. We acknowledge with thanks the British Society of Periodontology and Implant Dentistry for permission to use the figures in Appendix 3 and 4.

This book was originally inspired in collaboration with our original dear Senior Commissioning Editor, Caroline Connelly. We are very grateful to our current Managing Editor, Bhavya Boopathi, for her help, support and enthusiasm in bringing the book to fruition, to Monica Rogers, before her, for encouraging us to keep our momentum going with our beloved book, and to the wider Wiley team for their help in getting us to our publication goal. We wish to thank Devipriya Somasundaram for taking care of the Permissions for us and Holly Regan-Jones for her meticulous copyediting skills. It has been a joy to work with Adalfin Jayasingh, our Content Refinement Specialist and to see the printed magic he has created from the materials we have supplied him with. Susan Engelken and her team did a splendid job producing our front cover, and the ongoing support and advice from Fraser Dart in his role as Associate Editor has been very much appreciated. A huge amount of hard work has gone into the preparation and production of the second edition of *Periodontology at a Glance* and we acknowledge with gratitude the dedication and craftsmanship of all involved.

Dedications

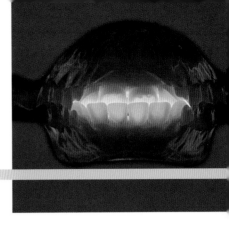

This book is dedicated to the memory of the late Bob Genco, who was our dear friend, colleague and co-editor of the first edition of *Periodontology at a Glance*. He was a true global icon who was revered in the world of periodontology and inspired us all. It was an honour to have known him and work with him. We are immensely proud of his contribution to our book and we look back fondly and with gratitude at his words of encouragement, wisdom and guidance throughout our publication journey together. We salute you, Bob Genco.

Professor Val Clerehugh wishes to thank her daughter Mary and son-in-law Adam, her sister and brother Carolyn and John, stepsons Jonathan and Antony, and all her family, for their love and support in the preparation of this book and for their encouragement, humour and cups of tea along the way. And always remembering Tony, Mum and Dad.

Dr Aradhna Tugnait would like to thank her husband Keith, daughter Adella and son Torrin for the magic of family: its support, delight and safe harbour. She would like to dedicate this book to them and to Mum, Dad and Anuja.

Professor Mike Milward wishes to thank his family, the team at Birmingham and the inspirational colleagues that he has worked with over many years.

Professor Iain Chapple wishes to thank his family and his team in Birmingham for their unwavering support.

Foundations

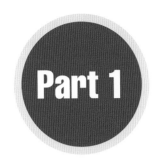

Part 1

Chapters

Overview

Part 1 lays the foundations for the book and covers the basic sciences relevant to periodontology. The chapters begin with the anatomy of the periodontium, then a concise schematic update of the 2018 classification of periodontal diseases, based on the 2017 World Workshop Classification of Periodontal and Peri-implant Diseases and Conditions (Chapter 2), followed by key aspects of periodontal epidemiology (Chapter 3). The next two chapters incorporate updates in our understanding of the role of plaque in the aetiology of periodontal diseases and plaque biofilm microbiology, including the principles of symbiosis and dysbiosis and the latest theories underpinning these (Chapters 4, 5), followed by core aspects of calculus (Chapter 6). The final three chapters in Part 1 present thoroughly updated but concise accounts of host defences, the development of periodontal disease and progression of periodontitis (Chapters 7–9).

1 Anatomy of the periodontium

Figure 1.1 Longitudinal section through part of a tooth showing healthy periodontal tissues.

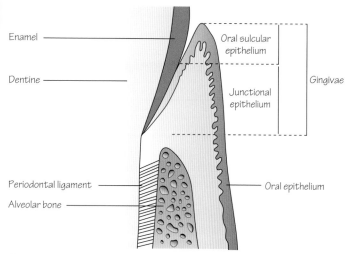

The gingiva is made up of the gingival epithelium and connective tissue.
The gingival epithelium comprises oral epithelium, oral sulcular epithelium and junctional epithelium.

Figure 1.2 Dentogingival fibres, alveolar crest fibres and circular fibres in the gingival connective tissue.

The four principal gingival fibre groups are:
- Dentogingival fibres
- Alveologingival fibres
- Circular fibres (shown in cross section)
- Transeptal fibres

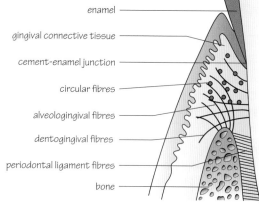

Figure 1.3 Interdental area showing transeptal and circular fibre groups in the gingival connective tissue.

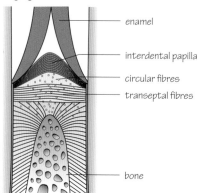

Figure 1.4 The periodontal ligament.

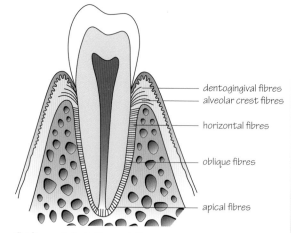

The four periodontal ligament fibre groups are:
- Alveolar crest fibres
- Horizontal fibres
- Oblique fibres
- Apical fibres

Figure 1.5 Bony fenestration and dehiscence.

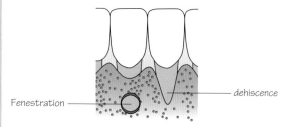

In most situations these areas of missing bone remain undetected as they are covered with soft tissue.
They may be clinically significant if associated with loss of soft tissue resulting in gingival recession (Chapter 32).

Periodontology at a Glance, Second Edition. Valerie Clerehugh, Aradhna Tugnait, Michael R. Milward, and Iain L. C. Chapple.
© 2024 John Wiley & Sons Ltd. Published 2024 by John Wiley & Sons Ltd.

The periodontal tissues form the supporting structures of the teeth. The principal components of the periodontium are shown in Fig. 1.1:
- Gingivae (including epithelium and connective tissue).
- Periodontal ligament.
- Cementum.
- Alveolar bone.

Gingivae

The gingivae in health are pink and firm with a knife-edge appearance, scalloped around the teeth. In certain ethnic groups the gingivae may be pigmented. In health, the gingival margin is a few millimetres coronal to the cement–enamel junction. The gingival sulcus (or crevice) is a shallow groove which may be between 0.5 and 3 mm in depth around a fully erupted tooth. The gingival tissues are keratinised and appear paler pink than sites of non-keratinised oral epithelium.

Gingival epithelium

The gingival epithelium comprises (Fig. 1.1):
- Oral epithelium (OE).
- Oral sulcular epithelium (SE).
- Junctional epithelium (JE).
The gingival sulcus is lined by SE and JE.

Oral epithelium
- The OE is an orthokeratinised, stratified, squamous epithelium.
- Surface cells lose their nuclei and are packed with the protein keratin.
- It presents an impermeable physical barrier to oral bacteria.
The basal layer of epithelial cells is thrown up into folds overlying the supporting connective tissue. These folds increase the surface area of contact between the epithelium and connective tissue and are known as rete ridges or rete pegs.

Oral sulcular epithelium
- There are no rete ridges.
- Cells are keratinised but still have nuclei (parakeratinised).

Junctional epithelium
- The JE forms a specialised attachment to the tooth via:
  - a hemidesmosomal layer within the JE cells;
  - a basal lamina produced by the epithelial cells.
- The JE is non-keratinised and has a very fast turnover of cells (2–6 days compared to 1 month for OE).
- The most apical part of the JE lies at the cement-enamel junction in health.
- The JE at its widest point is 20–30 cells thick coronally.
- The JE tapers until it is only one cell in width apically.
- The JE is permeable with wide intercellular spaces through which cells and substances can migrate (such as bacterial toxins or host defence cells).
- Migration of the JE from its position in health apically onto the root cementum indicates a loss of periodontal attachment and progression to the disease state of periodontitis.

Gingival connective tissue

The gingival connective tissue (or lamina propria) is made up of collagen fibre bundles called gingival fibres, around which lie ground substance, fibroblasts, blood and lymph vessels and neural tissues. The four fibre groups are shown in Figs 1.2 and 1.3.

Periodontal ligament

The periodontal ligament forms the attachment between the cementum and alveolar bone. It is a richly vascular connective tissue within which lie bundles of collagen fibres; these are divided into four groups based on their position (Fig. 1.4).

Within the ligament are mechanoreceptors that provide sensory input for jaw reflexes. Cells from the periodontal ligament are involved in the formation and remodelling of alveolar bone and cementum. The periodontal ligament acts to dissipate masticatory forces to the supporting alveolar bone and its width, height and quality determine a tooth's mobility.

Cementum

Cementum is a mineralised tissue overlying the root dentine. It does not undergo physiological remodelling but is continuously deposited throughout life. Cementum is classified into two types:
- Acellular.
- Cellular.

Acellular cementum

Acellular cementum forms on root dentine during root formation and tooth eruption. Fibres inserted from the periodontal ligament are mineralized within the cementum and are known as Sharpey's fibres and are abundant in acellular cementum.

Cellular cementum

Cellular cementum lies over the acellular cementum. It contains cells called cementocytes which lie in lacunae. The cellular cementum layer is thicker in the apical region of the root where it is between 0.2 and 1 mm thick.

Alveolar bone

- The walls of the sockets are lined with a layer of dense bone called compact bone, which also forms the buccal and lingual/palatal plates of the jaw bones.
- In between the sockets and the compact jaw bone walls lies cancellous bone that is made up of bony trabeculae.
- The compact bone plates of the jaws are thicker on the buccal aspect of the mandibular molars and thinnest on the labial surface of the mandibular incisors.
The thickness of the compact bone layer is relevant to the choice of local analgesia techniques as the anaesthetic solution passes through bone to reach the nerve supply. The thin bone, particularly in the lower incisor region, can manifest as incomplete bony coverage in the form of fenestrations and dehiscences (Fig. 1.5).

The tooth sockets are lined with compact bone within which the principal fibres of the periodontal ligament are inserted. This area of bone can appear as a dense white line called the lamina dura on a radiograph.

Key points
- Gingivae
  - JE forms the specialised attachment to the tooth
  - The most apical part of JE lies at the cement–enamel junction in health
  - Supported by connective tissue containing collagen fibre bundles
- Periodontal ligament
  - Forms attachment between the cementum and bone
- Cementum
  - Mineralised and deposited continuously
- Alveolar bone
  - Compact and cancellous bone
  - Periodontal ligament fibres inserted into compact bone lining the tooth sockets

2 Classification of periodontal diseases

Box 2.1 World Workshop 2018 Classification of Periodontal and Peri-implant Diseases and Conditions

An up-to-date classification:
- allows the clinician to be aware of the full range of periodontal and peri-implant diseases and conditions that can affect the patient.
- provides a basis for the diagnosis and subsequent management of the patient.

The 2018 classification[1] in Figures 2.1–2.8
- derives from the 2017 World Workshop on the Classification of Periodontal and Peri-implant Diseases and Conditions (Caton *et al*., 2018), which was convened jointly by the European Federation of Periodontology (EFP) and American Academy of Periodontology (AAP)
- replaces the previous 1999 classification scheme (Armitage, 1999).
- was intended to align and update the classification with current understanding of periodontal and peri-implant diseases and conditions.
- comprises three main categories of periodontal diseases and conditions, and includes four categories of peri-implant diseases and conditions that were introduced for the first time (Fig. 2.1).

Figure 2.1 2018 Classification of periodontal and peri-implant diseases and conditions. Source: Adapted from Caton *et al*. (2018).

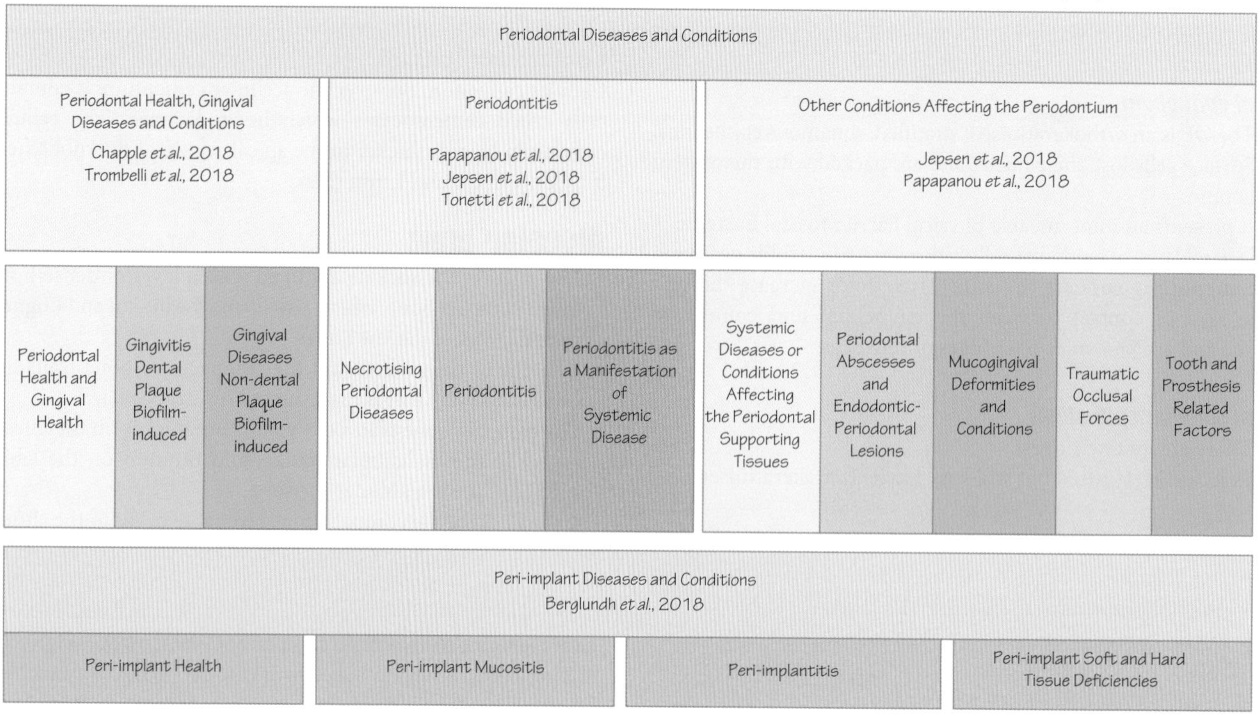
Periodontal Diseases and Conditions
Periodontal Health, Gingival Diseases and Conditions
Chapple et al., 2018
Trombelli et al., 2018
Periodontitis
Papapanou et al., 2018
Jepsen et al., 2018
Tonetti et al., 2018
Other Conditions Affecting the Periodontium
Jepsen et al., 2018
Papapanou et al., 2018
Periodontal Health and Gingival Health
Gingivitis Dental Plaque Biofilm-induced
Gingival Diseases Non-dental Plaque Biofilm-induced
Necrotising Periodontal Diseases
Periodontitis
Periodontitis as a Manifestation of Systemic Disease
Systemic Diseases or Conditions Affecting the Periodontal Supporting Tissues
Periodontal Abscesses and Endodontic-Periodontal Lesions
Mucogingival Deformities and Conditions
Traumatic Occlusal Forces
Tooth and Prosthesis Related Factors
Peri-implant Diseases and Conditions
Berglundh et al., 2018
Peri-implant Health
Peri-implant Mucositis
Peri-implantitis
Peri-implant Soft and Hard Tissue Deficiencies

1 Foot note: Although the World Workshop took place in 2017, the proceedings were published in 2018. To avoid confusion, the official decision was made to call it 'the 2018 classification' henceforth whilst acknowledging it emanated from 'the 2017 World Workshop on the Classification of Periodontal and Peri-implant Diseases and Conditions'. This convention of nomenclature will be adopted throughout Periodontology At A Glance, edition 2.

Periodontology at a Glance, Second Edition. Valerie Clerehugh, Aradhna Tugnait, Michael R. Milward, and Iain L. C. Chapple.

Figure 2.2 (a) 2018 Classification: periodontal health and gingivitis – dental plaque biofilm induced. Source: Adapted from Chapple *et al*. (2018), Table 2. (b) Abridged 2018 classification: gingival diseases: non-dental plaque induced. Source: Adapted from Chapple *et al*. (2018),Table 2. For unabridged version, see Appendix 1.

(a)

Periodontal health:

A. Clinical health on an intact periodontium

B. Clinical gingival health on a reduced periodontium

    i. Stable periodontitis patient

    ii. Non-periodontitis patient

Gingivitis - dental plaque biofilm-induced:

Intact periodontium
Reduced periodontium in non-periodontitis patient
Reduced periodontium in successfully treated periodontitis patient

A. Associated with plaque biofilm alone

B. Mediated by systemic or local risk factors

    i. Systemic risk factors (modifying factors)

        (a) Smoking

        (b) Hyperglycaemia

        (c) Nutritional factors

        (d) Pharmacological agents (prescription, non-prescription and recreational)

        (e) Sex steroid hormones

            Puberty

            Menstrual cycle

            Pregnancy

            Oral contraceptives

        (f) Haematological conditions

    ii. Local risk factors (predisposing factors)

        (a) Dental plaque biofilm retention factors (eg prominent restoration margins)

        (b) Oral dryness

C. Drug-influenced gingival enlargement

(b)

Gingival diseases: non-dental plaque-induced:

A. Genetic/developmental disorders

    i. Hereditary gingival fibromatosis

B. Specific infections

    i. Bacterial origin

    ii. Viral origin

    iii. Fungal origin

C. Inflammatory and immune conditions

    i. Hypersensitivity reactions

    ii. Autoimmune diseases of skin and mucous membranes

    iii. Granulomatous inflammatory lesions (orofacial granulomatoses)

D. Reactive processes

    i. Epulides

E. Neoplasms

    i. Premalignancy

    ii. Malignancy

F. Endocrine, nutritional & metabolic diseases

    i. Vitamin deficiencies

G. Traumatic lesions

    i. Physical/mechanical trauma

    ii. Chemical (toxic) burn

    iii. Thermal insults

H. Gingival pigmentation

    i. Melanoplakia

    ii. Smoker's melanosis

    iii. Drug-induced pigmentation (antimalarials, minocycline)

    iv. Amalgam tattoo

Figure 2.3 (a) 2018 Classification of periodontitis. (b) 2018 Classification of necrotising periodontal diseases (NPDs). Source: Adapted from Papapanou *et al.* (2018), Table 2.

(a)

- Necrotising periodontal diseases
- Periodontitis
- Staging and Grading required
- Periodontitis as a manifestation of systemic disease
- Rare systemic disorders like Papillon-Lefèvre Syndrome with early presentation of severe periodontitis are grouped as 'Periodontitis as a Manifestation of Systemic Disease' and classified by primary systemic disease
- Other systemic conditions eg neoplasms affecting the periodontium independent of plaque-induced periodontitis are grouped as 'Systemic Diseases or Conditions that Affect the Periodontal Supporting Tissues' (see Fig 2.4, also Appendix 2)
- All should follow the primary disease classification according to the International Statistical Classification of Diseases and Related Health Problems (ICD) codes

Note: Clinical cases of periodontitis without characteristics of necrotising periodontitis or that are not a manifestation of systemic disease should be diagnosed as 'periodontitis' and further characterised with Staging and Grading

(b)

Category	Patients	Predisposing conditions	Clinical condition
Necrotising periodontal diseases in chronically, severely compromised patients	In adults	HIV+/AIDS with CD4 counts <200 and detectable viral load	NG, NP, NS, Noma. Possible progression
		Other severe systemic conditions (immunosuppression)	
	In children	Severe malnourishments	
		Extreme living conditions	
		Severe (viral) infections	
Necrotising periodontal diseases in temporarily and/or moderately compromised patients	In gingivitis patients	Uncontrolled factors: stress, nutrition, smoking, habits	Generalised NG. Possible progression to NP
		Previous NPD: residual craters	
		Local factors: root proximity, tooth malposition	Localised NG. Possible progression to NP
	In periodontitis patients	Common predisposing factors for NPD	NG. Infrequent progression
			NP. Infrequent progression

Key: Necrotising Gingivitis (NG); Necrotising Periodontitis (NP), Necrotising Stomatitis (NS)

Figure 2.4 2018 Classification of systemic diseases and conditions that affect the periodontal supporting tissues. Source: Abridged from Jepsen *et al.* (2018), Table 1, which was adapted from Albandar *et al.* (2018). See Appendix 2 for unabridged version and ICD-10 codes.

1. Systemic disorders that have a major impact on loss of periodontal tissues by influencing periodontal inflammation	2. Other systemic disorders that influence the pathogenesis of periodontal diseases	3. Systemic disorders that can result in loss of periodontal tissues independent of periodontitis
1.1 Genetic disorders	Diabetes mellitus Obesity Osteoporosis Rheumatoid arthritis or osteoarthritis Emotional stress and depression Smoking (nicotine dependence) Medications	**3.1 Neoplasms**
1.1.1 Diseases associated with immunologic disorders Eg Down Syndrome; Papillon-Lefèvre Syndrome; Chediak-Higashi Syndrome; severe neutropenia (congenital or cyclic)		Primary neoplastic diseases of the periodontal tissues
1.1.2 Diseases affecting the oral mucosa and gingival tissue		Eg Oral squamous cell carcinoma; odontogenic tumours; or other primary neoplasms of the periodontal tissues
1.1.3 Diseases affecting the connective tissues Eg Ehlers-Danlos Syndromes (types IV, VIII)		Secondary metastatic neoplasms of the periodontal tissues
1.1.4 Metabolic and endocrine disorders Eg Hypophosphatasia		
1.2 Acquired immunodeficiency diseases Eg Acquired neutropenia, HIV infection		**3.2 Other disorders that may affect the periodontal tissues**
1.3 Inflammatory diseases		

Figure 2.5 2018 Classification of other conditions affecting the periodontium: periodontal manifestations of systemic diseases and developmental and acquired conditions. Source: Adapted from Caton *et al.* (2018), Table 4.

Systemic diseases or conditions that affect the periodontal supporting tissues (Albandar et al., 2018, Jepsen et al., 2018)	See Fig 2.4 and Appendix 2
Other periodontal conditions (Papapanou et al., 2018, Herrera et al., 2018)	Periodontal abscesses (Fig 2.6)
	Endodontic-periodontal lesions (Fig 2.7)
Mucogingival deformities and conditions around teeth (Cortellini and Bissada 2018)	Gingival phenotype
	Gingival/soft tissue recession
	Lack of gingiva
	Decreased vestibular width
	Aberrant frenum/muscle position
	Gingival excess
	Abnormal colour
	Condition of exposed root surface
Traumatic occlusal forces (Fan and Caton 2018)	Primary occlusal trauma
	Secondary occlusal trauma
	Orthodontic forces
Prostheses and tooth-related factors that modify or predispose to plaque-induced gingival diseases/periodontitis (Ercoli and Caton 2018)	Localised tooth-related factors (Fig 2.8)
	Localised dental prostheses-related factors (Fig 2.8)

Figure 2.6 2018 Classification of periodontal abscesses based on aetiological factors involved. Source: Adapted from Papapanou *et al.* (2018), Table 4.

Periodontal abscess in periodontitis patients (in a pre-existing periodontal pocket)	Acute exacerbations	Untreated periodontitis	
		Non-responsive to therapy periodontitis	
		Supportive periodontal therapy (SPT)	
	After treatment	Post-Professional Mechanical Plaque Removal (PMPR)	
		Post-surgery	
		Post-medications	Systemic antimicrobials Other drugs: nifedipine
Periodontal abscess in non-periodontitis patients (not mandatory to have a pre-existing periodontal pocket)	Impaction		Dental floss, orthodontic elastic, toothpick, rubber dam, popcorn hulls
	Harmful habits		Wire or nail biting and clenching
	Orthodontic factors		Orthodontic forces or cross-bite
	Gingival overgrowth		
	Alteration of root surface	Severe anatomic alterations	Invaginated tooth, dens evaginatus or odontodysplasia
		Minor anatomic alterations	Cemental tears, enamel pearls or developmental grooves
		Iatrogenic conditions	Perforations
		Severe root damage	Fissure or fracture, cracked tooth syndrome
		External root resorption	

Figure 2.7 2018 Classification of endodontic-periodontal lesions. Source: Adapted from Papapanou *et al.* (2018), Table 3.

Endo-periodontal lesions with root damage	Root fracture or cracking	
	Root canal / pulp chamber perforation	
	External root resorption	
Endo-periodontal lesions without root damage	Endo-periodontal lesions in periodontitis patients	Grade 1 - narrow deep periodontal pocket in 1 tooth surface
		Grade 2 - wide deep periodontal pocket in 1 tooth surface
		Grade 3 - deep periodontal pockets in >1 tooth surface
	Endo-periodontal lesions in non-periodontitis patients	Grade 1 - narrow deep periodontal pocket in 1 tooth surface
		Grade 2 - wide deep periodontal pocket in 1 tooth surface
		Grade 3 - deep periodontal pockets in >1 tooth surface

Figure 2.8 2018 Classification of factors related to teeth and to dental prostheses that can affect the periodontium. Source: Adapted from Jepsen *et al.* (2018), Table 4.

Factors related to teeth/dental prostheses that can affect the periodontium	
Localised tooth-related factors that modify or predispose to plaque-induced gingival diseases/periodontitis	Tooth anatomic factors
	Root fractures
	Cervical root resorption, cemental tears
	Root proximity
	Altered passive eruption
Localised dental prosthesis-related factors	Restoration margins placed within the supracrestal attached tissues
	Clinical procedures related to the fabrication of indirect restorations
	Hypersensitivity/toxicity reactions to dental materials

Key points

- The current 2018 classification derives from the 2017 World Workshop on Classification of Periodontal and Peri-implant Diseases and Conditions and replaces the previous 1999 International Classification
- The 2018 classification:
  - defines periodontal health for the first time, as well as plaque-biofilm induced gingivitis and non-dental-plaque-induced gingival conditions
  - provides a new classification for periodontitis, including Staging and Grading
  - includes categories for periodontitis as a manifestation of systemic diseases and systemic diseases and conditions that affect the periodontal supporting tissues
  - updates other conditions affecting the periodontium
  - classifies peri-implant health, peri-implant mucositis, peri-implantitis and peri-implant soft and hard tissue deficiencies for the first time
- Knowledge of the current classification provides a basis for subsequent diagnosis and management of periodontal and peri-implant diseases and conditions

3 Periodontal epidemiology

Figure 3.1 (a) Definition of epidemiology. (b) Definitions of epidemiological terms. Source: Last (2001)/Oxford University Press.

(a)

Epidemiology is the study of the distribution and determinants of health-related states or events in specified populations, and the application of this study to the control of health problems

(b)

Study	includes	Surveillance, observation, hypothesis testing, analytical research and experiments
Distribution	refers to	Analysis by time, place and classes of persons affected
Determinants	are the	Physical, biological, social, cultural and behavioural factors that influence (periodontal) health
Health-related states or events	include	(Periodontal) diseases, causes of morbidity, behaviour such as tobacco use, reactions to preventive regimes, and provision and use of health services
Specified populations	are	Those with identifiable characteristics
Application of this study to the control of health problems	makes explicit	The aim of epidemiology is to promote, protect, and restore (periodontal) health

Figure 3.2 (a) Types of periodontal epidemiology. (b) Descriptive, analytical and pragmatic studies. (c) Cross-sectional and longitudinal studies. (d) Case–control and case–cohort studies. (e) Clinical trial phases. (f) Types of trial. (g) Hierarchy of research evidence.

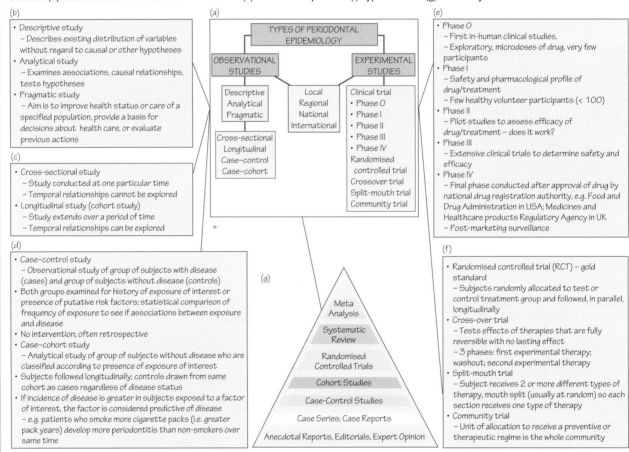

(b)
- Descriptive study
  - Describes existing distribution of variables without regard to causal or other hypotheses
- Analytical study
  - Examines associations, causal relationships, tests hypotheses
- Pragmatic study
  - Aim is to improve health status or care of a specified population, provide a basis for decisions about health care, or evaluate previous actions

(c)
- Cross-sectional study
  - Study conducted at one particular time
  - Temporal relationships cannot be explored
- Longitudinal study (cohort study)
  - Study extends over a period of time
  - Temporal relationships can be explored

(d)
- Case–control study
  - Observational study of group of subjects with disease (cases) and group of subjects without disease (controls)
- Both groups examined for history of exposure of interest or presence of putative risk factors; statistical comparison of frequency of exposure to see if associations between exposure and disease
- No intervention; often retrospective
- Case–cohort study
  - Analytical study of group of subjects without disease who are classified according to presence of exposure of interest
- Subjects followed longitudinally; controls drawn from same cohort as cases regardless of disease status
- If incidence of disease is greater in subjects exposed to a factor of interest, the factor is considered predictive of disease
  - e.g. patients who smoke more cigarette packs (i.e. greater pack years) develop more periodontitis than non-smokers over same time

(a)
TYPES OF PERIODONTAL EPIDEMIOLOGY

OBSERVATIONAL STUDIES

Descriptive / Analytical / Pragmatic

Cross-sectional / Longitudinal / Case–control / Case–cohort

Local / Regional / National / International

EXPERIMENTAL STUDIES

Clinical trial
- Phase 0
- Phase I
- Phase II
- Phase III
- Phase IV

Randomised controlled trial

Crossover trial

Split-mouth trial

Community trial

(g)
Meta Analysis
Systematic Review
Randomised Controlled Trials
Cohort Studies
Case-Control Studies
Case Series; Case Reports
Anecdotal Reports, Editorials, Expert Opinion

(e)
- Phase 0
  - First in-human clinical studies,
  - Exploratory, microdoses of drug, very few participants
- Phase I
  - Safety and pharmacological profile of drug/treatment
  - Few healthy volunteer participants (< 100)
- Phase II
  - Pilot studies to assess efficacy of drug/treatment – does it work?
- Phase III
  - Extensive clinical trials to determine safety and efficacy
- Phase IV
  - Final phase conducted after approval of drug by national drug registration authority, e.g. Food and Drug Administration in USA; Medicines and Healthcare products Regulatory Agency in UK
  - Post-marketing surveillance

(f)
- Randomised controlled trial (RCT) – gold standard
  - Subjects randomly allocated to test or control treatment group and followed, in parallel, longitudinally
- Cross-over trial
  - Tests effects of therapies that are fully reversible with no lasting effect
  - 3 phases: first experimental therapy; washout; second experimental therapy
- Split-mouth trial
  - Subject receives 2 or more different types of therapy, mouth split (usually at random) so each section receives one type of therapy
- Community trial
  - Unit of allocation to receive a preventive or therapeutic regime is the whole community

Figure 3.3 Common terms in epidemiology.

Prevalence	Number or % of affected subjects in population with disease at defined threshold
Extent	Number or % of affected teeth or sites with disease at defined threshold
Severity	How advanced disease is. May be bands of severity, e.g. 1–2 mm clinical attachment loss (CAL) is mild; 3–4 mm is moderate; 5+ mm is severe. May be mean mouth data, e.g. mean severity of CAL = 3.4 mm
Incidence	Number of new cases of disease at a defined threshold that appear in a population over a predetermined period of time
Threshold of disease	Level of disease being studied, e.g. clinical attachment loss of 2 mm; e.g. probing depths of 6 mm or more

Periodontology at a Glance, Second Edition. Valerie Clerehugh, Aradhna Tugnait, Michael R. Milward, and Iain L. C. Chapple.
© 2024 John Wiley & Sons Ltd. Published 2024 by John Wiley & Sons Ltd.

Figure 3.4 Attributes of a good periodontal index.

Attributes of a good index are that it should be:
- Valid (i.e. measures what it purports to measure)
- Reliable (i.e. can be reproduced if re-measured)
- Quick
- Simple
- Acceptable to the examiner and subject and use minimum equipment
- Amenable to statistical analysis

Figure 3.5 The Gingival Index. Source: Löe & Silness (1967)/ John Wiley & Sons.

Code 0	Normal gingiva
Code 1	Mild inflammation. Slight change in colour, slight oedema. No bleeding on probing
Code 2	Moderate inflammation. Redness, oedema and glazing. Bleeding on probing
Code 3	Severe inflammation. Marked redness and oedema, ulceration. Spontaneous bleeding

Figure 3.7 Factors influencing probing accuracy.

- Probing force
- Probe angulation
- Thickness of probe (thick tip diameter of probe will underestimate compared with thin probe)
- Accuracy of probe markings
- Examiner experience
- Degree of inflammation of tissues (tendency to overestimate if inflamed)
- Presence of subgingival calculus or anatomical feature (may impede probing)
- Location of probing (anterior easier than posterior, buccal more reproducible than palatal/lingual sites)

Figure 3.8 UK Adult Dental Health Survey 2009, showing the prevalence of pockets and CAL.

UK Adult Dental Health Survey 2009 6,469 dentate adults examined (representing population) using CPITN methodology:
- 37% had shallow pockets 4 mm – 5 mm
- 7% had deep pockets 6 mm – 8.5 mm
- 1% had very deep pockets ≥ 9 mm

Of adults aged ≥ 55 years examined for CAL :
- 66% had CAL ≥ 4 mm
- 21% had CAL ≥ 6 mm
- 4% had CAL ≥ 9 mm

Figure 3.6 (a) Clinical attachment loss (CAL) and probing depth (PD). (b) CAL and recession.

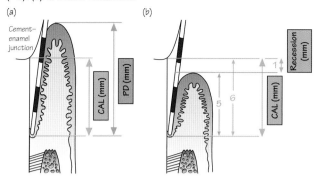

Figure 3.9 US NHANES 2009–14 prevalence of periodontitis by (a) CDC/ AAP case definitions, (b) CAL and (c) PPD. Source: Modified from Eke *et al*. (2018,) Figs 1–3, with permission of Elsevier.

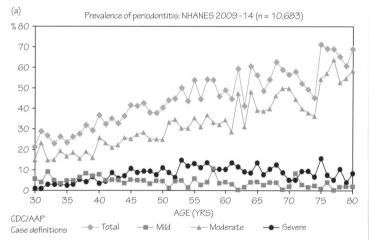

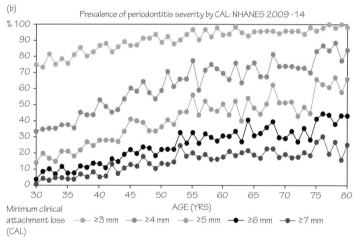

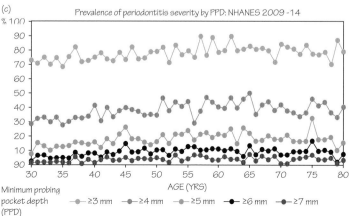

Epidemiology is the study of the distribution and determinants of health-related states or events in specified populations, and the application of this study to the control of health problems (Fig. 3.1).

Types of periodontal epidemiology

There are different types of periodontal epidemiology (Fig. 3.2). There is a hierarchy of research evidence that can be gleaned from different study types and statistical analyses (Fig 3.2g). Periodontal epidemiological studies seek to understand the natural course of the different periodontal diseases and the factors that influence their distribution (Fig. 3.3). Causative and risk factors (Chapters 10, 11 and 14) need to be established in order to determine the aetiology and determinants of disease development. Evidence-based research is important to establish the effectiveness of treatment methods and products and preventive regimes for periodontal diseases at a population level.

Ultimately, the particular research question and the aims and objectives of the study determine the type, design, size and duration of the epidemiological study.

Methodology

Periodontal indices

Measuring periodontal disease involves the use of a periodontal index (Fig. 3.4). There is no single periodontal index that satisfies all the desirable requirements in every type of study and many exist (Barnes *et al.*, 1986).

Gingival indices

In the 1960s, the Gingival Index was introduced in which the codes used mixtures of signs of inflammation: colour change, oedema, bleeding on probing and ulcerations (Fig. 3.5) – it is a compound index. Although widely used, assigning a code is difficult if not all signs are present or if signs from two codes occur. Dichotomous indices (presence or absence of the condition) are alternatives, e.g. bleeding on probing.

Plaque indices

Plaque indices have faced similar problems. The Plaque Index (Löe & Silness, 1967) assesses plaque thickness at the gingival margin. Other indices use disclosing solutions and measure plaque area (e.g. the Turesky modification of the Quigley–Hein Index), while yet others, like the O'Leary Plaque Index, simply record presence or absence but count the per cent of sites affected (Barnes *et al.*, 1986).

Periodontal indices

Russell's Periodontal Index was reported in 1956 and was the first index to be used widely. This was followed by Ramfjord's Periodontal Disease Index in 1959, which introduced the method for measuring clinical attachment loss (CAL). This has been the gold standard and basis of epidemiological clinical recording ever since (Fig. 3.6).

Other recordings may involve periodontal probing pocket depths (PPD) and recession (Fig.3.6). Ethical issues around limiting radiation doses can restrict the use of radiographic measurements. Technological advances enable digital manipulation of images; subtraction radiography allows detection and measurement of small bone changes.

Recording

Full mouth recording of data provides the most information, but some partial recording systems – although generally underestimating disease levels – have been incorporated into large-scale epidemiological studies in order to increase the sample size whilst retaining key information. UK and US national surveys have used this approach.

Other recording issues relate to operator measurement errors – many factors influence probing accuracy (Fig. 3.7). Also, it is important to remember that the periodontal tissues themselves are biologically active and therefore subject to change.

Statistical management

It is essential to distinguish between association and causation. Confounding variables also need to be taken into account, i.e. when the variable is not of primary interest but may affect the study results anyway. Due to measurements of multiple sites within the mouth and repeated recordings over time in some types of study, careful appraisal of data management options is necessary. In addition to the more conventional tests, multilevel modelling and structural equation modelling offer useful approaches for periodontal epidemiology (Tu *et al.*, 2008).

WHO Global Oral Data Bank

The World Health Organization (WHO) has a long tradition of epidemiological survey methodology and has encouraged countries to conduct surveys in a standardised way via its manual 'Oral Health Surveys – Basic Methods'. The WHO Global Oral Data Bank collates the epidemiological data gathered from such surveys (Nazir *et al.*, 2020). The Community Periodontal Index of Treatment Needs (CPITN) originally proposed by the WHO as an index to evaluate treatment needs in populations was renamed the Community Periodontal Index (CPI) to denote its use as an epidemiological tool although it does have limitations (Leroy *et al.*, 2010). In the fifth edition of the manual in 2013, the CPI was modified so that instead of being sextant based, assessment of gingival bleeding and pockets was for all teeth present using the WHO CPI probe; presence of calculus was not recorded as it is not a disease *per se*; CAL was recorded on index teeth 17, 16, 11, 26, 27, 36, 37, 31, 46, 47. For epidemiological studies, children under 15 years of age continued to be excluded from PPD/CAL probing measurements.

Global epidemiology

Population studies confirm the link between plaque and gingivitis. Adults worldwide exhibit gingival bleeding and inflammation. Gingivitis precedes periodontitis and there are no data to suggest that periodontitis develops in the absence of gingival inflammation.

- Incipient (Stage 1) periodontitis can begin in adolescents (Chapter 41).
- Mild to moderate periodontitis (Stage 1 or 2) is widespread in adults based on representative population samples from national studies but severe disease (Stage III) or very severe periodontitis (Stage IV) is less prevalent (Figs 3.8, 3.9).
- The 2009 UK Adult Dental Health Survey showed that since 1998 there has been an overall reduction in the prevalence of pocketing ≥4 mm from 55% to 45%, possibly linked to improved plaque control, but pocketing ≥6 mm had

increased from 6% to 9%, perhaps due to retaining teeth for longer (White *et al.*, 2011, 2012).

- The 2009–14 US National Health and Nutrition Examination Surveys (NHANES) showed that 42.2% of adults ≥30 years had periodontitis, comprising 34.4% with mild/moderate periodontitis and 7.8% with severe periodontitis. The prevalence was highest among current smokers, adults who did not use dental floss regularly and those who had not visited the dentist in the previous six months; it co-occurred with diabetes and increased numbers of missing teeth but not with obesity. These data provided the best estimates of periodontitis prevalence in the US but costs may be prohibitive for future surveillance (Eke *et al.*, 2018).

- There is variation in the prevalence of severe periodontitis reported globally, ranging from: 11.2% (Kassebaum *et al.*, 2014); then 10% (Frencken *et al.*, 2017), in a comprehensive systematic review, and more recently, 19%, representing more than 1 billion cases worldwide (Chen *et al.*, 2021; WHO, 2022). The review concluded that study heterogeneity and methodological issues hamper comparisons across studies over time and that geographic variation and time trends of the incidence and prevalence of periodontitis cannot be drawn from the available evidence.

- Consensus on a definition of what constitutes a periodontitis case is key (Borrell & Papapanou, 2005).

- The AAP/CDC case definition for epidemiological surveillance and the EFP case definition for risk factors research have both been used widely. Both definitions were found to be complementary for surveillance of severe diseases but not for mild/moderate periodontitis (Eke *et al.*, 2012).

- A consensus definition was adopted at the 2017 World Workshop on Classification of Periodontal and Peri-implant Diseases and Conditions (see Fig. 9.6): a patient is a periodontitis case in the context of clinical care if: (1) interdental CAL is detectable at ≥2 non-adjacent teeth, or (2) buccal or lingual CAL ≥3 mm with pocketing >3 mm is detectable at ≥2 teeth but the observed CAL cannot be ascribed to non-periodontitis-related causes (Tonetti *et al.*, 2018; Papapanou *et al.*, 2018). Inherent in the consensus definition is the understanding that there would be bone loss at ≥2 non-adjacent teeth in a periodontitis case. While an individual case should be further characterised by staging and grading (Chapter 36), it was acknowledged that specific considerations are needed for epidemiological surveys where threshold definition is likely to be based on measurement errors (Tonetti *et al.*, 2018).

Key points
- There are different types of epidemiological study
- There is no single ideal periodontal index
- The type of study and index depend on the study aims and objectives
- CPI and other epidemiological data have highlighted differences in global disease prevalence and severity

4 Role of plaque in the aetiology of periodontal diseases

Figure 4.1 (a) Stages and (b) design of classic experimental gingivitis study in humans. Source: Adapted from Loe *et al.* (1965).

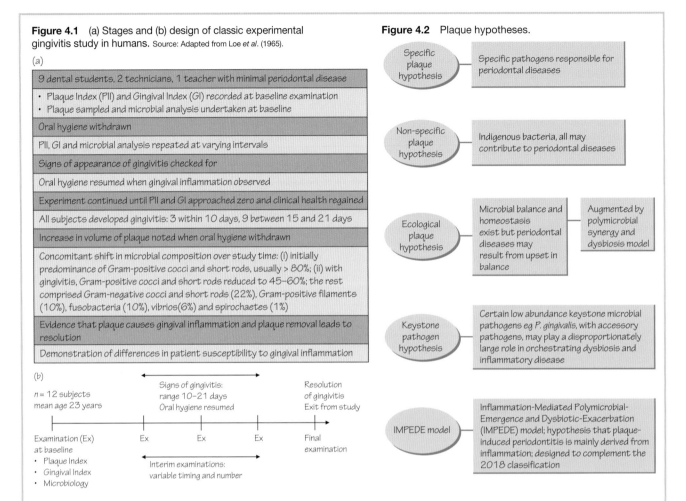

(a)

9 dental students, 2 technicians, 1 teacher with minimal periodontal disease
• Plaque Index (PlI) and Gingival Index (GI) recorded at baseline examination • Plaque sampled and microbial analysis undertaken at baseline
Oral hygiene withdrawn
PlI, GI and microbial analysis repeated at varying intervals
Signs of appearance of gingivitis checked for
Oral hygiene resumed when gingival inflammation observed
Experiment continued until PlI and GI approached zero and clinical health regained
All subjects developed gingivitis: 3 within 10 days, 9 between 15 and 21 days
Increase in volume of plaque noted when oral hygiene withdrawn
Concomitant shift in microbial composition over study time: (i) initially predominance of Gram-positive cocci and short rods, usually > 80%; (ii) with gingivitis, Gram-positive cocci and short rods reduced to 45–60%; the rest comprised Gram-negative cocci and short rods (22%), Gram-positive filaments (10%), fusobacteria (10%), vibrios(6%) and spirochaetes (1%)
Evidence that plaque causes gingival inflammation and plaque removal leads to resolution
Demonstration of differences in patient susceptibility to gingival inflammation

(b)

n = 12 subjects
mean age 23 years

Examination (Ex)
at baseline
• Plaque Index
• Gingival Index
• Microbiology

Signs of gingivitis:
range 10–21 days
Oral hygiene resumed

Interim examinations:
variable timing and number

Ex   Ex   Ex

Resolution
of gingivitis
Exit from study

Final
examination

Figure 4.2 Plaque hypotheses.

Specific plaque hypothesis	Specific pathogens responsible for periodontal diseases
Non-specific plaque hypothesis	Indigenous bacteria, all may contribute to periodontal diseases
Ecological plaque hypothesis	Microbial balance and homeostasis exist but periodontal diseases may result from upset in balance — Augmented by polymicrobial synergy and dysbiosis model
Keystone pathogen hypothesis	Certain low abundance keystone microbial pathogens eg *P. gingivalis*, with accessory pathogens, may play a disproportionately large role in orchestrating dysbiosis and inflammatory disease
IMPEDE model	Inflammation-Mediated Polymicrobial-Emergence and Dysbiotic-Exacerbation (IMPEDE) model; hypothesis that plaque-induced periodontitis is mainly derived from inflammation; designed to complement the 2018 classification

Table 4.1 Stages of plaque biofilm formation.

Stage	Plaque biofilm formation
1 Acquired pellicle formation	Host and bacterial molecules, salivary proteins, glycoproteins, lipds, bacterial glycans and enzymes are adsorbed onto the tooth surface, leading to formation of a surface-conditioning film, the acquired pellicle
2 Transport	Transport of bacteria to the pellicle occurs via natural salivary flow, Brownian movement or chemotaxis. Adsorption of coccal bacteria onto the pellicle occurs within 2 hours – pioneer species include *Neisseria*, *Streptococcus sanguis*, *S. oralis* and *S. mitis*, also Gram-positive rods, mainly *Actinomyces*
3 Reversible attachment	Long-range physicochemical interactions lead to reversible adhesion between the microbial cell surface and the pellicle involving van der Waals attractive forces and electrostatic repulsion
4 Irreversible attachment	Adherence of reversibly attached cells can become irreversible if adhesins on early bacterial colonisers bind to complementary receptors in the acquired pellicle. Once attached, these early colonisers divide and form microcolonies whose metabolism begins to modify the local environment
5 Secondary colonisation	Co-aggregation/co-adhesion of late colonisers to the already attached bacteria via adhesin–receptor interactions results in an increasingly diverse microflora, i.e. microbial succession
6 Maturation	Muliplication of attached organisms leads to confluent growth and biofilm maturation, facilitating interbacterial interactions (both synergistic and antagonistic) and formation of a biofilm matrix of extracellular polymers
7 Detachment	Detachment of bacteria if they sense adverse environmental changes allows colonisation at new sites

Periodontology at a Glance, Second Edition. Valerie Clerehugh, Aradhna Tugnait, Michael R. Milward, and Iain L. C. Chapple.
© 2024 John Wiley & Sons Ltd. Published 2024 by John Wiley & Sons Ltd.

Figure 4.3 Climax microbial community in plaque biofilm showing the diverse range of microbial forms. Source: Courtesy of Professor P. Marsh.

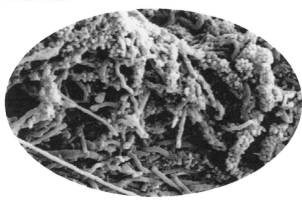

Figure 4.4 Noran Odyssey confocal laser scanning microscope image of intact one-week-old plaque biofilm formed *in vivo* using the Leeds *in situ* device. The image shows the three-dimensional structure and variations in biofilm density; biomasses of bacteria are pink; voids, channels and spaces are dark areas. Image achieved by volume rendering of a series of x-y (horizontal) sections. Scale bar = 50 μm. Source: Courtesy of Dr S. Wood (Wood *et al.*, 2002).

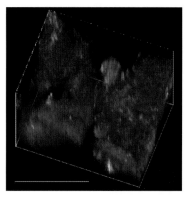

Figure 4.5 Schematic of ecological plaque hypothesis. Source: Adapted from Marsh (2022), Figure 1.5.4.

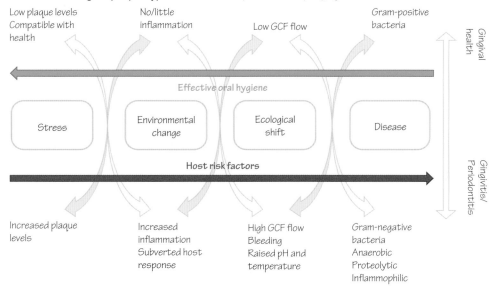

Figure 4.6 Keystone pathogen-induced dysbiosis and periodontal disease. Source: Adapted from Hajishengallis *et al.* (2012), Figure 2.

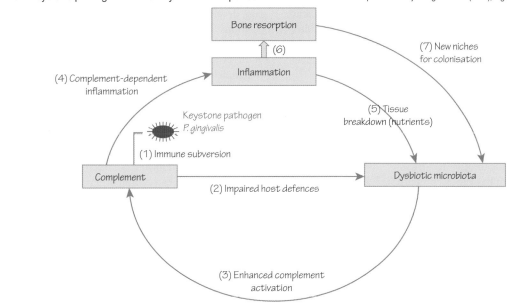

Figure 4.7   Inflammation-Mediated Polymicrobial-Emergence and Dysbiotic-Exacerbation (IMPEDE) model. Source: Adapted from Van Dyke *et al.*, (2020), Figure 1.

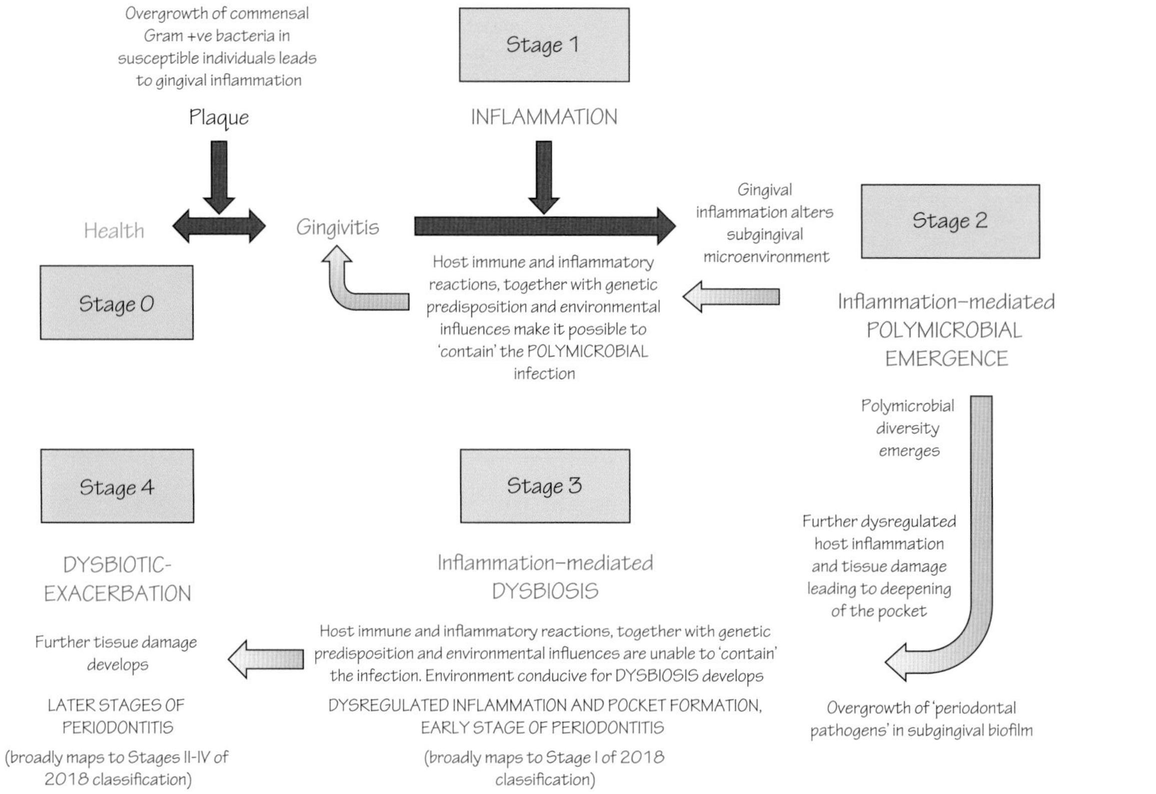

Plaque as a biofilm

Since the classic experimental gingivitis study (Loë *et al.*, 1965), the role of dental plaque as the key aetiological agent in gingivitis has been acknowledged (Fig. 4.1). Nowadays, plaque is considered a good example of a biofilm and different hypotheses of its role in the aetiology of periodontal diseases have evolved (Fig. 4.2).

Plaque as a biofilm

Dental plaque has been defined as a diverse community of micro-organisms found on the tooth surface as a biofilm, embedded in an extracellular matrix of polymers of host and microbial origin. Biofilms are defined as matrix-embedded microbial populations, adhering to each other and/or to surfaces or interfaces (Marsh, 2005). The production of extracellular polymers forms a functional matrix.

Formation and properties

Biofilm formation involves several stages (Table 4.1) before the diverse climax community is derived (Fig. 4.3). Microbial homeostasis is critical. Breakdown may occur due to host defence, local, systemic or other factors.

Plaque as a biofilm has various properties.

- It is spatially and functionally organised in a complex three-dimensional structure with pores and channels running through it (Fig. 4.4).
- The physical architecture protects it from desiccation and phagocytosis.
- It is less susceptible to antibiotics (see later).
- Structure and function are directly influenced by the biological properties and anatomy of the surface to which it attaches so

each biofilm has a unique, characteristic microbial composition reflecting the local environment.

- Growth in biofilms can have a direct effect on gene expression – many organisms have a radically different phenotype following attachment to a surface or host receptor, co-adhesion with other organisms or binding to a host protein. Indirect effects on gene expression may be due to an altered environment (e.g. pH, sugar concentration). Altered gene expression can also reduce the sensitivity of the biofilm to antibiotics.
- Close proximity of different species provides an opportunity for multiple types of synergistic and antagonistic interactions, e.g. development of food chains; physically close cell–cell associations, e.g. corncob/test-tube brush structure; antagonism between competing species; cell–cell signalling.
- Cell–cell communication can take place in various ways, for example via (i) horizontal gene transfer; (ii) small diffusible peptides; (iii) quorum sensing, using signalling compounds to regulate gene expression; (iv) autoinducer 2, which mediates messages between Gram-positive and Gram-negative species in a mixed species community; (v) cross-talk between host cells and bacteria.
- Physiological heterogeneity: micro-organisms of the same microbial species can exhibit different physiological states in a biofilm, even if in very close proximity to each other.
- Spatial and environmental heterogeneity: bacterial metabolism in plaque leads to varying gradients that are crucial to microbial growth, and these varying environments for pH, oxygen tension, redox potential and nutrients give sufficient heterogeneity for diverse organisms with different metabolic and growth needs that seem incompatible with each other to co-exist at the same site.

- Community life style supports a wider habitat range for growth and synergistic properties. The early colonisers alter the local environment and facilitate attachment and growth of later, sometimes more fastidious, micro-organisms, which leads to microbial succession and increased metabolic diversity and efficiency. Nearby cells can produce neutralising enzymes (β-lactamase) that protect susceptible micro-organisms against antimicrobials or environmental stress. The properties of the plaque biofilm community are greater than the individual components of the biofilm.
- Pathogenic synergism: the remit of a pathogen is to damage the host tissue and the benefit of being in a biofilm community is the synergistic enhancement of the virulence potential of individual subgingival microbes. There are various points at which the pathogenic potential can be influenced: microbial adherence, acquisition of nutrients from the host, multiplication, overcoming or evasion of host defences, tissue invasion and finally tissue damage.

Plaque hypotheses

Specific plaque hypothesis

The specific plaque hypothesis (Loesche, 1976, 1979) centres around the philosophy that periodontal diseases have a specific microflora associated with them, such as necrotising gingivitis (Chapter 39) and the severe form of periodontitis (Grade C, Stage IV) with molar/incisor pattern affecting young people, previously known as localised aggressive periodontitis (*Aggregatibacter actinomycetemcomitans*) (Chapter 35). Elimination of the specific bacteria leads to disease resolution, usually with the adjunctive use of systemic antibiotics.

Non-specific plaque hypothesis

This plaque hypothesis (Theilade, 1986) embraces the notion that if plaque biofilm develops undisturbed, it will grow in volume and change in composition from essentially aerobic Gram-positive cocci and rods located supragingivally to Gram-negative cocci and rods that are increasingly anaerobic as plaque extends subgingivally; filaments, fusobacteria, spirils and spirochaetes are also found. The microbiota produce virulence factors that lead to tissue inflammation/destruction. Plaque biofilm removal by effective toothbrushing or control by pharmacological agents restores the original supragingival microbiota and also influences the subgingival domain.

Ecological plaque hypothesis

According to the ecological plaque hypothesis (Marsh 1991, 1994, 2022; Naginyte et al., 2019, see Fig. 4.5), biofilm accumulation facilitates the growth of obligate anaerobes, inducing an inflammatory host response which causes local environmental changes subgingivally (increased flow of GCF and resultant increase in pH and temperature). If this fails to clear the microbial challenge then GCF can inadvertently act as a source of nutrients for the fastidious and potentially pathogenic species found in inflamed pockets. This favours the growth of Gram-negative proteolytic and obligately anaerobic species, leading to an ecological shift in the microbiota which is likely to provoke more inflammation (dysbiosis). These organisms are referred to as 'inflammophilic' in that they can tolerate and even benefit from the host response.

Keystone pathogen hypothesis

The polymicrobial synergy and dysbiosis (PSD) model augments the ecological plaque hypothesis by placing more emphasis on damage caused by the deregulated inflammatory response while reinforcing the concept that the change in the subgingival environment will drive dysbiosis (Lamont & Hajishengallis, 2015). According to the keystone pathogen hypothesis, certain key pathogens like *P. gingivalis*, even at low abundance, supported by accessory pathogens such as *S. gordonii*, can disproportionately orchestrate inflammatory disease by remodelling a normally benign synergistic microbiota into a dysbiotic state (Hajishengallis et al., 2012). Based on the PSD model, the host response is initially subverted by keystone pathogens, assisted by accessory pathogens, and is subsequently overactivated by pathobionts, which are organisms that promote pathology under conditions of disrupted host homeostasis (Lamont et al., 2018) (Fig. 4.6). Effective disease control strategies would need to identify and target factors driving the selection of these pathogens.

The keystone pathogen hypothesis is not widely held to be a front-runner of the various plaque hypotheses. However, temporal and spatial analyses of subgingival plaque help to explain the disproportionate effect of periodontal pathogens like *P. gingivalis* and *Treponema denticola* on dysregulation of the host defences, leading to accelerated attachment loss despite only appearing to constitute a small proportion of the overall microbiota at the base of a deep periodontal pocket (Van Dyke et al., 2020). Furthermore, it has been suggested that the levels of periodontal pathogens or "dysbiotic signature" of subgingival plaque may be a useful biomarker/predictor of disease site activity and imminent progression (Meuric et al., 2017; Van Dyke et al., 2020).

IMPEDE model

More recently, a new unifying hypothesis called the 'Inflammation-Mediated Polymicrobial-Emergence and Dysbiotic-Exacerbation' (IMPEDE) model has been proposed (Van Dyke et al., 2020) which is designed to integrate into and complement the 2018 classification derived from the 2017 World Workshop of Periodontal and Peri-implant Diseases and Conditions. According to this model, plaque-induced periodontitis is mainly derived from inflammation. IMPEDE has 5 stages (Fig 4.7): 0, health; 1, inflammation (associated with an overgrowth of commensal plaque bacteria); 2, emergence of inflammation induced polymicrobial diversity, triggering dysbiosis; 3, dysregulated inflammation and pocket formation (maps to initial Stage I periodontitis in the 2018 classification); 4, inflammation-mediated dysbiosis and further tissue damage (broadly maps to the later stages II-IV periodontitis in the 2018 classification).

Key points
- Plaque is a biofilm which is key in the aetiology of periodontal diseases
- Biofilm forms in stages and has various properties
- Various plaque hypotheses have evolved: specific, nonspecific, ecological, keystone pathogen, and the IMPEDE model

5 Plaque biofilm microbiology

Table 5.1 Advantages/disadvantages of different methods of examining plaque microbial composition.

Method	Advantages	Disadvantages
Microscopy	Recognises morphological types Determines spatial arrangements of organisms More recent novel, sophisticated applications, e.g. atomic force microscopy gives very high image resolution	Slow and labour intensive Precise speciation using immunological or hybridisation methods only possible for a few species in the sample
Culture – predominant	Can detect unrecognised species Provides cultures for further analysis Useful for antibiotic sensitivity testing	Very labour intensive Expensive Some uncultivable species Difficult to culture spirochaetes
Culture – selective media	Can detect specific species	As above Need to know which species to study Few suitable media Limited species identification
Culture – novel	Can cultivate novel, previously unculturable bacteria Characterisation will further understanding of oral microbiome in health and disease	Time-consuming Requires expertise, novel methodology Only a few novel taxa may be successfully cultivated
Immunofluorescence, ELISA	Quite specific[a] Rapid Cheaper than culture Can distinguish species, give counts/proportions	Limited numbers of monoclonal or polyclonal antibodies available Takes time to develop Relatively small numbers can be run
PCR (Polymerase chain reaction)	Reasonable sensitivity[b] Quite specific With appropriate primers can detect very small numbers of species present Rapid	Dichotomous (i.e. detects presence/absence, not quantities) Expensive Depends on amplification Not suitable for large numbers of species in large numbers of samples
Real-time PCR	Quantitative Greater sensitivity than PCR	Relatively slow As above, limited numbers can be processed
DNA–DNA hybridisation	Quantitative Low likelihood of cross-reactions with other species	Only detects species for which probes are available Modest numbers of species for modest number of samples
Checkerboard DNA–DNA hybridisation	Quantitative Can use whole sample without dilution or amplification by PCR Large numbers of species and samples Inexpensive Rapid	Only detects species for which probes are available Samples must be of appropriate size Possible cross-reactions if inappropriate sample size
16S rRNA gene sequencing	Mainstay of sequence-based bacterial analysis for decades Detection of cultivable and uncultivable species From 2008, comparison with the Human Oral Microbiome Database enabled phenotypic, phylogenetic information (www.ehomd.org)	Traditional method was expensive, laborious, time-consuming Small numbers of samples until advent of next-generation sequencing (NGS) enabled high-throughput sequencing of full 16S gene with adequate accuracy
NGS, e.g. Illumina's MiSeq	Allows for ultra-high-volume studies of genetic material in samples Dramatic increase in speed and reduced cost Has increased understanding of oral microbiome Useful technologies	Vast data generation and increased publication of data create inherent challenges for data analysis and interpretation Caution to avoid DNA contamination
Metagenomics Metatranscriptomics	Insights into genetic composition of microbial community – 'who is there'. Culture independent Allows study of actively transcribed genes, gene expression changes, i.e. 'what they are doing'	Complex datasets generated and requires computational biology, but great opportunities to further knowledge in both fields

[a] Specificity is the ability to correctly determine the absence of organism(s).
[b] Sensitivity is the ability to correctly identify the presence of organism(s).

Periodontology at a Glance, Second Edition. Valerie Clerehugh, Aradhna Tugnait, Michael R. Milward, and Iain L. C. Chapple.
© 2024 John Wiley & Sons Ltd. Published 2024 by John Wiley & Sons Ltd.

Figure 5.1 Atomic force microscope image of live *Streptococcus salivarius* (NCTC 8618) trapped in a pore in a track-etched polycarbonate membrane under phosphate-buffered saline. x–y dimensions = 774 nm. Work funded by the Medical Research Council, UK. Source: Courtesy of Dr R. Turner.

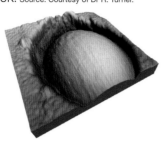

Figure 5.2 Microbial complexes. Source: Adapted from Socransky *et al.* (1998), Fig. 14.

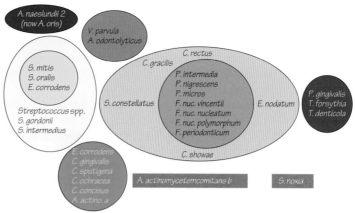

Figure 5.3 Health-associated, core and periodontitis-associated species from the subgingival microbiome appearing in ≥3 different 16S rRNA gene sequencing studies. Source: Adapted from Curtis *et al.* (2020), Fig. 5.

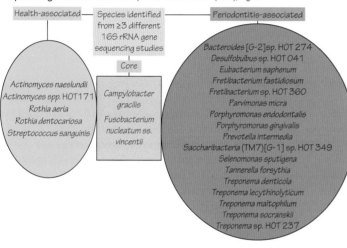

Figure 5.4 (a) Koch's original postulates, subsequently adapted by Falkow (1988). (b) Definitions of: (i) pathogen; (ii) virulence determinants of pathogen.

(a)

- According to Koch's postulates for a pathogen to cause disease, it must:
  - Be isolated from every case of disease
  - Not be recovered from cases of other types of disease, or non-pathogenically
  - Induce disease in experimental animals after isolation and repeated growth in pure culture

(b)

i) Pathogen
- An organism which reproduces and persists on or within another species by breaching or destroying a cellular or humoral host barrier (Falkow, 1988)

ii) Virulence determinants of pathogen
- Those gene products which facilitate colonisation, growth and survival within the diseased host organism and spread to a new host (Curtis *et al.*, 2005)

Figure 5.5 Stages for pathogens to exhibit virulence and cause infection/disease.

- Colonise
  - Attach eg by adhesins, fimbriae; co-aggregation
  - Multiply using available nutrients eg protease production, food chains, bacteriocins
  - Compete successfully against species trying to occupy site
  - Evade host defences eg via capsule, leukotoxin, neutrophil-receptor blocker
- Produce factors that cause tissue damage
  - Directly eg enzymes, bone resorbing factors, cytotoxins
  - Indirectly via inflammatory response
- Release and spread

Figure 5.6 Stages of bacterial pathogenicity and examples of virulence factors for *Aggregatibacter actinomycetemcomitans* (*A.a*). Stage 1: adhesins, autotransporter proteins and fimbriae have a role in attachment; Poly-N-acetylglucosamine (PGA) may be involved in autoaggregation and is resistant to phagocytosis and antimicrobial peptides. Stage 2: bacteriocins inhibit beneficial species allowing pathogens to multiply. Stage 3: *A.a.* produces factors that inhibit neutrophil chemotaxis and are immunosuppressive to immunoglobulin G (IgG) and IgM; leukotoxin is a powerful virulence factor that destroys neutrophils and macrophages. Stage 4: only a few bacteria have this property to penetrate (invade) tissues, possibly via cytolethal distending toxins and ApiA (an outer membrane protein produced by *A.a.*). Stage 5: *A.a.* activates T-helper cells and B-cells to incite bone loss and produces collagenases that degrade collagen and periodontal ligament; lipopolysaccharide (endotoxin) activates the host to secrete mediators that lead to bone resorption,

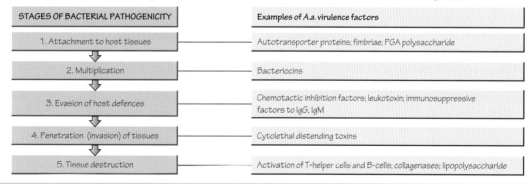

The expanded Human Oral Microbiome Database lists over 770 oral bacterial species, 58% of which are officially named, 16% unnamed but cultivated and 26% uncultured phylotypes. Subgingivally, microbial communities contain bacteria, archaea, fungi and viruses, but bacteria predominate with 500+ species present (Kilian *et al.*, 2016; Curtis *et al.*, 2020). Fewer species colonise at individual's sites.

Plaque biofilm bacteria can attach to tooth surfaces, periodontal tissues (sulcular, junctional or pocket epithelium lining), connective tissues (if access is gained via ulcerated pocket epithelium) or other bacteria already attached to surfaces. Hence, many pathways exist for oral bacteria to exert their effects. Teeth are predisposed to microbial accumulation as they are solid, non-shedding structures.

Microbiological techniques

Various ways of investigating plaque microbial composition have evolved, each with advantages and disadvantages (Socransky & Haffajee, 2005; Teles *et al.*, 2006; Zarco *et al.*, 2012; Kilian *et al.*, 2016; Krishnan *et al.*, 2017), including the following (Table 5.1):

- Microscopy (Fig. 5.1).
- Culture: novel methods have been developed to isolate and grow novel strains, such as use of siderophores and helper strains (Vartoukian *et al.*, 2016).
- Immunofluorescence: enzyme-linked immunofluorescence assay (ELISA) uses specific antibody to detect bacterial antigens (species specific).
- Polymerase chain reaction (PCR):
  - uses a DNA polymerase to amplify a piece of DNA by *in vitro* enzymatic replication rather than in living cells like *Escherichia coli*
  - can amplify a single or a few copies of a piece of DNA and generate millions of copies quickly.
- Real-time PCR: can view the increase in amount of DNA as it is amplified.
- DNA–DNA hybridisation:
  - measures the degree of genetic similarity between pools of DNA sequences
  - is usually used to determine the genetic distance between two species
  - allows species to be arranged in a phylogenetic tree.
- Checkerboard DNA–DNA hybridisation: provides a simultaneous quantitative analysis of 40 microbial species against up to 28 mixed samples on a single membrane.
- 16S rRNA gene sequencing: involves amplification, cloning and sequencing of extracted DNA segments encoding the 16S rRNA gene (which is unique to the species) using PCR.
- Next-generation sequencing (NGS): encompasses massively parallel, modern high-throughput sequencing technologies that read the sequence of millions of short fragments of DNA or RNA at the same time.
- Metagenomics: involves the study of environmental microbial communities using a suite of genomic tools to directly access their genetic content without prior cultivation of microbes in the laboratory. It detects all microorganisms in a sample.
- Metatranscriptomics: *techniques used to study the gene expression of microbes within natural environments* – the metatranscriptome reveals the taxonomic composition and active functions of a complex microbial community.

Microbial composition of plaque biofilm in health and disease

In a classic study using whole genomic DNA probes and checkerboard DNA–DNA hybridisation on 13 261 plaque samples from 185 subjects, Socransky *et al.* (1998) identified five bacterial complexes to which they assigned colours red, orange, green, yellow and purple (Fig. 5.2):

- Red complex: associated with periodontitis, deeper pockets and bleeding on probing.
- Orange complex: also found in deeper pockets; more diverse; often precedes the red complex.
- Grey outlier: *Aggregatibacter actinomycetemcomitans* serotype b and *Selenomonas noxia*.
- Dark purple outlier: *Actinomyces naeslundii* genospecies 2 (reclassified as *A. oris* in 2009) sometimes joined by purple complex.
- Dark purple and yellow (streptococci): early colonisers, followed by green complex; host compatible: associated with health.
- Purple complex: species closely associated; possible bridge to orange, then red complex.

Health

Findings from early microscopic and culture studies of microbial composition have been largely corroborated but extended by the advent of studies using 16S rRNA gene sequencing.

In health, the bacteria in the gingival crevice are predominantly Gram-positive including *Streptococci* spp. (*S. mitis*, *S anginosus*) and rods of the species *Actinomyces* (*A. odontolyticus*, *A. naeslundii*, *A. georgiae*), *Rothia* (*R. dentocariosa*, *R. aeria*) and *Corynebacterium* (*C. matruchotti*, *C durum*). Gram-negative genera include *Neisseria*, *Lautropia* (*L. mirabilis*), *Haemophilus*, *Capnocytophaga* (*C. ochracea*), *Fusobacterium* (*F. nucleatum*), *Prevotella* (*P. melaninogenica*, occasionally *P. nigrescens*) and *Veillonella* (*V. parvula*). Spirochaetes have also been detected (*T. vincentii*, *T. denticola*, *T. maltophilum*, *T. lecithinolytum*) (Marsh, 2016, 2022). The ecology is strongly influenced by GCF.

Gingivitis

The classic experimental gingivitis model (Chapter 4) using culture techniques showed an increase in the proportion of *Actinomyces* spp., capnophylic (especially *Capnocytophaga* spp.) and obligately anaerobic Gram-negative bacteria on withdrawal of oral hygiene and development of gingivitis. The consensus is that no specific pathogens are associated with gingivitis (Marsh, 2016, 2022) although subsequent experimental gingivitis protocols using 16S rRNA gene sequencing have refined knowledge (Schincaglia *et al.*, 2017).

Periodontitis

The transition from gingivitis to periodontitis is associated with a big shift in the composition of the subgingival microflora, with increased diversity and greater proportions of proteolytic, obligately anaerobic Gram-negative bacteria which are difficult to recover, grow and identify. Culture-independent metagenomic techniques have led to the discovery of novel bacteria, some uncultivable and unnamed. Evidence about which organisms may play an active role in periodontitis has been conflicting and different studies often highlight different species. However, microbial function may prove to be more relevant/important in disease pathogenesis than the mere presence/name of the organism.

Seventeen species were listed as strongly periodontitis associated from several 16S rRNA gene sequencing studies reviewed by Curtis *et al.* (2020) (Fig. 5.3), including the original 'red complex trio' (*T. denticola*, *P. gingivalis*, *Tanneralla fosythia*) (Fig. 5.2). Further, *Filifactor alocis* was deemed moderately periodontitis associated in a systematic review (Pérez-Chapparro *et al.*, 2014). Health-associated species are still present in periodontitis and vice versa, reinforcing the view that dysbiosis results from changes in dominant species rather than from colonisation of new species. *C. gracilis* and *F. nucleatum* ss. *vincentii* are classified as core species since they are consistently detected and have unchanged proportions (around 25% of the biomass) in health and disease.

Drivers of dysbiosis

Drivers of dysbiosis (see Figs 4.5, 4.6) include: (i) increased GCF in the transition from health to disease which promotes enrichment of proteinase-rich taxa associated with periodontitis; (ii) changes in oxygen as taxa associated with health/gingivitis have higher oxygen tolerance than anaerobic periodontitis-associated taxa; (iii) tissue disruption and presence of blood cells since periodontitis-associated species like black-pigmented anaerobes use haemoglobin-derived haemin as an iron source; (iv) an individual key pathogen like *P. gingivalis* can exert major dysbiosis effects via its ability to disable and deregulate host immune and inflammatory systems, especially complement (Curtis *et al.*, 2020).

The concept that periodontitis is the result of outgrowth of a small number of pathogenic species which become dominant in disease has been replaced by the concept that in health, the microbiome and inflammatory response are in bidirectional balance (homeostasis) whereas in periodontitis there is bidirectional imbalance and dysbiosis, with microbiome changes and expression of bacterial virulence factors.

Virulence factors

It is difficult to translate the original Koch's postulates of causation of disease by a pathogen (Fig. 5.4) to periodontal diseases, but these were adapted by Falkow (1988). For a periodontal pathogen to cause disease it must be able to: (i) colonise; (ii) produce factors that cause host tissue damage; (iii) release and spread (Fig. 5.5).

It has been suggested that many so-called virulence factors might be considered 'survival factors' since they do not constitute factors for pathogenicity and damage but rather for living and growth in deep, inflamed periodontal pockets (Dahlen *et al.*, 2019). An exception is the leukotoxin produced by *A. actinomycetemcomitans* and its JP2 genotype which has been shown to cause destruction; *A. actinomycetemcomitans* truly fulfils the designation 'putative periodontal pathogen' (Fig. 5.6).

Key points
- There are over 770 oral microbial species, 26 % of which are uncultivated and 16% unnamed
- Various techniques have evolved to identify bacteria, each with advantages and disadvantages
- Microbial composition alters from health to disease
- In health, the microbiome and inflammatory response are in bidirectional balance (homeostasis)
- In periodontitis, there is bidirectional imbalance (dysbiosis)
- Pathogens use a variety of mechanisms to exert damage

6 Calculus

Table 6.1 Differences between supragingival and subgingival calculus.

	Supragingival calculus	Subgingival calculus
Location	Coronal to gingival margin	Apical to gingival margin within gingival sulcus or periodontal pocket
Distribution	Adjacent to openings of salivary ducts: • lingual of mandibular incisors (sublingual duct) • buccal of maxillary second molar (parotid duct)	No predilection for particular parts of mouth Approximal and lingual sites more affected than buccal sites
Appearance	Creamy-white colour May become nicotine stained in smoker	Brownish-black due to haemorrhagic elements from gingival crevicular fluid and black pigments from calcified anaerobic rods
Morphology	Undifferentiated morphology – amorphous deposit	Variable: • ledges or rings around tooth, especially on the cementenamel junction • on root surface(s) as crusty, spiny, nodular formations, thin veneers, fern-like arrangements or individual islands • supragingival on subgingival deposits
Detection	Visible clinically Detection enhanced by air drying, which gives chalky appearance	By probing – tactile sensation enhanced by using ball end of WHO 621 probe If deposit is located at entrance to pocket: • it may be visible as dark shadow under the gingival margin • by directing air jet from three-in-one syringe at entrance to pocket, it may be possible to retract the gingiva and see deposit directly Following gingival recession, subgingival deposit may become located supragingivally and be easily visible Radio-opaque calculus 'wings' may be visible on approximal sites on radiographs
Formation	Nucleation and crystal growth are heterogeneous Calcification is heterogeneous Deposit builds up in layers with variable mineral content in the layers	Nucleation and crystal growth are heterogeneous Calcification is more homogeneous (uniform) than supragingival calculus Deposit builds up in layers, each with similarly high mineral density
Mineral content and source	Mean of 37% by volume (range 16–51% in the different layers) Derived from saliva	Mean of 58% by volume (range 32–78% in the different layers) Derived from gingival crevicular fluid
Composition	70–80% inorganic salts Mainly calcium, phosphate (lower ratio than subgingival calculus) Small amounts of magnesium, sodium, carbonate and fluoride. Regular distribution of fluoride Traces of other elements Organic matrix constitutes 15–20% of dry weight: protein (55%), lipid (10%) and carbohydrate	Greater concentration of calcium, magnesium and fluoride than in supragingival calculus Higher calcium to phosphorus ratio than in supragingival calculus Irregular distribution of fluoride
Crystal type	Mostly octacalcium phosphate and hydroxyapatite Some whitlockite Only a little brushite In the presence of low pH and high calcium to phosphorus ratio, brushite appears first in newly formed calculus but as it matures, it transforms to hydroxyapatite or whitlockite and is therefore rarely seen	Whitlockite is the major constituent; it develops under anaerobic, alkaline conditions in the presence of magnesium, zinc and carbonate and contains small amounts magnesium (3%) Hydroxyapapatite is also present Octacalcium phosphate present in the ledge/ring formations of subgingival calculus is typically found just under the gingival margin No brushite

Periodontology at a Glance, Second Edition. Valerie Clerehugh, Aradhna Tugnait, Michael R. Milward, and Iain L. C. Chapple.
© 2024 John Wiley & Sons Ltd. Published 2024 by John Wiley & Sons Ltd.

Figure 6.1 Supragingival calculus on the lingual of the mandibular anteriors and premolars, near the opening of the sublingual (Bartholin's) duct, showing nicotine stains from tobacco smoking.

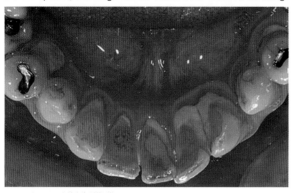

Figure 6.3 Supragingival calculus on the buccal of UL7 opposite the opening of the parotid (Stensen's) duct.

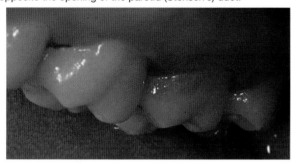

Figure 6.5 Ring (ledge) formation of subgingival calculus exposed on the buccal CEJ of UR3 and UR2 in a 35-year-old Asian female with severe periodontitis following clinical attachment loss and recession; dark shadows of subgingival calculus are visible on UR1.

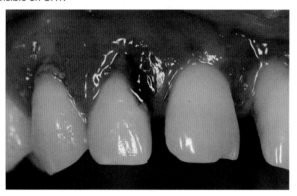

Figure 6.7 Ledges of subgingival calculus exposed at the palatal gingival margin of UR1 and UR2 following reduction in swelling/inflammation after instigating oral hygiene and interdental brushing, but prior to subgingival PMPR.

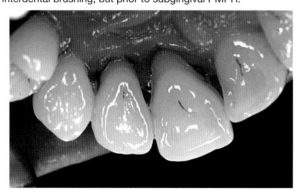

Figure 6.2 Gross deposits of supragingival calculus in a male of Asian ethnicity.

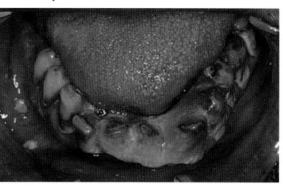

Figure 6.4 (a) Crusty, spiny, nodular deposits of subgingival calculus on an extracted tooth root. (b) Ring (ledge) formation of subgingival calculus around the CEJ on an extracted molar stained with Gomori's stain. The periodontal fibres are stained turquoise.

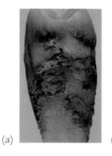 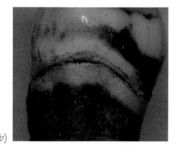

(a)   (b)

Figure 6.6 Thin veneers of subgingival calculus exposed on the labial of LR2 and distobuccal of LR1 following reduction in swelling/inflammation in a 28-year-old female undergoing subgingival PMPR; oral hygiene not optimal yet.

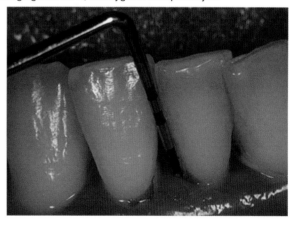

Figure 6.8 Subgingival calculus exposed on the mesial of UR4 following reduction in swelling/inflammation after instigating oral hygiene and interdental brushing, but prior to subgingival PMPR

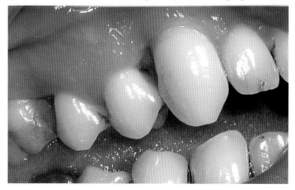

Figure 6.9 (a,b) Bitewing radiographs showing calculus 'wings' on the approximal surfaces of most teeth of this patient with periodontitis.

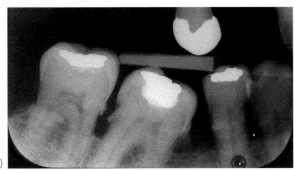
(a)

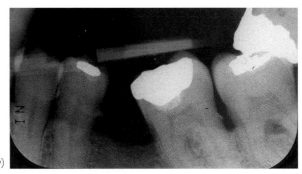
(b)

Dental calculus is defined as the calcified or calcifying deposits that are found attached to the surfaces of teeth and other solid structures in the oral cavity. Supragingival calculus has been extensively studied, particularly in the 1960s and 1970s, whilst subgingival calculus and its formation and composition have been studied much less. There are many differences between the two types (Roberts-Harry & Clerehugh, 2000; Jin & Yip, 2002) (Table 6.1).

Formation of calculus

Calculus formation is always preceded by plaque formation. Initially, pellicle forms on the tooth surface or irregular root cementum and when this calcifies, the calcified crystals create a strong bond to the surface affected, especially on the cementum at the sites of previous insertions of Sharpey's fibres. Implant surfaces tend to be smoother, therefore calculus may be less adherent.

The plaque accumulations become the organic matrix for subsequent mineralisation of the deposit. Small crystals appear in the intermicrobial matrix between the bacteria; first, the matrix becomes calcified and then the bacteria become mineralised. Supragingival calculus formation can occur within 12 days of supragingival professional mechanical plaque removal (PMPR), by which time up to 80% of the inorganic content may be present. However, the development and maturation of the crystal composition can take place over a long period.

Mineralisation requires nucleation of crystal seeds then crystal growth. The ions for supragingival calculus derive from saliva. Plaque forms the environment for the heterogeneous nucleation of calcium and phosphate crystals, which occurs even with a transient supersaturation of the ions. A rise in pH and salivary flow rate influences the supersaturation of saliva and is therefore instrumental in calculus formation. Other ions may be incorporated into the structure, depending on the conditions. Acidic phospholipids and specific proteolipids in cell membranes have a role in microbial mineralisation. Gingival crevicular fluid yields the calcium, phosphate and proteins for subgingival calculus to form. Nucleation inhibitors (e.g. magnesium) and crystal growth inhibitors present in some salivary proteins or dentifrices can influence calculus formation.

Crystal types

There are four different crystal types of calcium phosphate, which are found in differing proportions in supragingival and subgingival calculus (Table 6.1).

- Octacalcium phosphate: $Ca_8H_2(PO_4)_6 \times 5H_2O$.
- Hydroxyapatite: $Ca_{10}(PO_4)_6(OH)_2$:
  - where other cations capable of substituting for calcium Ca^{2+} are strontium Sr^{2+}, lead Pb^{2+}, potassium K^+ and sodium Na^+
  - where carbonate CO_3^- or hydrogen phosphate HPO_4^- can replace phosphate ions PO_4^-
  - where chloride $Cl-$ or fluoride $F-$ can replace the hydroxyl ion $OH-$.
- Whitlockite: $b\text{-}Ca_3(PO_4)_2$. This is sometimes called magnesium-containing β-tricalcium phosphate as magnesium can substitute for calcium.
- Brushite (dicalcium phosphate dihydrate): $CaHPO_4 \times 2H_2O$.

Morphology

Supragingival calculus

Supragingival calculus forms as an amorphous, creamy coloured mass building up in layers on the buccal of the maxillary molars or the lingual of the mandibular anterior teeth. It can readily become stained, e.g. by nicotine (Figs 6.1–6.3).

Subgingival calculus

Crusty, spiny, nodular deposits and ledge- or ring-type deposits are common (Roberts-Harry *et al.*, 2000) (Table 6.1; Figs 6.4, 6.5). At a microscopic level, well-aligned ribbon-shaped octacalcium phosphate crystals are probably formed by filamentous organisms and account for the formation of ledge-type deposits. They may represent a transitional calculus between supragingival and subgingival deposits as they are exposed to both saliva and gingival crevicular fluid.

Individual islands of calculus are thought to represent nucleation sites in early calculus formation. Superficially located deposits, including thin, smooth veneers, which are more difficult to detect by tactile sensation, can become visible near the gingival margin following reduction in gingival oedema and inflammation once plaque control improves or treatment is under way – this makes their subsequent removal easier (Figs 6.6–6.8). Radiographs should be routinely checked for calculus deposits that appear like radio-opaque 'wings' on proximal surfaces – small deposits will not be visible (Fig. 6.9).

Pathogenicity

Plaque always forms on top of calculus. The plaque biofilm that forms over the smooth crystalline surface of supragingival calculus contains filamentous organisms. Supragingival calculus is often associated with gingivitis and gingival recession. Subgingival calculus has an irregular, porous surface covered by a plaque biofilm that contains cocci, rods and filaments and which can act as a reservoir for periodontal pathogens and endotoxin. The presence of subgingival calculus and its plaque layer has been associated with the subsequent development of periodontitis and higher rates of disease progression in adolescents and adults.

Subgingival calculus composition and ethnicity

Studies have shown that the prevalence of subgingival calculus is greater in certain ethnic groups, including Asians. It has been found that Indo-Pakistani subjects have significantly less magnesium in apical deposits of subgingival calculus than white caucasians (Roberts-Harry et al., 2000). It is hypothesised that this makes their calculus more insoluble and helps explain the tenacious nature of the calculus and its greater accretion.

Anti-calculus dentifrices

Anti-calculus dentifrices work on the principle of crystal growth inhibition to prevent the formation of supragingival calculus and have not been shown to be effective against subgingival deposits, e.g. triclosan with pyrophosphate and co-polymer; zinc citrate.

Key points

- Calculus is always covered by a plaque biofilm
- Supragingival calculus:
  - forms near the openings of the salivary ducts
  - has its mineral content derived from saliva
  - is associated with gingivitis and recession
- Subgingival calculus:
  - has no predilection for particular parts of the mouth
  - has its mineral content derived from gingival crevicular fluid
  - is detected by probing, direct vision or on radiographs
  - has different morphological types
  - has ethnic variation in prevalence and composition
  - is associated with subsequent periodontitis

7 Host defences

Figure 7.1 NFκB signalling via PAMP binding.

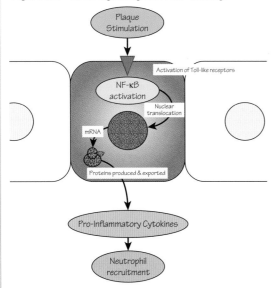

Figure 7.2 Neutrophil surface receptors. Different ligands all trigger ROS production via NADPH-oxidase (respiratory burst). *HMP – hexose-monophosphate shunt; GP – glutathione peroxidase; GR – glutathione reductase; SOD – superoxide dismutase; PKC – protein kinase-C; GSH – reduced glutathione; GSSG – oxidised glutathione.*

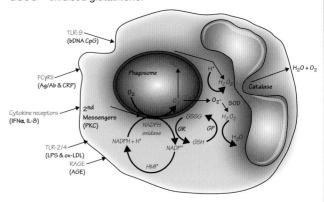

Figure 7.3 (a) Process of NET formation and release. (b) Photomicrograph of NETs (stained with for Sytox Green, fluorescent stain).
Source: Philippa White et al./with permission of John Wiley & Sons.

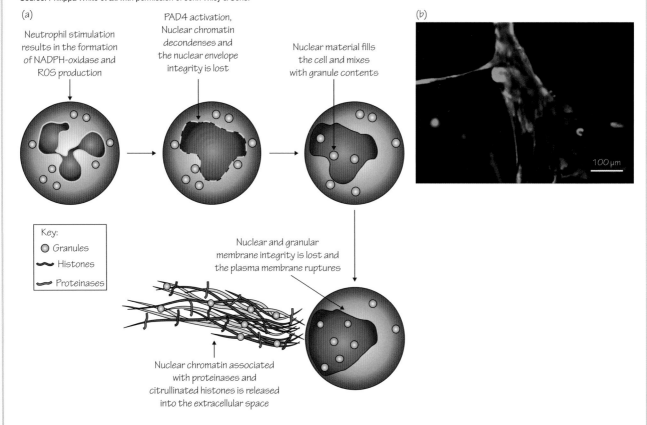

Figure 7.4 Process of neutrophil recuitment from blood vessels into tissues.

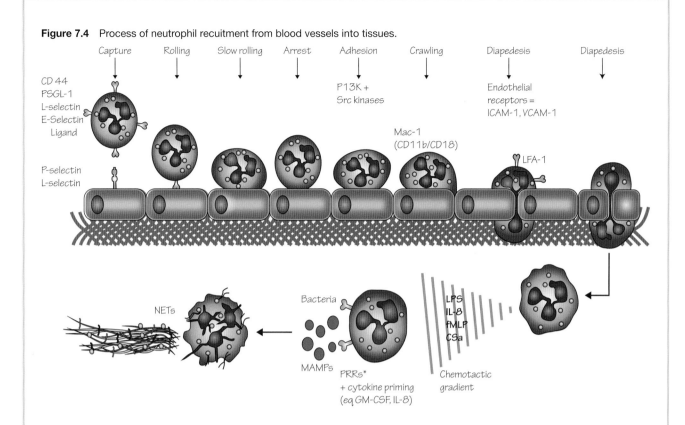

Figure 7.5 Contemporary model of neutrophil contribution to periodontal tissue damage.

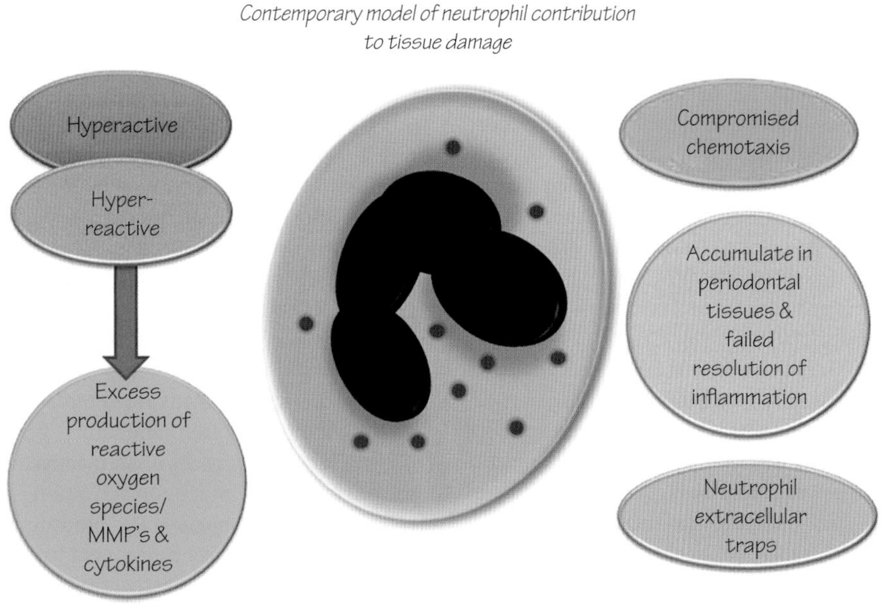

*Contemporary model of neutrophil contribution
to tissue damage*

Hyperactive

Hyper-reactive

Excess production of reactive oxygen species/ MMP's & cytokines

Compromised chemotaxis

Accumulate in periodontal tissues & failed resolution of inflammation

Neutrophil extracellular traps

Figure 7.6   T-cell types and cytokines. Th0: naïve T-cells; Treg: T-regulatory cells.

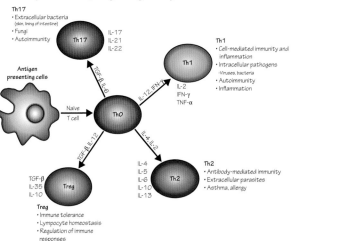

The host response to colonising periodontal bacteria is complex and stratified in nature, governed partly by the maturity of the periodontal biofilm and partly by an individual's genetic code, which is modified by lifestyle factors such as smoking, glycaemia, adiposity and stress. More recently, 'epigenetic' factors have been identified as playing an important role in host defence, and essentially involve posttranslational modifications made to proteins by bacterial or host-derived enzymes which alter a protein's function or how it is viewed by our immune system (friend or foe).

There are two major arms to the host response – the innate or 'non-specific' arm and the adaptive or 'specific' arm.

Recent changes in our understanding of host–microbial interactions include the following:

- The realisation that periodontal health requires a health-promoting biofilm that co-exists symbiotically with a balanced and proportionate host response – 'symbiosis'.
- That if the biofilm is allowed to accumulate without disruption or regular removal, pathogenic species can take advantage of an overly reactive host defence response and use components of that response transported via gingival crevicular fluid (GCF) to sustain their growth and proliferation – 'dysbiosis' (Lamont & Hajishengallis, 2015).
- That acute inflammation is protective, but should 'auto-resolve' as part of an active process whereby host cells, particularly neutrophils, produce short chain fatty acids (called lipoxins) which change the behaviour of other immune cells such as macrophages in order to actively resolve the inflammation (Chapter 9) – 'pro-resolving lipid mediators'.
- That failure of host pro-resolution mechanisms can result in chronic inflammation where the host's attempts at healing a periodontal wound (angiogenesis and fibrosis) occur simultaneously with continued inflammation and result in frustrated healing, i.e. granulation tissue formation, repair and scarring, rather than natural resolution and regeneration.
- There are many aspects of neutrophil behaviour that can become dysfunctional and potentially cause periodontitis (see later).
- The recognition that neutrophils can return from microbial exposure within tissues via circulation to bone marrow, to influence inflammation-induced epigenetic, metabolic and transcriptomic alterations to myeloid stem cell populations. The resulting mature neutrophils effectively undergo 'training' as haemopoietic stem cells during myelopoiesis and are released in a state of high alert with a hyperreactive phenotype (Mitroulis et al., 2018).

Innate immunity

Epithelial defences

Historically, epithelium was thought to function solely as a physical barrier to protect internalised vital organs from the external environment. In the periodontal tissues, the epithelial barrier is important in preventing bacterial ingress in to the underlying connective tissues; epithelial mesenchymal transition (EMT) has been reported to cause epithelial breakdown and is induced by periodontal pathogens resident in the mature plaque biofilm. EMT causes a shift in the phenotype/genotype of epithelial cells to cells exhibiting a more mesenchymal type structure, resulting in compromised epithelial barrier integrity. This allows bacterial ingress and the downstream inflammatory sequalae that are characteristic factors in the pathogenesis of periodontitis.

In addition to their function as a barrier, epithelial cells are now known to play an active role in innate immune defence, responding to stimulation (e.g. by bacteria) via 'pattern recognition receptors' (PRRs) that recognise highly conserved 'microbe/pathogen-associated molecular patterns' (MAMPs/PAMPs) and which when engaged activate second messengers that trigger gene expression and synthesis and release of chemokines, which generate a proinflammatory response. The best characterised PAMPs are the Toll-like receptors (TLRs) which when activated produce a range of downstream biological responses leading to activation of the proinflammatory gene transcription factor NF-κB. NF-κB is present in an inactive form (bound to IκB) in the cell cytoplasm and, upon activation, splits from its inhibitor, translocates to the nucleus and binds to DNA where it activates gene transcription. The subsequent messenger RNA is exported to ribosomes where it is transcribed into a range of proinflammatory cytokines and chemokines which are subsequently excreted from the cell and induce a range of downstream proinflammatory sequelae, most notably neutrophil recruitment to the site of challenge (Milward et al., 2007) (Fig. 7.1).

In the periodontal tissues, the sulcular or pocket epithelium is intimately related to the plaque biofilm and when stimulated by periodontal pathogens (P. gingivalis and F. nucleatum), activates NF-κB and downstream cytokine production, e.g. especially interleukin (IL)-8, IL-1, tumour necrosis factor (TNF)-α, IL-17 and cytokine-induced neutrophil chemoattractant-2. In addition, host defence proteins, such as α- and β-defensins, are released. This suggests a key role for sulcular and junctional epithelium in the initiation and propagation of the periodontal lesion.

Neutrophilic polymorphonuclear leukocytes (neutrophils)

Neutrophils (PMNs) are the dominant inflammatory immune cell in the periodontium, comprising 95% of leukocytes infiltrating the gingival crevice. They are packed with a cytotoxic arsenal of proteolytic enzymes (e.g. serine proteases like elastase) within various forms of granule/lysosome, and reactive oxygen species (ROS), and are capable of synthesising chemokines (IL-8, MIP-1α) and cytokines (IL-1, IL-6) and producing other defensive proteins such as S100A8/9 molecular chaperones. PMNs are known to survive up to 5.4 days in the circulation and are now recognised to comprise various different subsets that respond differently to different signals, providing wide heterogeneity (Van Staveren et al., 2018).

There are three forms of neutrophil-mediated killing, triggered by ligation of TLRs (innate immunity), FcΥ receptors (specific B-cell immunity), or various other receptors (Fig. 7.2).

- Phagocytosis – regarded as safe killing, where engulfed bacteria are exposed to ROS and enzymes within the safe confines of the phagosome, prior to neutrophils undergoing programmed cell death (apoptosis) and safe removal by macrophages (efferocytosis).
- Extracellular degranulation – unsafe killing, where release of ROS and enzymes into the extracellular tissue space is associated with substantial collateral host tissue damage.
- NETosis (Neutrophil Extracellular Trap) formation – release of decondensed nuclear DNA decorated with antimicrobial peptides (AMPs) (Fig. 7.3). NETosis is a very recent discovery but may be a double-edged sword as human DNA is autoimmunogenic and evidence is emerging that autoantibodies are produced against NET DNA when present in human tissues. Neutrophils are recruited into tissues (Fig. 7.4) in response to bacterial molecules and also host factors are released to combat infection such as complement.

Other recent discoveries that may underpin neutrophil-mediated periodontal tissue damage are summarised in Fig. 7.5 and include the following.

- Hyperactivity and -reactivity of PMNs in periodontitis patients in terms of release of ROS, enzymes like elastase and also cytokines such as IL8 (Matthews et al., 2007; Ling et al., 2015).
- Defective chemotaxis of periodontitis neutrophils in terms of speed, velocity of movement and also accuracy of movement towards chemotactic stimuli (Roberts et al., 2015).
- Reduced NET removal (White et al., 2016).

Adaptive/specific immunity

Cell-mediated immunity

Cell-mediated immunity involves T-cells whose microbial receptor, the 'T-cell receptor', is fixed to its surface, meaning that receptor–microbe engagement has to be mediated by the cell – thus 'cell mediated'. Following presentation of antigen, undifferentiated T-lymphocytes (TH0) form various T-cell types, principally T-helper cells (TH-1, TH-2, TH-17) and T-regulatory cells (Tregs), as well as the T-cytotoxic cell which directly lyses bacteria. The various functions of the different TH cells are summarised in Fig. 7.6 but are largely dictated by the types of cytokines they produce. TH-1 cells are generally regarded as proinflammatory (IFn-γ, TNF-α) and TH-2 cells modulate TH-1 activity, being anti-inflammatory (IL-4, IL-10), and facilitate B-cell differentiation into antibody-producing plasma cells. More recently, TH-17 cells (IL-17, IL-21, IL-22) have received a lot of attention as they control PMN homeostasis (synthesis, release from bone marrow, extravasation to tissues and apoptosis), interact with complement and are also potently osteoclastogenic.

Overall, T-cells are associated with stable periodontal lesions, perhaps because the T-cytotoxic cell is extremely specific in its targeting of bacteria and directly lyses cells, whereas the B-cell system relies upon less discriminating PMNs for pathogen clearance and, as discussed, PMNs in periodontitis patients appear dysfunctional.

Humoral immunity

This is directed towards antibody production and involves B-cells (plasma cells). In Latin, the word 'humor' means a fluid or secretion, hence the release and transport of immunoglobulins (antibody) freely in blood and tissue fluids comprises 'humoral immunity'.

- Tissue macrophages (e.g. epithelial Langerhans cells) process microbial antigens and transport them to lymph nodes, where they present antigen in association with their MHC class II surface antigens as 'altered self' to circulating lymphocytes which recognise the specific antigen and undergo clonal expansion.
- B-lymphocytes differentiate into plasma cells that secrete antibody against that specific antigen under the control of TH-1 lymphocytes (Fig. 7.6).
- Antibody production is protective, particularly IgG and IgA, although different immunoglobulin isotypes vary in their efficacy (IgG1, 2, 3, 4 and IgA1, 2).
- Antibody may be produced systemically or locally to aggregate micro-organisms; stop them from adhering to epithelium; work with complement to lyse bacteria (opsonisation); work with neutrophils for opsonisation, phagocytosis and safe killing.
- Antibody titres vary between individuals and also before and after treatment; in general, they rise after therapy. Antibody avidity (strength of binding to bacteria) also varies.
- High levels may indicate either a positive immune response or an inability of the body to eliminate the pathogen.
- The end of the antibody that binds the bacteria is the 'Fab' (fragment that is antigen binding) end, which is specific to that antigen. The distal end is the 'Fc' component and this is consistent and bound by the Fc receptor (FcγR) of the PMN, which then effects phagocytosis and safe killing.

Mediators

Mediators are soluble chemical messengers that regulate/provide a link between the inflammatory response, the immune response and tissue damage. Their actions are short-lived, potent and subject to rapid inactivation, and include the following.

- Cytokines, e.g. proinflammatory (IL-1, IL-6, IL-17, TNF-α); anti-inflammatory (IL-4, IL-10, IL-13); and transforming growth factor-β (both pro- and anti-inflammatory).
- Prostaglandins, e.g. PGE-2 (responsible for bone resorption, neutrophil chemotaxis, vascular permeability and dilation).
- Matrix metalloproteinases (proinflammatory, degrade connective tissue).

Key points
- Periodontal health requires a balanced immune-inflammatory response that is in symbiosis with heath-promoting bacteria.
- The PMN is the dominant inflammatory cell in periodontal tissues and whilst it is vital to acute inflammation, which is protective, it can also become dysfunctional and induce tissue damage.
- Innate and adaptive immune responses are intended to be protective but collateral tissue damage is believed to be the major cause of periodontal tissue destruction.
- Innate immunity involves an intact bioactive epithelium, GCF and inflammatory response.
- Adaptive/specific immunity comprises humoral and cell-mediated responses.
- Mediators link the inflammatory and immune responses and the PMN bridges both responses.
- Failed resolution of acute inflammation leads to chronic inflammation and periodontitis.

8 Development of periodontal disease

Figure 8.1 'Causal pie theory' – examples of component causes of plaque-induced periodontitis. Source: Chapple *et al.* (2017), Fig. 1/John Wiley & Sons.

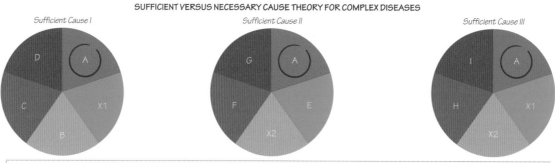

SUFFICIENT VERSUS NECESSARY CAUSE THEORY FOR COMPLEX DISEASES

Sufficient Cause I   *Sufficient Cause II*   *Sufficient Cause III*

Causal Pies. Each combination is sufficient for the disease to develop. "A" is a necessary cause because it is present in every pie. The rest (X1, X2, C, etc...) are component causes that could belong to different sufficient causes or appear as a joint element (eg. sufficient cause III).

Figure 8.2 Pristine gingiva.

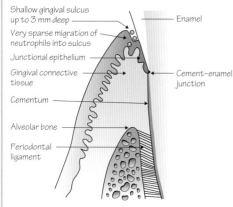

- Shallow gingival sulcus up to 3 mm deep
- Very sparse migration of neutrophils into sulcus
- Junctional epithelium
- Gingival connective tissue
- Cementum
- Alveolar bone
- Periodontal ligament
- Enamel
- Cement–enamel junction

Figure 8.3 An initial lesion.

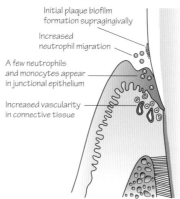

- Initial plaque biofilm formation supragingivally
- Increased neutrophil migration
- A few neutrophils and monocytes appear in junctional epithelium
- Increased vascularity in connective tissue

Figure 8.4 Clinically healthy gingiva in a 19-year-old female.

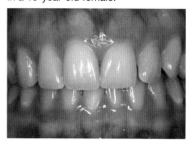

Figure 8.5 An early lesion.

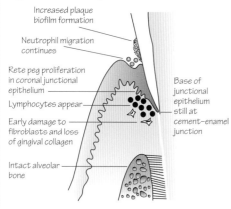

- Increased plaque biofilm formation
- Neutrophil migration continues
- Rete peg proliferation in coronal junctional epithelium
- Lymphocytes appear
- Early damage to fibroblasts and loss of gingival collagen
- Intact alveolar bone
- Base of junctional epithelium still at cement–enamel junction

Figure 8.6 An established lesion.

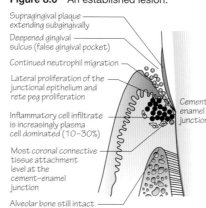

- Supragingival plaque extending subgingivally
- Deepened gingival sulcus (false gingival pocket)
- Continued neutrophil migration
- Lateral proliferation of the junctional epithelium and rete peg proliferation
- Inflammatory cell infiltrate is increasingly plasma cell dominated (10–30%)
- Most coronal connective tissue attachment level at the cement–enamel junction
- Alveolar bone still intact
- Cement–enamel junction

Figure 8.7 Clinical image of plaque-induced gingivitis.

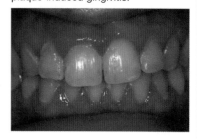

Periodontology at a Glance, Second Edition. Valerie Clerehugh, Aradhna Tugnait, Michael R. Milward, and Iain L. C. Chapple.
© 2024 John Wiley & Sons Ltd. Published 2024 by John Wiley & Sons Ltd.

Figure 8.8 An 'advanced' lesion (note 'advanced' here is a descriptor of the histological stage, not a descriptor of clinical severity) showing Stage-I periodontitis: true shallow periodontal pockets (4–5 mm); CAL of 1–2 mm; and early alveolar bone loss (horizontal), with the formation of a supra-bony pocket.

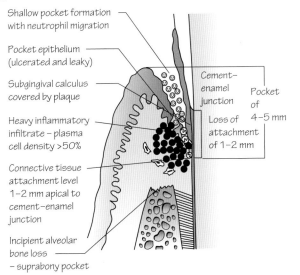

- Shallow pocket formation with neutrophil migration
- Pocket epithelium (ulcerated and leaky)
- Subgingival calculus covered by plaque
- Heavy inflammatory infiltrate – plasma cell density >50%
- Connective tissue attachment level 1–2 mm apical to cement–enamel junction
- Incipient alveolar bone loss – suprabony pocket
- Cement–enamel junction
- Pocket of 4–5 mm
- Loss of attachment of 1–2 mm

Figure 8.9 Patient with moderate periodontitis showing swollen, inflamed gingivae with blunted margins and loss of contour; deep periodontal pockets ≥6 mm and CAL of 3–4 mm were present in this patient.

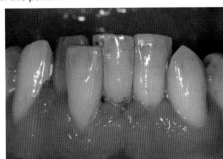

Gingivitis is ubiquitous, with the majority of the world population showing some level of gingival inflammation. Gingival inflammation is also a prerequisite for periodontitis to develop, although gingivitis does not always develop into periodontitis and progression is dependent upon individual host susceptibility, governed by risk factors such as genetic predisposition, smoking or hyperglycaemia in type 2 diabetes. Importantly, 26-year longitudinal data demonstrated that consistent site-specific gingival inflammation is associated with 70% more attachment loss and deeper pockets, as well as significantly greater tooth loss (Schätzle *et al.*, 2003, 2004).

Periodontitis is a complex multifactorial disease, and as such it has no single cause. Pathogenic bacteria (within a dysbiotic plaque) are a prerequisite for periodontitis, but are not sufficient on their own to 'cause' it; if they were, everyone would develop periodontitis, which is not the case (Chapter 9). Complex diseases rarely have a single cause, but have multiple 'component causes' and these may differ in number and magnitude of influence from one person to the next. Initial gingival inflammation causes a dysbiotic plaque community which influences a series of inflammatory-immune events, whose efficacy in restoring the microbial/host symbiosis is influenced by other component causes, also referred to as risk factors. Component causes of periodontitis are largely host-dependent variables and if the magnitude of their influence exceeds a certain threshold, periodontitis develops. A dysregulated and excessive host response is believed to cause the majority (80%) of periodontal tissue damage. This 'causal pie theory' of complex diseases was proposed by Rothman (2002) (Fig. 8.1).

Our current treatment strategies therefore aim to correct risk factors and minimise plaque levels (bacterial load) in order to reduce the inflammatory response to a proportionate one. A White Paper by the Economist Intelligence Unit (EIU) modelled the financial return on investment (ROI) of focusing resources on eliminating incident gingivitis versus a current model of 'business as usual', for six European countries, over 10 years.

The model demonstrated country-specific savings of between €8–32 billion and ROIs of 15–60 Euros for every Euro invested in managing gingivitis and preventing periodontitis (EIU, 2021).

Histological stages of development from health to gingivitis to periodontitis (Page & Schröeder, 1976)

Health

'Pristine' gingival health (Fig. 8.2) is characterised by pink gingivae which are uniform in colour, stippling, knife edge gingival margins, triangular interdental papillae, absence of bleeding or suppuration, probing depths ≤3 mm and no swelling. This clinical picture is almost a myth as the vast majority of the population show some level of gingival inflammation clinically. Patients who practise meticulous standards of oral hygiene can achieve 'clinical health' which permits up to 10% of bleeding sites according to the 2018 classification of 'clinical health' (Chapple *et al.*, 2018). Some inflammation also remains visible at a histological level (Figs 8.3, 8.4) as part of a 'proportionate' inflammatory-immune response that exists symbiotically with a health-promoting biofilm (Kilian *et al.*, 2016) (Chapter 7).

Initial lesion

Inflammation begins within 24 hours of plaque accumulation, resulting in vasodilation of the local vasculature and increased gingival crevicular fluid (GCF) flow. This inflammatory response is initiated by bacterial stimulation of sulcular epithelial cells that are intimately associated with the plaque biofilm via pattern recognition receptors (e.g. Toll-like receptors) found on the cell membrane. The result is an activation of the key proinflammatory gene transcription factor "Nuclear Factor κB" (NF-κB) causing changes in gene expression and downstream proinflammatory cytokine production. Activation of this pathway

(Chapter 7) results in a range of proinflammatory sequelae, including increases in the inflammatory infiltrate. The proinflammatory infiltrate is characterised by:

- neutrophilic polymorphonuclear leukocytes (neutrophils/ PMNs) which migrate into the gingival tissues from the local circulation. Local activation of complement and chemokine release causes vasodilation, reductions in blood flow and increased expression of adhesion molecules (e.g. intercellular adhesion molecule 1 [ICAM1] and endothelial leukocyte adhesion molecule [ELAM 1]) on vascular endothelium, which facilitate PMN egress (diapedesis) from the circulation and migration through the periodontal tissues along chemotactic gradients (e.g. IL-8, LTB4, MIP-1α) into the gingival crevice
- low numbers of lymphocytes can be seen at this stage, which express cluster determinant 44 (CD44) on their cell surface, allowing their binding to connective tissue components
- appearance of small numbers of macrophages.

This cellular response develops in 2–4 days and at this point the gingival tissues appear to be clinically healthy.

Early gingival lesion

Following one week of plaque accumulation, the early lesion develops (Fig. 8.5), characterised by the following.

- Further accumulation of the cellular and humoral inflammatory infiltrate.
- The local blood vessels remain dilated, resulting in gingival redness, a classic characteristic of gingival inflammation.
- Increases in neutrophils and lymphocyte numbers; these cells are the predominant cellular response at this stage with few plasma cells present.
- Connective tissue changes are evident, with collagen loss and damage to fibroblasts.
- Changes can also be seen in the junctional/sulcular epithelium, with increased basal cell and rete ridge proliferation. Th-17 cells appear and release IL-17, which promotes formation of a barrier (pocket lining) epithelium by enhancing tight junctions, as opposed to the semi-permeable sulcular epithelium in periodontal health (Konkel & Chapple, 2022). The enhanced epithelial barrier function helps to prevent bacterial invasion. Loss of coronal epithelium can be seen along with subgingival extension of the plaque biofilm.

The early lesion can persist and may not necessarily progress to established gingivitis.

Established lesion

It is difficult to predict at what stage the established lesion develops (Figs 8.6, 8.7), but histologically it is characterised by the following:

- Increased GCF flow, moving from a passive transudate that facilitates immune surveillance to secreted exudate carrying the immune response to the biofilm.
- Further increases in the inflammatory infiltrate arise, with the neutrophil remaining the predominant cell. Migration from the peripheral circulation to the periodontal lesion increases and neutrophils accumulate in the periodontal tissues.
- At this stage, plasma cells make up only 10–30% of the inflammatory infiltrate.
- Further damage to the connective tissues can be seen with increasing levels of injury to fibroblasts and loss of collagen, releasing damage-associated molecular peptides (DAMPs) that

stimulate further PMN chemotaxis for wound debridement. Connective tissue loss allows space for the accumulation of the inflammatory infiltrate.

- Changes to the epithelium continue with more pronounced rete ridges as the permeable junctional epithelium becomes less well attached to the tooth surface and transforms to a barrier pocket lining epithelium, influenced by IL-17. This allows further subgingival extension of the pathogenic biofilm and the resulting pocket epithelium shows increased permeability and areas of ulceration may develop.

At this stage, the clinical signs of gingivitis can be seen which include redness, swelling and bleeding, and the various inflammatory components, such as haemoglobin, act as nutrient sources for key pathogens like *P. gingivalis*.

The established lesion may remain stable or progress to periodontitis dependent on host susceptibility, the influence of various risk factors and/or clinical intervention.

Advanced lesion

As the gingival epithelium migrates apically, the gingival pocket deepens, allowing further apical extension of the plaque biofilm (Figs 8.8, 8.9). Histologically this lesion is characterised by the following:

- Further development of the inflammatory infiltrate with increased lateral and apical extension into the periodontal connective tissue attachment apparatus.
- Increased proportion of plasma cells which constitute >50% of the cell infiltrate.
- Irreversible tissue changes are seen, i.e. apical migration of junctional epithelium with 'true' pocket formation, loss of connective tissue and alveolar bone.
- Increased IL-17 by Th-17 cells stimulates myelopoiesis for PMNs in bone marrow.
- Hyperactivity and -reactivity of PMNs with respect to ROS, cytokine and proteolytic enzyme release (e.g. elastase) (Matthews *et al.*, 2007; Ling *et al.*, 2016).

As the advanced lesion develops, periodontal pockets and clinical attachment loss (CAL) increase. Initially, pockets are shallow (Stage-I periodontitis) (4–5 mm) with a CAL of 1–2 mm and a predominant horizontal pattern of bone loss and supra-bony pockets (base of pocket coronal to alveolar bone crest) (Fig. 8.8).

As the disease progresses, pockets become deeper (≥6 mm) and CAL increases (moderate loss 3–4 mm; severe >5 mm), associated with increasing levels of alveolar bone loss. At this stage, infra-bony pockets may be seen (base of pocket apical to alveolar bone loss) (Fig. 8.9; see also Fig. 35.1b).

The mature periodontal lesion is chronic in nature and characterised by the accumulation of inflammatory cells, frustrated healing and a 'non-resolving' chronic inflammation. The levels of damaging reactive oxygen species, proteolytic enzymes and matrix metalloproteinases released from host immune cells increase and local antioxidant defence systems become overwhelmed, resulting in oxidative stress which leads to further periodontal tissue breakdown via NF-κB and osteoclast activation.

There are considerable patient-based differences in how disease develops from health to gingivitis to periodontitis. This reflects the importance of the host response to the developing plaque biofilm and the influence of risk factors in disease pathogenesis.

Currently, clinical management strategies involve disrupting and reducing the biofilm to encourage re-establishment of health-promoting Gram-positive bacteria, and by damping down the exaggerated inflammation seen in susceptible patients. Future management may involve methods to directly modulate the aberrant inflammatory response alongside conventional treatment, such as the discovery of proresolution mediators (Serhan *et al.*, 2008).

Active lesion

The conversion of a stable advanced lesion to an active one is characterised by a change from a T-cell-dominated inflammatory infiltrate to a B-cell-dominant one (Seymour *et al.*, 1979), where the end effector cell is the neutrophil.

Key points
- Initial, early and established histological lesions represent different stages of gingivitis.
- The advanced histlogical lesion shows irreversible loss of periodontal tissues, i.e. periodontitis, and can be stable (T-cell dominant) or active (B-cell dominant).
- The time scale for transition between stages is variable and unpredictable, with no inevitable progress from gingivitis to periodontitis.
- Patient susceptibility modulated by risk factors is a key aspect of the development of periodontitis.
- Current treatment regimens aim to reduce plaque biofilm as a way of reducing the aberrant host response, but proresolution of inflammation approaches are under development.

9 Progression of periodontitis

Figure 9.1 (a) Random burst model of clinical attachment loss (CAL). (b) Examples of three sites (UR1, LL6 and UR6) showing random bursts of CAL over the patient's lifetime.

- Sites are categorised as active or inactive
- Bursts of activity are short – a few days or weeks
- One or more bursts can occur at each active site
- Occurrence of bursts is independent of the previous burst history

(a)

UR1: Slight CAL in random bursts from 1 to 2 mm between 15 and 80 years
LL6: Moderate CAL in random bursts from 2 to 4 mm between 15 and 80 years
UR6: Severe CAL in random bursts from 2 to 10 mm between 15 and 50 years when tooth is extracted

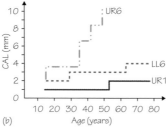

(b)

Figure 9.2 (a) Asynchronous multiple burst model of CAL. (b) Examples of three sites showing asynchronous bursts of CAL over the patient's lifetime.

- Multiple active sites break down within a relatively short period of time, with long periods of quiescence which can last months or years
  - periods of activity may be clustered around particular phases in a patient's life perhaps when stress, illness or some other periodontal risk factor comes into effect (i.e. transient)

(a)

UR1: Slight CAL in burst from 1 to 2 mm around 50 years
LL6: Moderate CAL in bursts from 2 to 4 mm around 50 years
UR6: Severe CAL in bursts from 2 to 10 mm mainly around 50 years when tooth is extracted

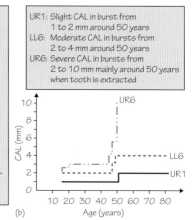

(b)

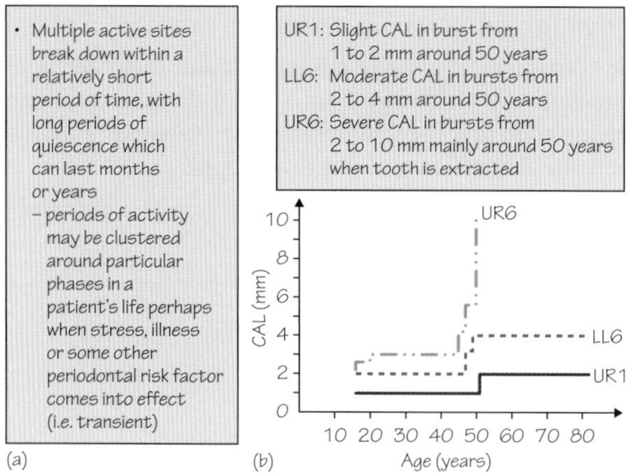

Figure 9.3 (a) Continuous rate model of CAL. (b) Examples of three sites showing different rates of continuous 'linear' CAL over the patient's lifetime.

UR1: Slight 'linear' CAL from 1 to 2 mm between 15 and 80 years
LL6: Moderate 'linear' CAL from 2 to 4 mm between 15 and 80 years
UR6: Severe 'linear' CAL from 2 to 10 mm between 15 and 50 years when tooth is extracted

- Sites are categorised as active or inactive
- Active sites break down at a constant rate
- Fluctuations in the rate of progression at an active site are possible

(a)

(b)

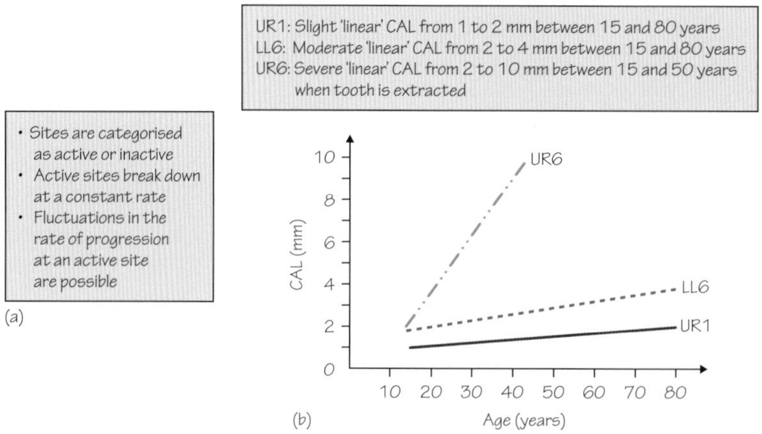

Figure 9.4 Contemporary model of host–microbe interactions in the pathogenesis of periodontitis. Source: Meyle & Chapple (2015), Fig. 1/John Wiley & Sons.

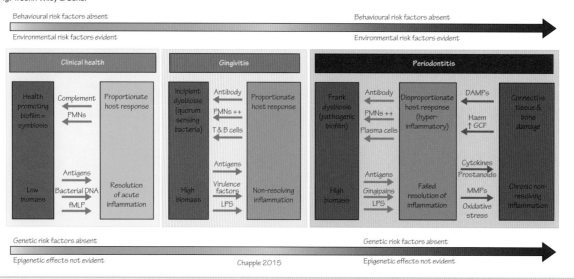

Periodontology at a Glance, Second Edition. Valerie Clerehugh, Aradhna Tugnait, Michael R. Milward, and Iain L. C. Chapple.
© 2024 John Wiley & Sons Ltd. Published 2024 by John Wiley & Sons Ltd.

Figure 9.5 Derivation of lipoxins from arachidonic acid. Source: Van Dyke (2011), Fig. 1/John Wiley & Sons.

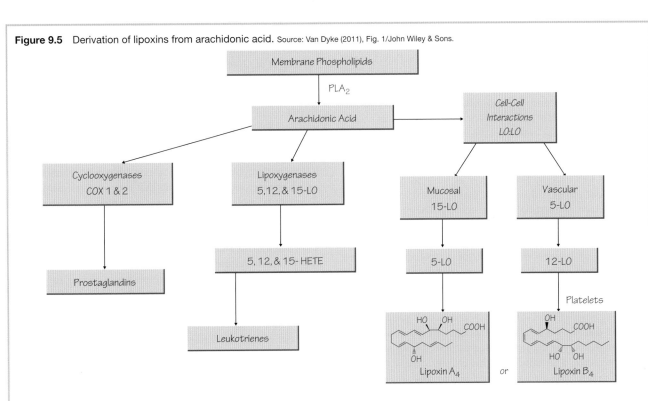

Figure 9.6 2017 World Workshop definition of a periodontitis case. Source: Papapanou *et al.* (2018)/John Wiley & Sons.

In the context of clinical care, a patient is a "periodontitis case" if:
1. Interdental CAL is detectable at ≥2 non-adjacent teeth, or
2. Buccal or oral CAL ≥3 mm with pocketing ≥3 mm is detectable at ≥2 teeth but the observed CAL cannot be ascribed to non-periodontitis-related causes such as:
   1) gingival recession of traumatic origin;
   2) dental caries extending in the cervical area of the tooth;
   3) the presence of CAL on the distal aspect of a second molar and associated with malposition or extraction of a third molar;
   4) an endodontic lesion draining through the marginal periodontium; and
   5) the occurrence of a vertical root fracture.
(Papapanou et al 2018)

Periodontal diseases comprise a large group of conditions that affect the periodontal tissues, the most common being inflammatory conditions initiated by an inflammation-driven dysbiotic plaque biofilm, specifically gingivitis and periodontitis. The factors that govern the progression of periodontitis are not fully understood and may differ from those risk factors or component causes that initiate the disease. There is consensus that gingival inflammation is a prerequisite for periodontitis to develop and progress (Chapter 8) and therefore managing gingivitis is a primary preventive strategy for periodontitis (Chapple *et al.*, 2015). Factors governing the recurrence of successfully treated periodontitis may also differ from those that initiate the primary disease or fuel its progression; however, it seems likely that the major risk factors are common to all three scenarios (initiation, progression and recurrence). Secondary prevention is the prevention of recurrent periodontitis.

Natural history of periodontitis

The natural history of any disease describes its course in the absence of any medical or surgical intervention, which in the case of periodontitis is tooth loss. Natural history may be studied at a population level, or at a patient, tooth or site level. Population studies are challenging as they require a population with no access to modern healthcare, either professional or personal care. The classic Sri Lankan tea worker studies of Löe and colleagues (1986) examined tea plantation workers longitudinally over 15 years. The tea workers had no access to modern medicine or dentistry and periodontitis progression was compared to that of a Norwegian control population. The Sri Lankans had higher levels of plaque and calculus and rates of progression varied.

- 11% showed no progression at all and appeared 'disease resistant'.
- 81% progressed at a moderate rate and had 'moderate risk'.
- 8% progressed at a rapid rate and were 'high risk'.

Today, these figures are regarded as being slightly on the high side due to the measurement methods employed and the definitions used for a 'case' or for assigning 'disease progression'. Contemporary epidemiology for disease prevalence (rather than progression) demonstrates that between 11.2% (Kassebaum *et al.*, 2014) and 19% (Chen *et al.*, 2021) of the world population has severe periodontitis and severe periodontitis is the sixth most prevalent human disease.

In the 1980s, Socransky and colleagues (1984) started to explore the progression of periodontitis at a site-specific level by measuring attachment loss in 22 periodontitis sufferers every two months for a year. They demonstrated that the disease progressed in a random pattern over time with bursts of activity and periods of quiescence – the so-called 'random burst hypothesis' (Fig. 9.1). A variant of this pattern of progression was shown by the same authors as 'multiple asynchronous bursts' (Fig. 9.2). However, this was disputed seven years later by Jeffcoat and Reddy (1991), who claimed that the definition of an 'episode' of attachment loss used by Socransky et al. (around 2.5 mm after measurement error) had created a mathematical model biased towards detecting bursts of disease activity. They employed an electronic periodontal probe accurate to 0.1 mm and, using smaller increments to define disease activity, demonstrated a linear pattern of progression in 76% of 30 patients examined (Fig. 9.3). Nevertheless, 24% still progressed non-linearly in their study and the debate remains unresolved.

In general, of the studies that followed, those that demonstrated a 'burst' model of activity monitored patients with untreated disease, whereas those that showed a predominantly linear progression monitored treated patients during periodontal maintenance. The authors of this chapter believe that both forms of progression are likely, but if risk factors are controlled and the disease is treated, then it is natural to expect progression during supportive care to be more predictable and thus predominantly linear, whereas untreated disease is more likely to progress in a non-linear and less predictable pattern.

Using multilevel modelling, Gilthorpe and colleagues (2003) concluded that the linear and burst theories are a manifestation of the same phenomenon, namely that loss of attachment progresses in some sites, while other sites improve, in a cyclical manner.

Pathogenic model of periodontitis progression

The classic model of periodontitis progression from a healthy state was defined by Page and Kornman (1997), but advances in knowledge over the last decade have led to a contemporary version of the original model being developed by Chapple (Meyle & Chapple, 2015). In this model (Fig. 9.4), progression from health to gingivitis and ultimately periodontitis is underpinned by genetic, epigenetic, lifestyle and environmental risk factors. In clinical health (as opposed to pristine health – Chapter 7), a symbiosis exists between a health-promoting biofilm and the host response, the two being in balance and self-sustaining. However, if the biofilm is allowed to accumulate, local conditions change and an 'incipient dysbiosis' develops whereby pathogenic bacteria start to emerge; the host response remains proportionate and a self-limiting chronic inflammatory state develops – gingivitis. In susceptible (high-risk) patients, the host response becomes exaggerated and disproportionate and an excessive release of various inflammatory molecules causes host tissue damage, the products of which become a substrate for pathogenic bacteria and a frank dysbiosis develops. Various virulence strategies of key pathogens like P. gingivalis conspire to drive further dysfunction in the host's inflammatory-immune response, which fails to eliminate the pathogens and restore a health-promoting biofilm. The inflammation becomes chronic in nature and fails to resolve without intervention, and periodontitis progresses.

Resolution of inflammation

Research over the last two decades by Serhan and Van Dyke (Serhan et al., 2008) led to the discovery of a novel class of small chain fatty acid signalling molecules, derived endogenously from arachidonic acid and called lipoxins (Fig. 9.5), alongside similar classes of pro-resolving lipid mediators derived from dietary omega-3 polyunsaturated fatty acids called resolvins, protectins and maresins (Van Dyke, 2011). These molecules are receptor agonists that bind to inflammatory cells and actively 'switch off' inflammation, by promoting a non-phlogistic phenotype in cells like macrophages, meaning that they stop releasing proinflammatory molecules and instead commence the removal of spent/apoptosing neutrophils and enhance clearance of periodontal pathogens at mucosal surfaces. Resolvin RVE1 has been shown in murine and rabbit models to actively switch off inflammation and to restore health and indeed a health-promoting biofilm. Moreover, these pro-resolution lipids appear to promote wound healing by regeneration rather than by repair. Progression of periodontitis is associated with failed pro-resolving mechanisms, and novel interventions employing topical applications of these natural mediators may not only prevent periodontal disease progression, but also appear to have the potential to regenerate lost periodontal attachment and bone. Their use in mouthrinse formulations has been shown to be safe (Hasturk et al., 2021).

Clinical studies of disease progression

Defining 'active' periodontitis has been a challenge for several decades and it seems more likely that saliva-based biosensor technologies hold the key to this in the future (Grant et al., 2022). However, currently, decisions concerning disease activity and progression in patients are governed by clinical outcomes from clinical trials. The principal measures employed are those of:
- probing pocket depth.
- bleeding from the base of the pocket.
- clinical attachment loss.

Clearly, disease progression in research studies is defined by progressive attachment loss but in clinical practice, attachment loss is rarely measured for reasons of practicality. A classic three-year prospective study by Westfelt and colleagues (1998) demonstrated that pockets ≥6 mm were more likely to progress than those of ≥5 mm and similar studies by Lang et al. (1990) demonstrated that bleeding on probing was one of the strongest indicators of progressive disease. They demonstrated a sensitivity of 20% in predicting 1 mm attachment loss over a two-year period and a 5% sensitivity for predicting a 2 mm attachment loss over that period. However, smoking was not fully controlled for in this study. More importantly, of those sites that did not bleed, 100% experienced no further attachment loss. Today, treatment aims to achieve non-bleeding pockets of 4 mm or less and these are defined as 'closed pockets', which have a very low risk of disease progression (Wennström et al., 2005).

Definition of progression and risk factors

It was concluded at the fifth European Workshop on Periodontology in 2005 that studies of risk factors and progression should use a consistent definition for a 'periodontitis case' and 'periodontitis progression' to improve consistency in data interpretation globally. The case definition for periodontitis was changed in 2018 to that illustrated in Fig. 9.6 (Papapanou et al., 2018). It should also be noted that in addition to the descriptors given for CAL, a case of periodontitis requires bone loss to be present at ≥2 non-adjacent teeth. Risk factors for periodontitis are discussed in Chapter 10, but in terms of disease progression, the most widely recognised factors are:

- major life events that create stress and where there are no coping behaviours in patients under stress.
- hormonal changes during pregnancy.
- hyperglycaemia in poorly controlled/undiagnosed diabetes
- smoking.
- secondary occlusal trauma.

Key points

- Most humans experience gingivitis but approximately 50% will develop some periodontitis and around 11.2–19% will experience severe periodontitis
- Factors governing progression of gingivitis to periodontitis remain poorly understood but involve development of a dysbiosis and hyperactive host immune-inflammatory response
- Resolution of inflammation has emerged as an important field and may contribute greater insights in the future concerning why periodontitis progresses in some patients and not others
- Sites most likely to progress are those with probing pockets >4 mm, bleeding and suppuration

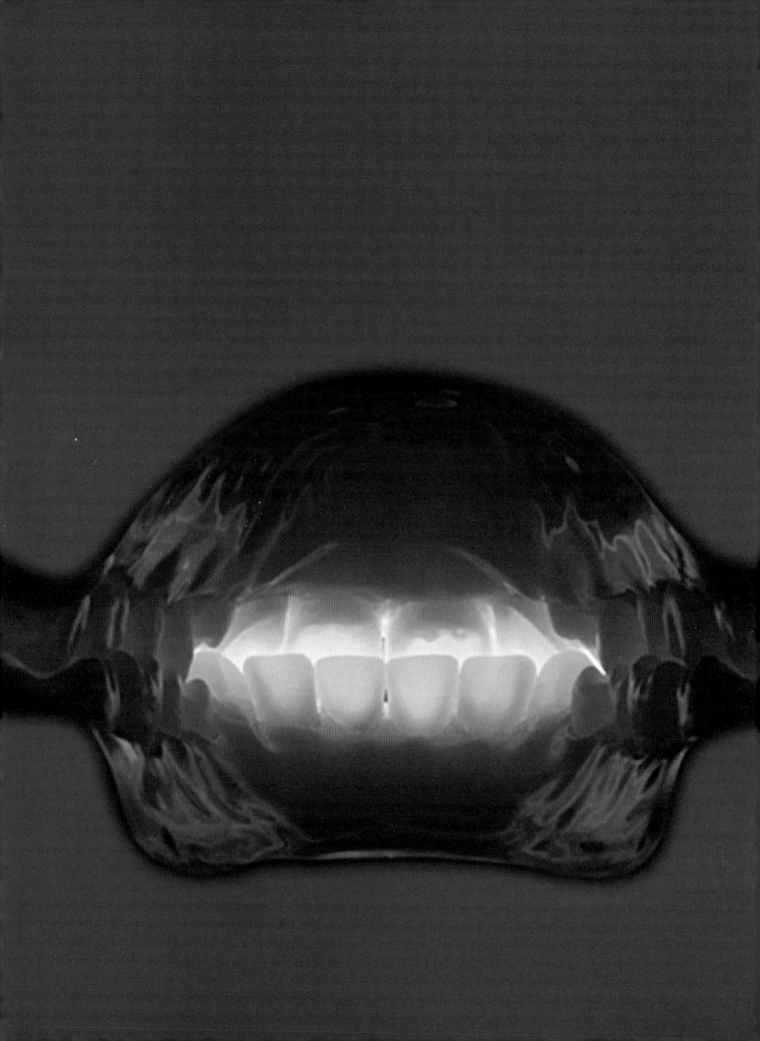

Risk and periodontal diseases

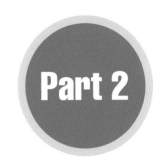

Part 2

Chapters

Overview

Part 2 starts with chapters on the current views of risk and the periodontal diseases (Chapter 10), systemic (or modifying) risk factors for periodontitis (Chapter 11) and the link between periodontal diseases and general health problems, including diabetes mellitus, atherosclerotic cardiovascular diseases, stroke, rheumatoid arthritis, chronic kidney disease, nosocomial respiratory infections, adverse pregnancy outcomes, Alzheimer disease and certain cancers (Chapter 12). The next chapter on the role of diet in periodontal diseases incorporates salient recommendations that healthcare professionals may counsel their patients on in respect of dietary calcium, reduced intake of refined sugars, increased antioxidant micronutrient intake and overall weight control (Chapter 13). The penultimate chapter addresses local (or predisposing) risk factors for periodontal diseases and the rationale to prevent, modify or eliminate them where possible (Chapter 14). The final chapter in Part 2 looks at occlusion and periodontal diseases, and while reinforcing the view that occlusal forces cannot initiate periodontal breakdown, provides up-to-date guidance on treatment, occlusal adjustment and management of tooth mobility (Chapter 15).

10 Risk and periodontal diseases

Figure 10.1 Interaction of periodontal microflora, the inflammatory response and risk factors.

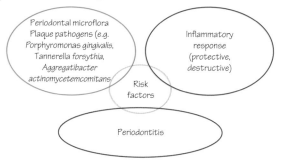

Table 10.2 Systemic risk factors and indicators for periodontal disease, based on current knowledge.

Risk factors	Risk indicators
Smoking	Low dietary calcium
Poorly controlled diabetes mellitus types 1 and 2	High and frequent intake of refined sugars
Race/ethnicity	Postmenopausal osteoporosis and osteopenia
Genetics	Visceral obesity
Ageing	Stress and inadequate coping
Polymorphonuclear leukocyte (neutrophil) function	
Socioeconomic status	
Glycaemia in people without diabetes	
Severe malnutrition (micronutrient deficiency)	

Table 10.1 Levels of evidence for risk factors in chronic diseases and characteristics of these studies which make the factors more convincing, and not likely to be spurious associations.

Type of study	Study characteristics
Cross-sectional or case–control studies	Confounding factors are eliminated or adjusted for in the analysis. Many assess dose response and specificity
Longitudinal epidemiological studies	Help establish temporality; may also be adjusted for confounding factors
Mechanism studies	Human or animal, as well as *in vitro* studies that demonstrate how the risk factors exert their effects in the causal pathway
Intervention studies	Effects are clinically meaningful. Important step in proving causality, and provide justification for risk modification in clinical practice

Figure 10.2 Pack-years of cigarette smoking and clinical attachment loss.

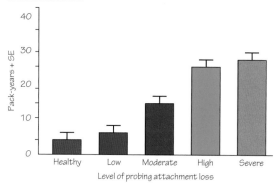

Figure 10.3 Periodontal disease and glycaemic control: cause or effect?

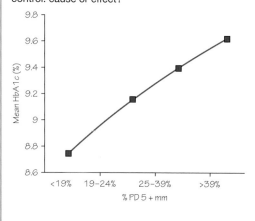

Table 10.3 Modification of risk factors for periodontal disease.

Factor	Modification
Risk factor	
Smoking	Smoking cessation
Diabetes	Improve glycaemic control
Risk indicator	
Low dietary calcium	Calcium supplementation
High dietary refined sugar intake	Reduce frequency and amount of sugar intake
Osteoporosis or osteopenia	Bone-sparing agents, calcium and vitamin D supplementation
Visceral obesity	Diet and exercise
Stress and inadequate coping	Stress reduction measures

Periodontology at a Glance, Second Edition. Valerie Clerehugh, Aradhna Tugnait, Michael R. Milward, and Iain L. C. Chapple.
© 2024 John Wiley & Sons Ltd. Published 2024 by John Wiley & Sons Ltd.

Periodontal diseases are associated with accumulation of dental biofilms and population of the subgingival area with a dynamic community of microbes, including anaerobic bacteria that express virulence factors. The term 'dysbiosis' is now employed to describe the emergence of pathogenic species from within a symbiotic and health-promoting biofilm, and dysbiosis is underpinned by gingival inflammation, in a circular manner. These virulence factors cause direct tissue destruction and trigger destructive host immunopathological responses. The effect of the subgingival microbiota is modified by the host since some individuals have large accumulations of dental plaque and suffer little periodontitis, while others have little plaque accumulation and suffer severe periodontitis.

It appears, then, that risk factors are important in periodontitis, determining who develops the disease, the severity of the disease, which sites in the dentition are affected and the rate of disease progression. Risk factors probably also influence the response to therapy and disease recurrence rates. In assessing risk, the probability that a disease outcome will occur following a particular exposure is estimated (Last, 2001).

What is a risk factor?

A risk factor can be an aspect of personal behaviour or lifestyle, an environmental exposure, or an inborn or inherited characteristic that changes the susceptibility to periodontal disease. Risk factors such as these affect the whole dentition and are called systemic risk factors. There are also local risk factors which increase biofilm accumulation at a specific site or tooth. In the 2018 classification of periodontal diseases and conditions, risk factors were categorised as 'predisposing factors' (local risk factors) and 'modifying factors' (systemic risk factors).

- On the basis of cross-sectional epidemiological evidence, putative risk factors are associated with disease after accounting for possible confounding factors (Last, 2001).
- Longitudinal studies can help determine if the presence of the factor precedes the onset of disease, which strengthens the evidence that the factor is truly related to the disease and not just a chance association.
- True risk factors are part of the causal chain or expose the host to the causal chain (Beck, 1998) and evidence for causality usually comes from human association studies in conjunction with animal and *in vitro* studies of mechanisms of action (Fig. 10.1).
- Finally, true risk factors will most often affect disease outcome if removed or moderated. This can be determined by randomised controlled trials where the risk factor is removed or reduced and the disease eliminated or reduced.

Different terms are used for factors associated with disease risk. Risk indicators are associated with an increased probability of disease, based on cross-sectional studies carefully designed to eliminate those confounders that may result in spurious associations. A risk indicator may also be called a probable or putative risk factor. If confirmed in longitudinal and intervention studies, and determined to be in the causal pathway, they would be called risk factors. There are other terms used, such as risk markers, which are attributes or exposures associated with an increased probability of the disease. Risk markers are not usually factors in the causal pathway but are indirectly associated with the true risk factor.

In summary, true risk factors are not only associated with the disease and precede the development of disease, they frequently accelerate disease progression or are associated with recurrence. They are shown to be in the causal pathway by studies of disease mechanisms, for which biological plausibility exists, and they most often show dose–response effects and specificity. Proof of the effect of reduction or modification of risk factors on the disease most often comes from randomised controlled trials (Table 10.1).

Types of risk factors for periodontal disease

There are two major classes of risk factors for periodontal disease.

1 *Predisposing or local factors* such as overhanging restorations and root caries that tend to allow for plaque accumulation and hence result in more periodontal disease (see also Chapter 14). Other local risk factors for periodontal disease include pocket probing depth, intra-bony pockets, especially involving furcations, and root canal infections.
2 *Modifying or systemic factors* affect the entire body, such as cigarette smoking, sub-optimally controlled diabetes mellitus and genetic factors, and are often most clearly expressed as increasing the severity of periodontal disease (Table 10.2).

Are risk factors modifiable?

Many risk factors are modifiable, including local factors such as overhanging restorations and systemic factors such as smoking. An overhanging restoration can be removed, and smoking can be eliminated by engaging in a smoking cessation programme. Other risk factors are currently non-modifiable, such as genetic factors.

Levels of exposure to risk factors – the threshold

Often risk factors have a clear dose response, i.e. the more exposure to the risk factor, the greater the susceptibility to the disease. This is the case for cigarette smoking. There is a direct linear relationship between the exposure to smoking, estimated by the number of pack-years of cigarette smoking, and the amount of alveolar bone loss, as seen in periodontal patients (Fig. 10.2). Also, there is a direct relationship between the level of plasma glucose in patients with diabetes and the severity of periodontal disease (Fig. 10.3). In many studies, well-controlled patients with diabetes appear to be at comparable risk for periodontal disease as those with no diabetes.

These observations bring up the concept of a threshold. For many risk factors, it is believed that there is a threshold below which the risk factor has a negligible clinical effect on the disease. For example, normal or near normal levels of blood glucose (or haemoglobin A1c <6.5%) in patients with diabetes appear to represent a threshold below which there is little increased risk of periodontitis, even in individuals diagnosed as suffering from diabetes.

Modification of risk factors is part of the management of periodontitis

It has been shown that glycaemic control in patients with diabetes and smoking cessation enhance the prognosis of treatment for periodontitis and are important measures to prevent recurrence of periodontal disease. Weight control, calcium supplementation, control of stress and enhancement of coping skills may also prove important in the management of risk for periodontal disease (Table 10.3).

It is clear that the removal of local risk factors such as overhanging restorations, restoration of root caries and reduction of periodontal pockets is important in the management of periodontal disease and particularly in preventing recurrence.

Key points

- Overgrowth of dental biofilm and the emergence of dysbiosis involving a community of pathogenic bacteria may be a necessary but not a sufficient cause of periodontitis
- Risk factors work to change the susceptibility or resistance of individuals to the disease-causing effects of dental biofilms
- Risk factors can be local (predisposing) or systemic (modifying)
- Risk factors are in the causal pathway and, if altered, will alter the course of periodontitis
- Evidence to establish true risk factors can come from population-based epidemiological studies – *in vitro* and *in vivo* studies of causality relating the risk factor to the disease causal pathways. Evidence can also be sought via intervention studies, which help establish whether or not risk modification will contribute to disease reduction
- Gingival inflammation can lead to dysbiosis within the dental plaque biofilm, which in turn influences the host immune-inflammatory response causing dysregulation and exaggerated inflammation that leads to tissue periodontal damage. This relationship is a circular one.

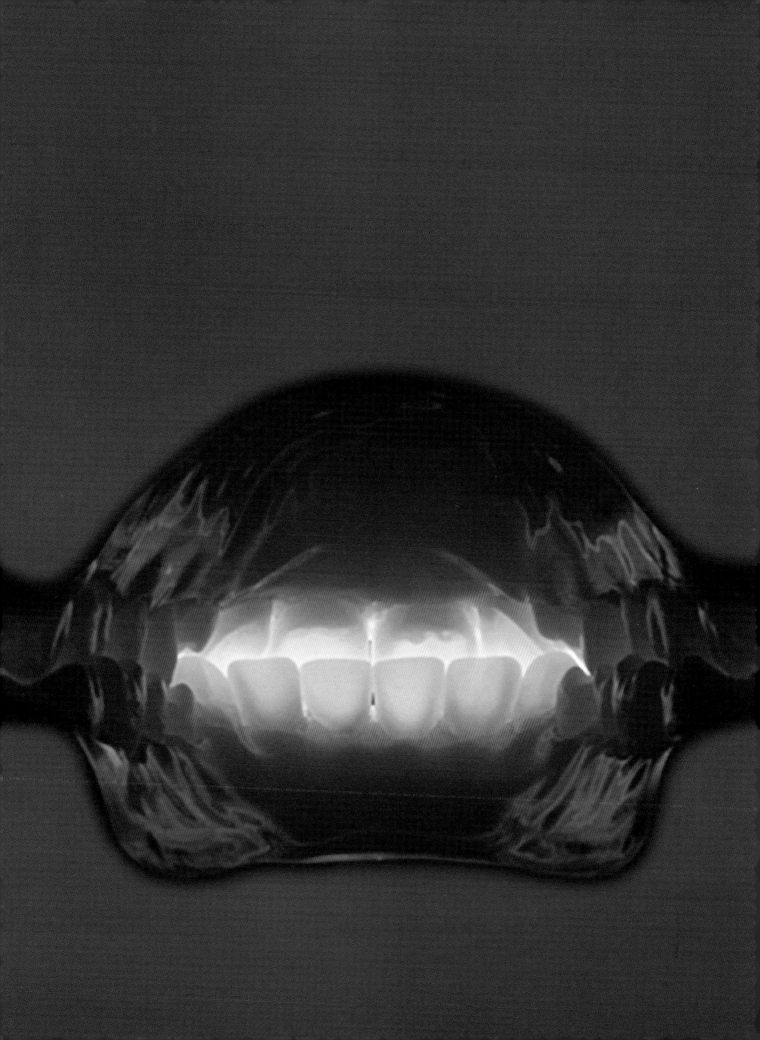

11 Systemic risk factors for periodontitis

Table 11.1 Systemic risk factors and indicators for periodontitis.

Systemic risk factors	Systemic risk indicators (potential risk factors)
Smoking	Low dietary calcium
Hyperglycaemia in diabetes mellitus type 1 and 2	High dietary refined carbohydrate intake
Obesity	Postmenopausal osteoporosis and osteopenia
Race	Stress and inadequate coping
Genetics	Hormonal influences
Ageing	Drugs (e.g. phenytoin, calcium channel blockers, immuno-suspension)
PMN function	
Socioeconomic status (low educational level)	
Glycaemia in people without diabetes	
Severe malnutrition (micronutrient deficiency)	

Figure 11.1 Local and systemic risk factors affecting the causal pathways in periodontal disease.

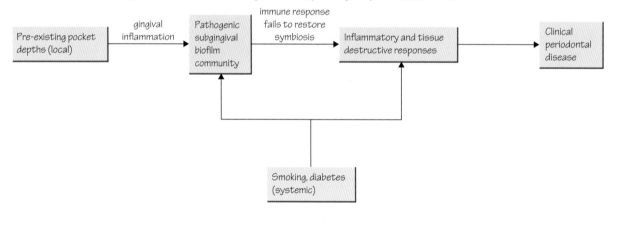

Periodontology at a Glance, Second Edition. Valerie Clerehugh, Aradhna Tugnait, Michael R. Milward, and Iain L. C. Chapple.
© 2024 John Wiley & Sons Ltd. Published 2024 by John Wiley & Sons Ltd.

Systemic risk factors for periodontal disease are referred to as 'modifying factors' in the 2018 classification system, because they generally modify the host response to microbial plaque accumulation rather than cause plaque build-up. In contrast to the local risk factors described in Chapters 10 and 14, systemic risk factors influence all periodontal tissues in an individual's dentition. Types of evidence required to establish risk factors in the causal pathway of a disease are discussed in Chapter 10.

Systemic risk factors and risk indicators for periodontitis

- Systemic risk factors include smoking, diabetes mellitus, obesity, race, genetic factors, male gender, polymorphonuclear (PMN) functional abnormalities, low socio economic status (SES), low educational level, high dietary intake of refined carbohydrates and severe malnutrition (Table 11.1).
- Based on current knowledge, systemic risk indicators or putative risk factors include low dietary calcium intake, postmenopausal osteoporosis and osteopenia, stress and inadequate coping, certain sex hormones and certain drugs such as calcium channel blockers and anti-siezure drugs such as phenytoin (Table 11.1).
- Regular dental visits, higher SES, anaemia and anti-allergy medications appear protective for periodontitis.
- Many of the risk factors for periodontitis especially smoking, also affect risk for peri-implant diseases.

Mechanisms by which systemic risk factors appear to operate

Tobacco smoking
In the more than 4000 components of tobacco smoke, there are many that exaggerate the inflammatory responses to periodontal pathogens and others that suppress the immune response (Fig. 11.1). Local effects of smoking also include direct toxic effects to cells, thermal effects, increased stain and calculus, and effects on the subgingival microbiome. There are also adverse effects of smoking on bone tissue, resulting in reduced bone mineral density. Clinical features of smokers are illustrated in Chapter 37.

Diabetes
Both type 1 and type 2 diabetes, when poorly controlled are thought to lead to increased risk of infections, and of periodontitis, by impairing protective immune responses and interfering with wound healing. The hyperglycaemia is associated with a hyperinflammatory state associated with activated protein kinase C and advanced glycation end products (AGEs) from glycation of proteins. These adverse processes likely lead to increased tissue destruction and greater levels of infection in those with diabetes compared to those without diabetes, as well as delayed and poorer healing due to the effects of AGEs on protein structure and blood flow. There is evidence for an altered subgingival microflora in subjects with diabetes.

Obesity
The adverse effects of obesity appear to be associated with the production of adipokines and cytokines by adipose tissue and by macrophages in adipose tissues. These proinflammatory molecules lead to a hyperinflamed state, which appears to increase tissue destruction triggered by periodontal and other pathologies. Some of the inflammatory mediators produced by adipose tissue, such as tumour necrosis factor (TNF)-α are thought to also bring about insulin resistance, which leads to diabetes and, in turn, an increased risk for periodontitis.

Genetic factors
Twin studies suggest a significant contribution of genetic factors to periodontal disease risk. However, it is clear that periodontitis is a complex disease resulting from the interaction of multiple gene loci, as well as environmental and behavioural factors influencing the deleterious effects of the subgingival microbiota. Currently, over 40 genetic associations have been reported between single nucleotide polymorphisms in candidate genes and periodontitis. However, these are often weak and not reproducible and differ among racial and ethnic groups. Genetic polymorphisms detected in an ever increasing number of pathways suggest that periodontitis is affected by many genes, each contributing a small percentage to the overall risk of periodontitis.

Dietary calcium
Low dietary calcium is associated with increased periodontal bone loss in both men and women. The mechanism may involve reduced bone mineral density which, in turn, renders the alveolar bone supporting the teeth more susceptible to periodontal inflammation.

Dietary refined carbohydrate intake
It is now widely recognised that diets high in refined carbohydrate intake and frequency of intake drive systemic inflammation (Chapple, 2009; Dommisch et al., 2018). This arises from the direct effect of glucose on metabolism resulting in mitochondrial stress and leakage of oxygen radicals, and also from the formation of AGEs. AGEs form when glucose binds to proteins like collagen and haemoglobin and are irreversible. There are receptors for AGEs, called RAGEs, which when bound by AGEs activate inflammatory cascades in key immune cells like neutrophils. A so-called 'hyperinflammatory state' results, which affects the periodontal tissues and contributes to tissue damage.

Osteopenia and osteoporosis in postmenopausal women
A complex set of pathways, which affect bone mineral density, occur at menopause and it is likely that those brought about by

reduced oestrogen levels lead to bone resorption outpacing bone deposition, which sets the stage for more advanced periodontal bone loss. Calcium supplementation and bone-sparing agents have shown modest effects in reducing tooth loss in older adults, suggesting that the modification of osteopenia may have a beneficial effect on alveolar bone.

Stress and inadequate coping

Chronic stress and adequate coping mechanisms appear to have many deleterious effects on the host, including suppression of the immune response with increased susceptibility to infections, including periodontitis.

Ageing

Previously, older age was not considered a risk factor for periodontitis, more that as people age, their lifetime accumulation of risk factors is likely to increase. However, it is now widely believed that ageing is associated with 'immune senescence' – a situation where the immune response becomes less specific and targeted, therefore less efficient and more indiscriminate (Hazeldine et al., 2015). The latter results in ineffective elimination of pathogens and increased collateral host tissue damage. In addition, as we age, epigenetic changes can arise in tissues, whereby 'damage-associated molecular signatures' are retained in those tissues, and epigenetic modifications are passed onto daughter cells during mitosis. This can result in disease recurrence arising more rapidly as the tissues are sensitised. In addition, innate immune cells like neutrophils undergo 'myeloid cell training', whereby the experience of encountering pathogens is transmitted to stem cells in bone marrow during myelopoiesis, resulting in the production of daughter neutrophils that are in a state of 'high alert' and which overreact to subsequent stimuli, even if they are different from the original pathogenic stimulus.

Low socioeconomic status

For most chronic non-communicable disease, low educational and income levels are often associated with increased risk for disease. One possible mechanism may be increased stress with lack of locus of control in individuals of low SES. Another is reduced access to dental care in those of lower SES, since it is well known that lack of regular dental visits increases the risk for periodontitis. Another possible explanation is lack of adequate oral hygiene, diets rich in refined sugars, higher levels of smoking and other risk factors which may result from cultural differences or lack of adequate knowledge about healthy behaviours.

Clinical studies to assess the effects of risk factor modification on the initiation and progression of periodontitis

It is clear that smokers are more difficult to treat, and many cases have been termed as 'refractory' to treatment. It is also clear that increased rates of implant failures are found among smokers. It has been found that subgingival antimicrobial agents sometimes give an added periodontal treatment benefit in smokers over that achieved in non-smokers. Smokers are known to heal poorly and many clinicians will not perform periodontal surgical, regenerative or implant procedures on heavy smokers until they demonstrate success in smoking cessation programmes.

Several studies show that patients with diabetes, especially if uncontrolled, heal more slowly and have more postoperative complications than those without diabetes after periodontal treatment. However, those patients with diabetes who have good glycaemic control most often heal at a similar rate and suffer no more complications than those who are non-diabetic after periodontal therapy. It is also clear that those with diabetes and periodontitis have a tendency for the periodontitis to recur more often after treatment, again especially in those who have poorly controlled diabetes. Hence, more frequent maintenance intervals and more intense attention to recurrent periodontitis and its prevention are often necessary in patients with diabetes mellitus. Collaboration with the patients' physician in maintaining good glucose control is gaining in importance in management of periodontal patients with diabetes.

PMN abnormalities

Neutrophils are key immune cells that bridge the innate and adaptive immune responses. They are primarily protective as key factors in acute inflammation, and in its resolution prior to tissue healing by regeneration. However, neutrophils can also become destructive when exposed to pathogenic stimuli with which they struggle to cope.

Neutrophil-mediated pathogen killing by phagocytosis is regarded as safe killing, but when the stimulus exceeds the ability of neutrophils to phagocytose, they can release toxic species extracellularly (degranulation), and this is associated with substantial host tissue damage. Peripheral blood neutrophils in periodontitis patients have been shown to be hyperactive in terms of oxygen radical release, and hyperreactive in terms of cytokine and oxygen radical release. The latter is in part due to 'immune training' but also to priming by periodontal pathogens and their virulence factors in the systemic circulation, prior to neutrophils entering periodontal tissues, when they 'overreact' to pathogenic stimuli. Moreover, periodontitis patient neutrophils exhibit poor chemotactic speed and accuracy, resulting in increased tissue transit times and exaggerating the collateral host tissue damage they cause.

Practice implications

It is clear that smoking cessation and diabetes control are important parts of the management of periodontal patients. Oral healthcare professionals can perform a great service to the patient by working with a physician in monitoring glycaemic control in diabetics and by instituting smoking cessation programmes in smokers. Likewise, physicians should refer patients with diabetes and suspected periodontitis to a dentist for a complete dental and periodontal examination. There are several studies which show that screening and monitoring for hyperglycaemia in the dental office is feasible and may result in great benefit to the patient. See Chapter 37 for details of smoking cessation programmes and Chapter 38 for management of patients with diabetes.

It has recently been proposed that risk factor modification has great value in affecting patients' susceptibility to periodontitis and hence contributes to long-term success of periodontal and implant therapy. The concept of modification of risk factors common to periodontal disease and associated systemic disease may benefit the management of not only periodontitis but also diabetes and heart disease. The common risk factors which can be addressed in the dental office include smoking cessation, reduction of consumption of added refined sugar in the diet, weight control and regular exercise.

Key points

- Systemic risk factors for periodontitis affect most, if not all, the tissues of the body. They may be modifiable (such as smoking) or non-modifiable (such as genetic factors)
- Reducing the effects of systemic risk factors is critically important in managing periodontitis
- Systemic risk factors may be associated with increased incidence, progression and recurrence of periodontitis. They may also affect the long-term prognosis of treatment
- Systemic risk factors are generally in the causal pathway and modify the expression of the disease by increasing susceptibility or decreasing resistance
- Present information supports the close monitoring of glycaemic control in patients with diabetes and instituting smoking cessation programmes as a key part of the management of periodontitis

12 Periodontal diseases and general health

Box 12.1 Non-plaque-induced gingival diseases and conditions.

- Genetic/developmental disorders
- Specific infections (bacterial, viral, fungal)
- Inflammatory and immune conditions (hypersensitivity reactions, autoimmune conditions, granulomatous inflammatory lesions)
- Reactive processes (epulides)
- Neoplasms (premalignancy and malignancies)
- Endocrine, nutritional and metabolic diseases
- Traumatic lesions (physical, chemical, thermal trauma)
- Gingival pigmentation

Box 12.2 Periodontitis as a manifestation of systemic diseases/conditions.

- Papillon-Lefèvre syndrome
- Haim–Munk syndrome
- Leukocyte adhesion deficiency
- Down syndrome
- Chediak–Higashi syndrome
- Ehlers–Danlos syndrome (types IV and VIII)

Box 12.3 Systemic diseases and conditions affecting periodontal tissues.

- Hypophosphatasia
- Histiocytosis X
- Granulomatosis with polyangitis (Wegener granulomatosis)
- Neoplasms

Figure 12.1 The effect of periodontal disease on glycaemic control: results from a two-year study. Source: Adapted from Taylor *et al.* (1996).

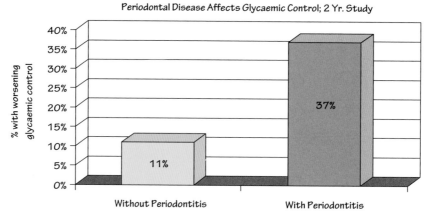

Figure 12.2 The effect of periodontal treatment on glycaemic control: results from a pilot randomised control study of 125 patients with type 2 diabetes mellitus showing the change in HbA1c at three months. PMPR, professional mechanical plaque removal.

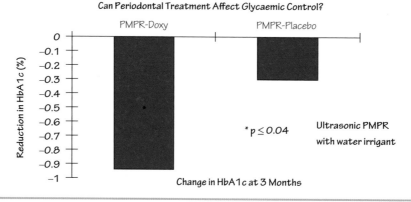

Periodontology at a Glance, Second Edition. Valerie Clerehugh, Aradhna Tugnait, Michael R. Milward, and Iain L. C. Chapple.
© 2024 John Wiley & Sons Ltd. Published 2024 by John Wiley & Sons Ltd.

Figure 12.3 Periodontal diseases and systemic disease – possible links.

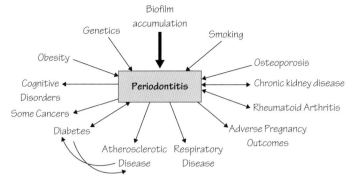

Figure 12.4 Proposed role of periodontitis in coronary heart disease (CHD) and cardiovascular disease (CVD).

Proposed Role of Periodontitis in CHD/CVD

Periodontal pathogens

Bacteraemia

Inflammatory mediators (TNFα, IL-6)

Immune responses

Endothelial dysfunction following invasion by periodontal pathogens

Liver

CRP

Neutrophils & cross-reacting antibodies

CHD/CVD

Figure 12.5 Scanning electron micrographs of bacteria in vascular biopsies from patients with periodontitis. (a) Area of aneurysmal wall with bacteria entangled in meshwork of delicate fibres. (b) Area of aneurysmal wall with bacteria entangled in meshwork of delicate fibres and remnants of intravascular plaque on aneurysmal wall. (c) Micro-organisms (rods) with remnants of intravascular plaque on aneurysmal wall. (d) Area of aneurysmal wall with bacteria entangled in meshwork of delicate fibres and remnants of intravascular plaque on aneurysmal wall. (e,f) Area of aneurysmal wall with coccus-shaped bacteria entangled in meshwork of delicate fibres and remnants of intravascular plaque on aneurysmal wall. Apparently, division of coccus-shaped bacteria is occurring. Delicate fibres are likely neutrophil extracellular traps (NETs).

Source: Armingohar et al. (2014), Fig. 1. Copyright © 2014 Zahra Armingohar et al. © 2014 Journal of Oral Microbiology, reprinted by permission of Informa UK Limited, trading as Taylor & Francis Group.

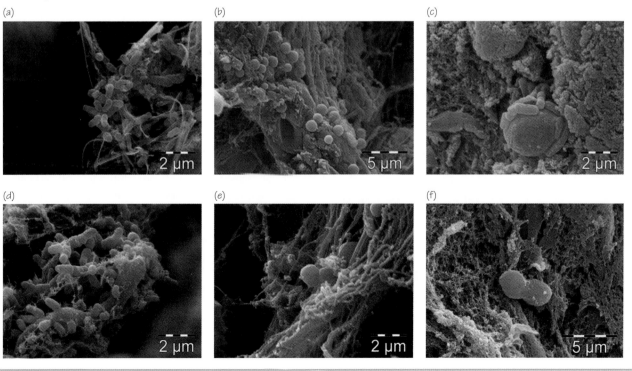

Systemic conditions and diseases may manifest within the periodontium. Conversely, periodontal diseases are also independently and significantly associated with premature mortality and with several non-communicable diseases of ageing.

The 2018 classification of periodontal diseases and conditions categorises systemic conditions that present within or impact upon the periodontal tissues into four groups:

- Non-plaque-induced gingival diseases and conditions.
- Systemic disorders having a major impact on loss of periodontal tissues by influencing periodontal inflammation.
- Other systemic disorders influencing the pathogenesis of periodontal inflammation (e.g. poorly controlled diabetes mellitus, obesity, osteoporosis, rheumatoid arthritis).
- Systemic disorders causing loss of periodontal tissues independently of periodontitis.

Other oral manifestations of systemic conditions include oral osteonecrosis seen in patients receiving head and neck radiation chemotherapies and intravenous bisphosphonates.

Gingival conditions are also associated with dermatological diseases such as pemphigus vulgaris, lichen planus and erythema multiforme. These 'non-plaque-induced gingival diseases and conditions' (Box 12.1) are broadly categorised into eight major groups and a more detailed list of subcategories is available in Table 2 of the World Workshop manuscript (Chapple *et al.*, 2018, page S75; see also Figs 2.2a,b and Appendix 1).

Periodontitis may manifest as a result of underlying systemic conditions that increase risk for plaque-induced periodontal tissue damage, through defects in neutrophil function or connective tissue structure and function. Such conditions are rare but Box 12.2 lists some of the more well-known examples.

There are also a number of systemic diseases and conditions that affect the periodontal tissues and/or present within them, but whose pathogenesis is not related to plaque accumulation or composition. Such conditions can be confused with or misdiagnosed as periodontitis, but their true aetiology is important to ascertain (Box 12.3).

Clinical implications of periodontal diseases for systemic health

The standard of care is to eliminate oral infection and inflammation, including periodontal disease, before initiating radiation therapy for head and neck cancers and before initialising intravenous bisphosphonate therapy. It is becoming clear that treatment of oral inflammation, including periodontitis, before instituting such therapies may reduce serious complications.

Importantly, treating periodontitis to a target of health has been shown to improve outcomes of diabetes, rheumatoid arthritis and surrogate measures of cardiovascular health, and is safe to undertake in such patient groups.

Periodontal diseases as risk factors for systemic conditions and diseases

The evidence for periodontal disease as a risk factor or as part of the causal pathway of several major chronic systemic diseases is accumulating. These include diabetes mellitus, atherosclerotic cardiovascular diseases, chronic kidney disease, rheumatoid arthritis nosocomial respiratory infections, adverse pregnancy outcomes, Alzheimer's disease and certain cancers.

Diabetes

Perhaps the strongest case for causation is in diabetes, where there is evidence that those patients suffering from diabetes types 1 and 2 who also have severe periodontal disease have poorer glycaemic control and increased complications of their diabetes (Fig. 12.1). Furthermore, treatment of periodontitis contributes to improving glycaemic control and reducing macrovascular and microvascular complications of diabetes (Fig. 12.2). There is now 12-month data available to demonstrate that optimal periodontal treatment can reduce HbA1c levels by 6%, equivalent to a second drug in a metformin regime (D'Aiuto *et al.*, 2020).

There is also evidence that those patients with diabetes who suffer from periodontal disease have increased risk of dying from cardiovascular disease or diabetic nephropathy.

These effects on systemic diseases are thought to be mediated largely by systemic inflammation as evidenced by elevated blood levels of C-reactive protein (CRP) and other acute phase proteins, and proinflammatory cytokines seen in patients with periodontitis. For example, the elevation of tumour necrosis factor (TNF)-α and interleukin (IL)-6 may well contribute to insulin resistance, a central pathological process in diabetes (Fig. 12.3).

Heart disease

There is strong evidence that periodontitis is associated with and precedes cardiovascular disease (Fig. 12.4). There is similar evidence for the association of periodontal disease with ischaemic stroke and peripheral artery disease (Herrera *et al.*, 2023). There are *in vitro* and animal studies showing that periodontal inflammation could be in the causal pathway of cardiovascular disease, mediated through induction of systemic inflammation and the effects of homing of oral bacteria to atheromas that occurs in periodontal patients (Fig. 12.5). These, in turn, are thought to contribute to atheroma formation, a central pathology in heart disease, ischaemic stroke and peripheral artery disease (Figs. 12.4, 12.5). Randomised controlled trials are needed to determine if and to what extent treating or preventing periodontal disease will have an effect on atherosclerotic conditions.

Respiratory infections

The association between poor oral hygiene and periodontal disease in institutionalised patients with respiratory infections such as pneumonia and bronchitis is well established. Furthermore, there are several small, randomised controlled trials that show that maintaining good oral hygiene in patients in intensive care units or nursing homes will reduce the incidence of respiratory infections, many of which are fatal. The mechanism is probably colonisation of the oral cavity of institutionalised patients by respiratory pathogens, which are aspirated, leading to respiratory infections. Increasingly, institutions that care for respiratory compromised patients provide regular oral hygiene measures to control nosocomial respiratory infection of oropharyngeal microbial origin. Recent evidence also supports a significant and independent association between periodontitis and chronic obstructive respiratory diseases, obstructive sleep apnoea, and COVID-19 complications. (Molina *et al.*, 2023).

Clinical implications

It is reasonable to treat periodontal disease in patients with diabetes, not only to save the dentition but also to help improve glycaemic control and possibly reduce other complications of diabetes. Furthermore, the institution of oral hygiene in patients who are institutionalised – in intensive care units or nursing homes – is justified to not only improve their oral condition but also possibly prevent or reduce respiratory infections.

The role of periodontal disease as either a complication of systemic diseases or as a risk factor for systemic diseases or conditions provides compelling reasons for complete periodontal care in high-risk patients. It also provides reason for dentists to expand their scope of activities and participate more fully as part of the healthcare team. Oral healthcare professionals see patients more often than physicians do, and see patients when they are well, putting them in the ideal place to risk assess patients for such systemic conditions and play a role in early case detection for conditions such as type 2 diabetes (Yonel *et al.*, 2023).

Finally, there is good reason for the dental profession to promote the control of risk factors common to both oral diseases and related systemic diseases, including smoking cessation, dietary control and reduction of refined sugar intake.

Key points

- Systemic diseases and conditions may present within the gingival tissues, e.g. diabetes, leukaemia, neutrophil disorders, dermatological diseases and medication side-effects
- Periodontal disease may contribute to several major chronic diseases including diabetes and its complications, atherosclerotic cardiovascular disease and respiratory infections
- There is strong evidence that periodontitis induces a systemic inflammatory response as evidenced by elevated levels of acute phase proteins, oxidative stress and proinflammatory cytokines. These may contribute to insulin resistance, atheroma formation and other adverse responses
- Clinical trials show that treating periodontitis can improve glycaemic control in diabetes. Other trials show a reduction in respiratory infections in institutionalised patients. Large randomised trials are needed to assess the extent to which periodontal intervention will affect these systemic conditions
- These associations between periodontal disease and several major chronic diseases, which are major causes of mortality and morbidity, call for urgency in the diagnosis, prevention and treatment of periodontal diseases, and for control of common risk factors
- Oral healthcare professionals have a role to play in the early case detection of type 2 diabetes

13 Diet and periodontal diseases

Figure 13.1 Amounts of milk and other food sources providing 300 mg of calcium. Source: Adapted from Weaver *et al.* (1999).

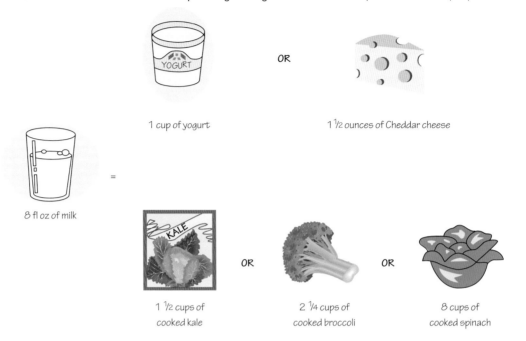

Figure 13.2 Odds ratio for periodontal disease (mean clinical attachment loss >1.5 mm) by level of dietary vitamin C intake after adjusting for age decade, gender, tobacco use and gingival bleeding in the National Health and Nutrition Examination Survey (NHANES) III (Nishida *et al.*, 2000b). Weights provided in NHANES III data were used, and tobacco use, age decade, gender and gingival bleeding were adjusted for using multiple logistic regression. Dietary vitamin C intake was divided into five categories, and odds ratios are presented using the highest intake group as a reference. CI, confidence interval.

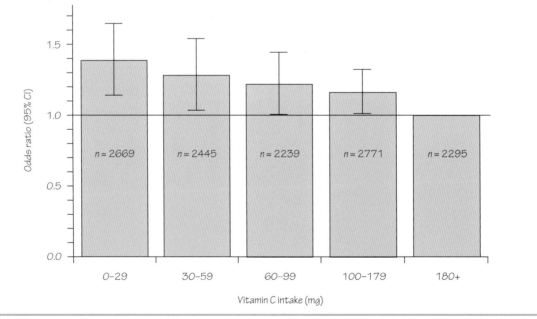

Table 13.1 Association of periodontal disease (mean clinical attachment loss of >1.5 mm) with calcium intake in males and females of different ages after adjusting for tobacco use status and gingival bleeding in the National Health and Nutrition Examination Survey (NHANES) III.

Age range	Male	Female
20–30 years		
Odds ratio[a]	1.84	1.99
95% CI	1.36–2.48	1.34–2.97
P value	<0.001	<0.001
N	2727	3348
40–59 years		
Odds ratio[a]	1.90	1.31
95% CI	1.41–2.55	0.85–2.03
P value	<0.001	0.2401
N	1675	1863
60+ years		
Odds ratio[a]	1.11	1.13
95% CI	0.71–1.71	0.86–1.48
P value	0.6582	0.4037
N	1422	1384

CI, confidence interval.
[a] Computer software and weights provided in NHANES III data were used, and odds ratios were adjusted for tobacco use (categorised as 'never', 'former' and 'current') and gingival bleeding in multiple logistic regression.
Source: Nishida et al. (2000a)/John Wiley & Sons.

Table 13.2 Recommended dietary allowance/adequate intake for dietary calcium.

Age	Calcium (mg/day)		
	Male	Female	Pregnancy and lactation
0–6 months[a]	200	200	
7–12 months[a]	260	260	
1–3 years	700	700	
4–8 years	1000	1000	
9–13 years	1300	1300	
14–18 years	1300	1300	1300
19–50 years	1000	1000	1000
51-70 years	1000	1200	
≥71 years	1200	1200	

[a] Adequate intake.
Source: Institute of Medicine (2011); National Institutes of Health, Office of Dietary Supplements (2022).

Figure 13.3 Health risks of too much calcium.

Tolerable upper intake limits for calcium (mg/day) (Institute of Medicine, 2011)

Age	Male	Female	Pregnancy and lactation
0-6 months	1000	1000	
7-12 months	1500	1500	
1-8 years	2500	2500	
9-18 years	3000	3000	3000
19-50 years	2500	2500	2500
≥ 51 years	2000	2000	

Higher levels can result in:
- Hypercalcaemia (serum levels > 10.5 mg/dL) and hypercalcuria (urinary calcium levels higher than 250 mg/day in females or 275 mg/day in males), although rare in healthy people
- Possible increased risk of cardiovascular disease and prostate cancer although not all studies confirm this (National Institutes of Health, Office of Dietary Supplements, 2022)

Calcium can react with certain medications including: digoxin, ciprofloxacin, tetracyclines, levothyroxine, lithium and thiazide diuretics

Calcium decreases the absorption of iron, zinc, magnesium and phosphorus

Figure 13.4 Government-recommended intake of vitamin C.

- United Kingdom: 40 mg/day
- World Health Organization: 45 mg/day
- Health Canada
  - Adult male, 90 mg/day
  - Adult female, 75 mg/day
- United States:
  - Adult male, 90 mg/day
  - Adult female, 75 mg/day
  - Smokers should take 35 mg/day more than above

In discussing the role of diet in periodontal disease, there are two main issues.

- The effect of diet on periodontal disease.
- The effect of tooth loss, which can impair mastication, leading to dietary intake changes.

The role of diet in periodontal disease

It is well known that nutritional status plays a major role in modulating the immune system, reducing inflammatory responses and maintaining tissue homeostasis. The studies of vitamin C deficiency and scurvy-associated gingivitis are well known, as are the devastating effects of severe malnutrition on the periodontium leading to diseases such as necrotising periodontitis. In the developed world, such severe deficiencies are rare. However, inadequacies in the diet have been found to be risk factors for periodontal disease.

- One is the effect of low dietary calcium, which is common in the population today. Low dietary intake of calcium (Fig. 13.1) increases the risk for periodontal disease in women under the age of 30 and men under the age of 60 years (Table 13.1). Furthermore, calcium supplementation, especially in postmenopausal women who show osteopenia or osteoporosis, has been shown to prevent tooth loss related to periodontal disease. Direct evaluation of calcium supplementation to reduce periodontal disease, however, has not been carried out.
- There are large population studies showing that low levels of vitamin C and other micronutrients in the diet increase the risk for periodontitis (Chapple et al., 2007) (Fig. 13.2). Supplementation trials with natural sources of micronutrients such as vitamin C have shown reductions in periodontal inflammation (Chapple et al., 2012; Amaliya, 2018; Graziani, 2018).
- With respect to dietary protective factors, it has been shown in large epidemiological studies that increased fibre in the diet is associated with less periodontal disease. The mechanism is not entirely clear, but it is known that increased fibre leads to slower gastric emptying, which reduces the glucose spike in blood and thus reduces the systemic inflammation caused by glucose intake within the diet. There is emerging evidence that high-fibre diets also affect the gut microbiome, leading to production of short-chain fatty acids with systemic anti-inflammatory activity.
- It is proposed that hypovitaminosis D is linked to more periodontitis, as well as to other conditions such as cancer, diabetes and cardiovascular disease. There is a need for large randomised clinical trials with vitamin D to determine the extent to which elevated dietary vitamin D in the diet would affect periodontal disease.

Dietary intervention in periodontal disease

Several studies have shown that dietary interventions, including soya isoflavones, vitamin C, fruit and vegetable extracts and omega-3 fatty acids, will improve periodontal status. Recent studies show that calorie restriction is associated with decreased periodontitis, probably due to reductions in the frequency and magnitude of glucose spikes within blood (Chapter 11). A recent study has shown that weight loss as well as exercise benefits the periodontal tissues.

Effects of adult tooth loss on diet

There are several studies that show that tooth loss in adults, especially if teeth are not adequately replaced, has effects on dietary intake. For example, tooth loss can lead to reduction of intake of foods that are hard to chew, such as carrots, leaf salads, whole grains, fruits and vegetables. Large epidemiological studies have shown that an overall reduction in fibre intake and an increase in consumption of refined sugar and fats are associated with tooth loss. The extent to which adequate dentures or implants improve mastication and moderate the diet is not clear. However, studies show that denture wearers, if trained properly in dietary requirements, will consume a diet similar to those with a natural dentition. However, overall, patients who wear conventional or even implant-supported dentures have a poorer diet and reduced masticatory function relative to dentate individuals.

The effects of high levels of refined sugar in the diet on dental caries are well known. Periodontal patients often suffer from gingival recession, exposing roots to the cariogenic microflora, and in these patients, a diet rich in refined sugar has been shown to increase root surface caries. This is especially true in individuals who experience a dry mouth, or who have decreased salivary flow associated with medications or smoking. There is emerging evidence that refined sugar consumption is also associated with increased periodontitis.

The role of diet in healing after periodontal treatment

The importance of adequate diet in healing after periodontal or peri-implant surgical procedures is frequently overlooked. Dietary intake may be transiently compromised by difficulty in chewing associated with postoperative pain and discomfort. Adequate nutrition should be dealt with by recommending soft foods that contain the macro- and micronutrients necessary for proper nutrition in the weeks after surgery.

Recommendations for dental patients

As part of the healthcare team, it is reasonable for oral healthcare professionals to advise patients on their diet, especially since there is clear evidence that refined sugars lead to increased coronal and root surface caries, and now also contribute to periodontitis. There is also evidence that obesity, as well as calcium and vitamin C deficiency, low dietary calcium intake and low levels of serum antioxidant micronutrients, contribute to the risk for periodontal disease. The well-known benefits of adequate dietary calcium, vitamin C and weight control as part of the overall health of the patient are important also in the justification for oral healthcare professionals to assist their medical colleagues in counselling patients on adequate nutrition.

Therefore, the following recommendations are made for the management of diet in adult dental patients.

- Reduced intake of refined sugars and limiting intake to mealtimes to reduce the frequency of blood glucose spikes, especially in those who have periodontitis, as well as those with gingival recession who are prone to root caries. This is also important in those who suffer from oral dryness associated with smoking or medications that reduce salivary flow.
- Proper intake of calcium. If dietary calcium is not at or near the recommended daily allowance (RDA) for the patient, calcium supplementation to bring them to the RDA should be recommended (Table 13.2; Figs 13.3, 13.4).
- Weight reduction for those who are overweight or obese, since obesity, especially visceral adiposity, is a risk factor for periodontal disease. Weight reduction may improve periodontal health, and it will clearly decrease the risk for several other chronic diseases such as diabetes and cardiovascular disease and hence will contribute to the overall health of the patient.

- Patients should include adequate fibre in the diet from fruits, vegetables and whole grains. The dentist should strive to provide an adequate dentition so that chewing these hard foods is possible.
- Reducing refined carbohydrate intake and increasing consumption of antioxidant micronutrients in fruits and vegetables will contribute to periodontal as well as systemic health.

Key points

- Diet may affect periodontal tissues, and tooth loss may affect diet
- There is evidence to suggest that inadequate dietary calcium and antioxidant micronutrients such as vitamin C leads to more periodontal disease
- Studies show that dietary calcium supplementation in postmenopausal women prevents tooth loss
- Tooth loss is associated with decreased dietary intake of fibre, and increased intake of refined sugars and fats
- It is recommended that oral healthcare professionals counsel their patients on dietary calcium, reduced intake of refined sugars, increased antioxidant micronutrient intake and overall weight control.

14 Local risk factors for periodontal diseases

Figure 14.1 Classification of local risk factors and tooth- and prosthesis-related factors. Source: Adapted from Caton *et al.* (2018), see Chapter 2 for detail.

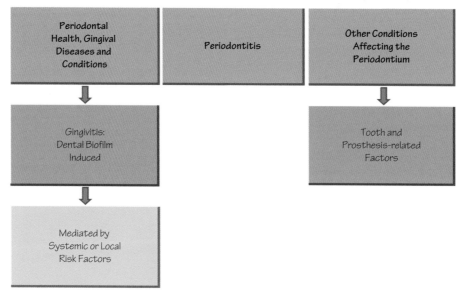

Figure 14.2 Classification of factors related to teeth and dental prostheses that can affect the periodontium. Source: Jepsen *et al.* (2017)/John Wiley & Sons.

A. Localised tooth-related factors that modify or predispose to plaque-induced gingival diseases/periodontitis
1. Tooth anatomical factors
2. Root fractures
3. Cervical root resorption, cemental tears
4. Root proximity
5. Altered passive eruption

B. Localised dental prosthesis-related factors
1. Restoration margins placed within the supracrestal attached tissues
2. Clinical procedures related to the fabrication of indirect restorations
3. Hypersensitivity/toxicity reactions to dental materials

Figure 14.3 An enamel pearl.

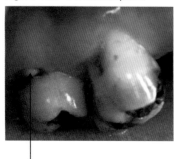

Enamel pearls are ectopic deposits of enamel that lie apical to the normal cement-enamel junction.

Figure 14.4 Overhanging restoration margins.

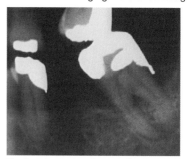

Overhanging restoration margins are seen on LL5 and particularly on the distal surface of LL7.

Figure 14.5 Subgingival crown margins.

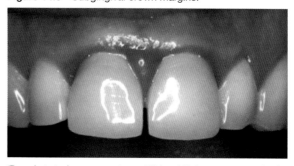

The subgingival crown margins on UR1 and UL1 are associated with gingival inflammation.

Periodontology at a Glance, Second Edition. Valerie Clerehugh, Aradhna Tugnait, Michael R. Milward, and Iain L. C. Chapple.

Figure 14.6 An overcontoured crown and subgingival calculus.

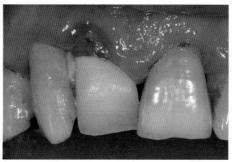

A crown on UR2 tries to mimic the appearance of a central incisor leading to an overbuilt mesial contour, plaque retention and gingival inflammation. Subgingival calculus can be seen for instance at the gingival margin of UL1, which acts as a plaque retention factor.

Figure 14.7 Minimising the periodontal consequences of restorative treatment.

- Matrix bands and wedges should be used when placing plastic restorations
- Contact areas should allow for the normal gingival papilla
- Supragingival margins are to be preferred where possible
- Where aesthetics are of concern margins should be placed no more than 0.5 mm into the gingival crevice
- Sufficient tooth reduction is required to avoid overbuilt crowns
- A good impression technique with use of gingival retraction cord should be used for indirect restorations
  - soft tissue injury can occur from placement of gingival retraction cords but healing is generally rapid if the gingivae are initially healthy
- Excess cement should be removed on the placement of indirect restorations
- Extracoronal restorations (and bridge pontics) should be contoured to facilitate plaque control and allow for the normal dimensions of the gingival tissues

Figure 14.8 (a) Poorly designed acrylic partial denture with gingival coverage (shown out of the mouth). (b) Partial denture *in situ*; interproximal plaque is visible. (c) Following removal of the denture, the gingivae can be seen to be reddened and inflamed.

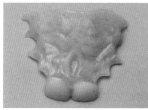

(a)

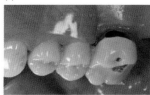

(b)

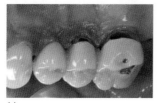

(c)

Figure 14.9 Partial denture with extensive gingival coverage.

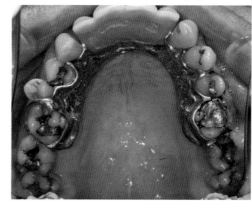

This upper cobalt chromium partial denture covers the palatal gingival margins which augments its role as a plaque retention factor.

Figure 14.10 Minimising the periodontal consequences of providing a partial denture.

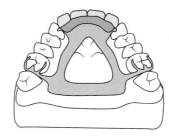

- Denture should be well supported with appropriate use of rest seats
- 3 mm clearance of the gingival margins should be provided where possible
- Denture design should be kept simple
- Partial dentures should be adequately maintained long term

Figure 14.11 Orthodontic appliance acting as a plaque retention factor.

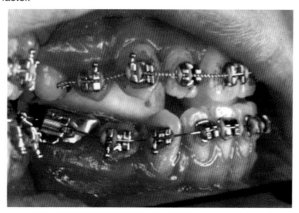

Figure 14.12 Supragingival calculus acting as a local plaque retention factor.

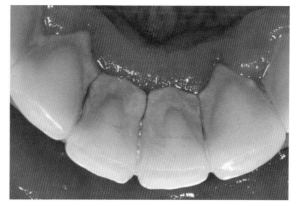

Local risk factors or predisposing factors can increase the risk of development and progression of periodontal diseases by acting as plaque retention factors. Local factors should be identified when carrying out a thorough dental examination of the patient and their removal or modification where possible should be included in the patient's management.

A large number of local factors have been raised as relevant to periodontal management. Figure 14.1 shows where local risk factors fit within the 2018 Classification of Periodontal Diseases and Conditions (see also Chapter 2, Figure 2.8), with Fig. 14.2 showing the classification of factors related to teeth and dental prostheses that can affect the periodontium as agreed in the 2018 Classification (Chapter 2). Some other local factors related to sites or specific teeth are also considered under the following headings.

- Anatomical factors.
- Restorations.
- Removable partial dentures.
- Orthodontic appliances.
- Root fractures and cervical root resorption.
- Calculus.
- Local trauma.
- Frenal attachments.
- Mouth breathing and lack of lip seal.

Anatomical factors

A number of anatomical variations may be associated with localised gingivitis and attachment loss.
- Enamel pearls or cervical enamel projections (Fig. 14.3).
- Cemental tears occur either within the cementum layer or as full-thickness separation of the cementum from the dentine.
- Developmental grooves are most commonly seen palatally on the upper lateral incisors.
- Furcation lesions can act to retain plaque, making sites harder to maintain.
- Untreated periodontal pockets and posttreatment residual pockets harbour subgingival plaque.

Tooth position

- Oral hygiene measures can be harder to implement where teeth are crowded with imbrication, rotations or marked angulation.
- Some malocclusions can cause direct soft tissue trauma (e.g. occlusion of the upper incisors on the lower labial gingivae in a marked class II division 2 malocclusion).
- Some studies have shown an association between tooth malalignment and loss of periodontal support (Jensen & Solow, 1989; Eismann & Prusas, 1990).
- Open contacts lead to greater food impaction and have been associated with increased pocketing and loss of attachment (Jernberg et al., 1983).

Restorations

- Subgingival restoration margins can be associated with gingivitis and attachment loss related to:
  - roughness of the restorative material and at the tooth–restoration interface due to increased plaque retention
  - overhanging restorative material (Fig. 14.4) (Parsell et al., 1997)
  - marginal discrepancies and exposed cement margins.

- Supracrestal tissue attachment (replacing the term 'biologic width') consists of the junctional epithelium and supracrestal connective tissue. Placement of subgingival restoration margins within the junctional epithelium and supracrestal connective tissue attachment can be associated with gingival inflammation (Fig. 14.5) or potentially recession may occur (Ercoli & Caton, 2018). It is not clear, however, whether these effects are caused by dental plaque, trauma, dental material toxicity or a combination of these.
- Overcontoured crowns are often associated with increased gingival inflammation (Fig. 14.6).
- Gingival recession is commonly associated with fixed prostheses.
- Optimal restoration margins within the gingival sulcus do not cause gingival inflammation if plaque control is of a high standard (Morris, 1989).

Restorations must be placed with great care to avoid the creation of local risk factors for periodontal disease (Fig. 14.7).

Removable partial dentures

Removable partial dentures (RPDs) can enhance plaque accumulation and increase the risk of periodontal diseases (Figs 14.8, 14.9). Proximal surfaces are most at risk. Factors to be considered to minimise the periodontal consequences of providing RPDs are shown in Fig. 14.10.

Orthodontic appliances

Fixed and removable orthodontic appliances may be worn for several years and can potentially have reversible or irreversible effects on the periodontal tissues (Chapter 30). Aspects to be aware of with the wearing of orthodontic appliances include the following.
- Access to interdental cleaning is usually compromised, leading to plaque accumulation.
- Components of the orthodontic appliances, especially bands, can lie close to the gingival margin, leading to plaque accumulation (Fig. 14.11).
- Good oral hygiene will minimise the effect on periodontal tissues.
- Coronal attachment loss can occur during orthodontic treatment (0.05–0.3 mm annually).

Root fractures and cervical root resorption

Vertical root fractures can be associated with periodontal lesions. Periodontal breakdown can occur at the site of cervical external root resorption where there is a communication with the oral environment (Andreasen, 1985).

Calculus

Supragingival and subgingival calculus act as local plaque retention factors (Figs 14.6, 14.12) (Van der Velden et al., 2006). The surfaces of the calculus offer large irregular areas harbouring plaque close to the gingival margins. These sites are also relatively sheltered from host defences. Much of periodontal therapy is directed at calculus detection and removal.

Local trauma

This can be associated with over-zealous tooth brushing or habits such as direct picking of the gingivae with a fingernail. The results may be gingival recession, attachment loss and bone loss.

Frenal attachments

A prominent frenum can act as a local plaque retention factor, reducing access for the patient's oral hygiene measures. Frenal pull acting directly on the gingival margin has been described as a factor in the development of gingival recession but the associated increased plaque retention may be of greater aetiological significance.

Mouth breathing and lack of lip seal

Mouth breathing and a lack of lip seal at rest can lead to dehydration of the oral tissues and higher levels of dental plaque. This results in greater gingivitis in the associated anterior region.

Key points

- Local or predisposing factors can act as risk factors for periodontal diseases
- Local factors act by increasing plaque retention, trauma, dental material toxicity or a combination of these
- Local factors should be prevented, modified or eliminated where possible

15 Occlusion and periodontal diseases

Figure 15.1 Diagnosis of occlusal trauma.

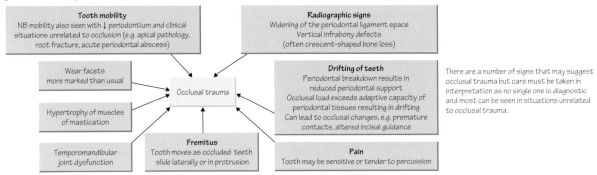

Tooth mobility
NB mobility also seen with ↓ periodontium and clinical situations unrelated to occlusion (e.g. apical pathology, root fracture, acute periodontal abscess)

Radiographic signs
Widening of the periodontal ligament space
Vertical infrabony defects
(often crescent-shaped bone loss)

Wear facets more marked than usual

Hypertrophy of muscles of mastication

Temporomandibular joint dysfunction

Fremitus
Tooth moves as occluded teeth slide laterally or in protrusion

Occlusal trauma

Drifting of teeth
Periodontal breakdown results in reduced periodontal support
Occlusal load exceeds adaptive capacity of periodontal tissues resulting in drifting
Can lead to occlusal changes, e.g. premature contacts, altered incisal guidance

Pain
Tooth may be sensitive or tender to percussion

There are a number of signs that may suggest occlusal trauma but care must be taken in interpretation as no single one is diagnostic and most can be seen in situations unrelated to occlusal trauma.

Figure 15.2 Tooth with healthy periodontal tissues: (a) prior to application of traumatic alternate mesial and distal occlusal forces, (b) following application of traumatic occlusal forces, and (c) following occlusal adjustment. Source: Lindhe *et al.* (2008)/John Wiley & Sons.

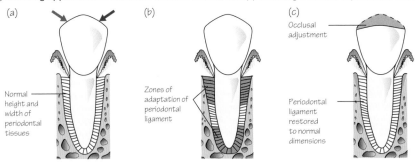

(a) Normal height and width of periodontal tissues

(b) Zones of adaptation of periodontal ligament

(c) Occlusal adjustment
Periodontal ligament restored to normal dimensions

Bone resorption occurs in response to traumatic, occlusal, 'jiggling-type' forces leading to a widened periodontal ligament space and increased tooth mobility. Resorption stops when this force has been compensated for. No apical migration of the junctional epithelium or loss of attachment is seen. After occlusal adjustment there is a reduction in width of the periodontium and in tooth mobility.

Figure 15.3 Tooth with reduced height of healthy periodontal tissues: (a) prior to application of traumatic occlusal forces, (b) following application of traumatic occlusal forces, and (c) following occlusal adjustment. Source: Lindhe *et al.* (2008)/John Wiley & Sons.

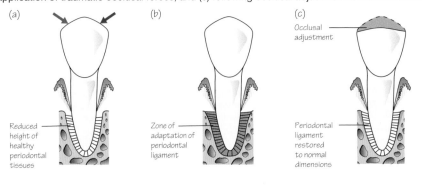

(a) Reduced height of healthy periodontal tissues

(b) Zone of adaptation of periodontal ligament

(c) Occlusal adjustment
Periodontal ligament restored to normal dimensions

Bone resorption occurs following the application of traumatic, occlusal, 'jiggling-type' forces as with the normal height of periodontium. Adaptation occurs as the periodontal ligament space widens without additional loss of attachment and the tooth mobility increases. After occlusal adjustment there is a reduction in width of the periodontium and in tooth mobility.

Figure 15.4 Tooth with periodontal disease: (a) prior to application of traumatic occlusal forces, (b) following application of traumatic occlusal forces, and (c) following occlusal adjustment. Source: Lindhe *et al.* (2008)/John Wiley & Sons.

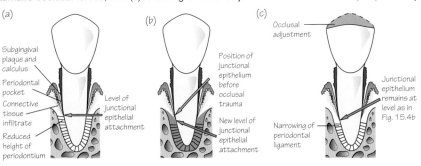

(a) Subgingival plaque and calculus
Periodontal pocket
Connective tissue infiltrate
Reduced height of periodontium
Level of junctional epithelial attachment

(b) Position of junctional epithelium before occlusal trauma
New level of junctional epithelial attachment

(c) Occlusal adjustment
Junctional epithelium remains at level as in Fig. 15.4b
Narrowing of periodontal ligament

Bone resorption occurs following the application of jiggling forces with the associated changes occurring within the zone occupied by the inflammatory infiltrate. If the tissues cannot adapt to the occlusal forces then bone loss, attachment loss and apical migration of the junctional epithelium are seen. In such a case, periodontal destruction is aggravated by the occlusal trauma. Treatment directed at the occlusal trauma alone may reduce tooth mobility with narrowing of the periodontal ligament. However, the plaque-induced periodontal lesion remains and the occlusal adjustment will not arrest the rate of further periodontal destruction.

Periodontology at a Glance, Second Edition. Valerie Clerehugh, Aradhna Tugnait, Michael R. Milward, and Iain L. C. Chapple.
© 2024 John Wiley & Sons Ltd. Published 2024 by John Wiley & Sons Ltd.

The periodontium attaches the tooth to the alveolar bone and dissipates the forces of occlusion to the surrounding tissues. If the occlusal load is abnormally high or the periodontium is reduced in height due to periodontal disease, then tissue changes may be seen (Lindhe *et al.*, 2008) and the lesion is termed occlusal trauma. Clinical and radiographic indicators of occlusal trauma are shown in Figure 15.1.

Tissue changes in response to occlusal load

Experiments in beagle dogs designed to mimic prolonged traumatic occlusion by applying alternate mesial and distal 'jiggling-type' trauma to a tooth (Lindhe & Ericsson, 1982) have shown the following.

- A healthy periodontium remodels in response to the occlusal forces.
- The periodontal ligament space widens if:
  - the periodontium is of normal height (Fig. 15.2a,b)
  - the periodontium is of reduced height due to past periodontal disease (Fig. 15.3a,b).
- The tooth shows non-progressive increased mobility.
- The periodontal ligament returns to its normal width following occlusal adjustment (Figs 15.2c, 15.3c).

It can be concluded from this that occlusal trauma does not initiate periodontal destruction.

When jiggling-type trauma is applied to a tooth with plaque-associated periodontal disease (Fig. 15.4a):

- there is remodelling of the periodontium
  and either:
- remodelling stops if the periodontium can adapt to the forces
- the tooth shows non-progressive increased mobility but no further loss of attachment
  or:
- remodelling may continue if the periodontium cannot adapt to the forces (Fig. 15.4b)
- the tooth may show progressive mobility and attachment loss with trauma from occlusion acting as a co-factor in periodontal destruction
- removal of the occlusal trauma alone may reduce tooth mobility but it will not stop the rate of further periodontal breakdown (Fig. 15.4c).

Similar work in monkeys by another research group found that there was no difference in the connective tissue attachment loss between animals with periodontitis alone and those with periodontitis and excessive occlusal forces, so occlusal trauma was not a co-factor in periodontal destruction (Polson & Zander, 1983). These conflicting results highlight the difficulties in using animal models and applying results to humans.

Nonetheless, both research groups found that the control of plaque in a lesion with periodontitis and occlusal trauma led to gains in attachment and bone levels but removal of the occlusal trauma had little effect.

The conclusion was that the successful treatment of periodontal disease will arrest periodontal destruction even if occlusal trauma persists.

Occlusal analysis and adjustment

Following identification of potential occlusal interferences and trauma, a detailed occlusal analysis may be carried out by mounting study models on a semi-adjustable articulator, usually in the retruded contact position as this position is reproducible. The teeth can then be examined for wear facets and tooth surface loss, tooth loss, rotations, drifting and tilting. The lateral and incisal guidance can be reviewed and premature contacts identified. Clinically, the muscles of mastication and temporomandibular joints should be assessed. The occlusion can be altered by selective grinding, restorative treatment or orthodontics.

Although many dentists have advocated occlusal adjustments as part of periodontal therapy, a Cochrane review (Weston *et al.*, 2008) concluded that there was insufficient evidence for occlusal intervention. A subsequent systematic review by Fox *et al.* (2012) concluded that the benefit of occlusal adjustment was not proven but also not detrimental. The position paper from the 2017 World Workshop on Classification found no evidence that traumatic occlusal forces can accelerate the progression of periodontitis in humans (Jepsen *et al.*, 2018). A recent systematic review by Dommisch *et al.* (2021) found that occlusal adjustment on teeth with mobility and/or premature contacts may lead to improved CAL. The ultimate decision to undertake occlusal adjustments for a patient will therefore be based on a thorough clinical evaluation of each individual case.

Management of tooth mobility

Treatment of periodontal disease

One of the signs of periodontal disease is tooth mobility in association with loss of the supporting tissues. Periodontal therapy should be instituted and following treatment, mobile teeth may respond with a reduction in mobility due largely to the reduction in inflammation of the supporting tissues. However, where significant support has been lost, the tooth is still likely to exhibit some mobility. Where mobility is not progressive or does not interfere with function, this mobility is generally acceptable to the patient.

Splinting

If function is compromised or the mobility is progressive, splinting can be considered. Temporary splinting can be used to increase patient comfort and facilitate the delivery of periodontal treatment (Dommisch *et al.*, 2021). A mobile tooth can be splinted to adjacent teeth using composite resin alone or with an orthodontic wire or composite fibre mesh. Debonding and the need to repair splints are common. A splint may act as a plaque retention factor, particularly across the interdental spaces, so excellent plaque control is needed to avoid worsening the periodontal condition.

Permanent splinting can be achieved by the construction of a removable splint or by linked crowns as described by Lindhe & Nyman (1979). Such restorations require significant tooth preparation and are technically demanding.

For a very mobile tooth, elective replacement by the provision of a cantilevered adhesive bridge or immediate partial denture may be considered.

Key points

- The periodontal tissues respond and adapt to occlusal loading even when there is reduced periodontal support following periodontal disease
- Occlusal forces cannot initiate periodontal breakdown
- The successful treatment of periodontal disease will arrest destruction even if occlusal trauma persists
- Where forces are too great for adaptation, teeth may become mobile or drift
- Occlusal analysis has a role in identifying occlusal interferences
- Occlusal adjustments can be made by selective grinding, restorative treatment or orthodontics
- Tooth mobility is seen in teeth with reduced periodontal support resulting from periodontal disease
- Splinting can be considered when tooth mobility is progressive or compromising function or patient comfort

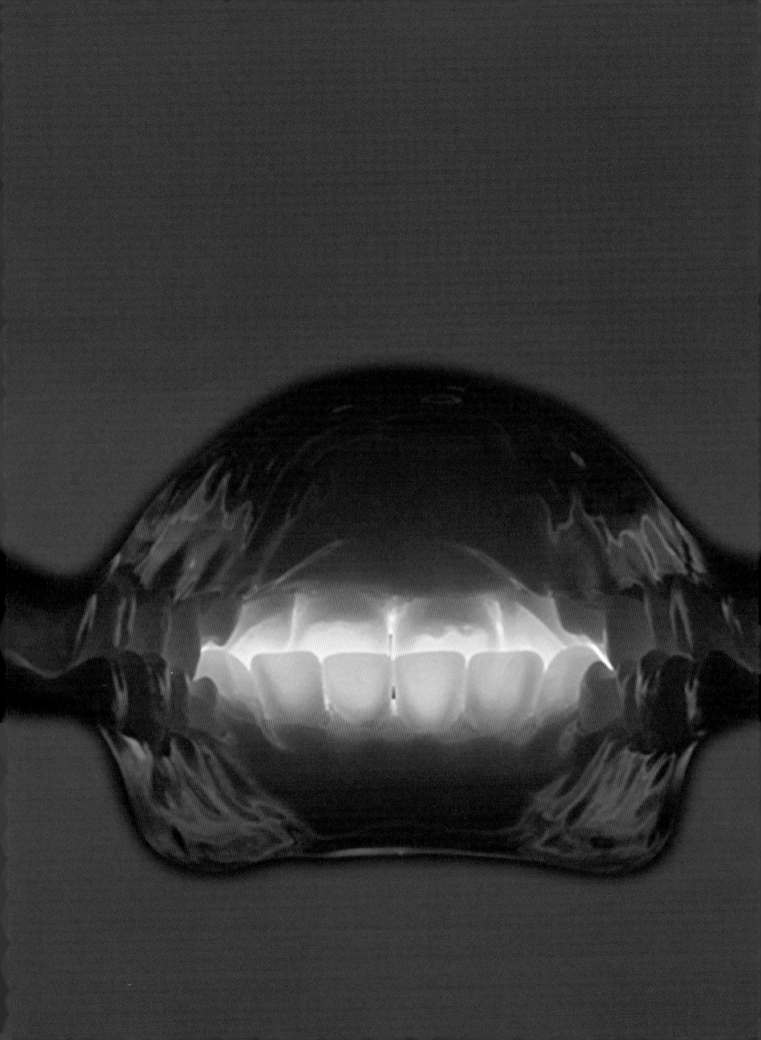

Reaching a periodontal diagnosis and treatment plan

Part 3

Chapters

Overview

Part 3 is targeted at reaching a periodontal diagnosis and treatment plan, beginning with the chapter on the key aspects of the periodontal history and examination in reaching a diagnosis, which signposts the reader to a useful clinical decision-making algorithm on reaching a definitive diagnosis in the context of the 2018 classification emanating from the 2017 World Workshop Classification of Periodontal and Peri-implant Diseases and Conditions. The next chapter (17) covers the role of periodontal screening, namely the Basic Periodontal Examination (BPE) in adults in the UK, and simplified BPE (sBPE) in children and adolescents; the American equivalent is Periodontal Screening and Recording (PSR). How the UK implementation guidance of the 2018 classification has been mapped to the BPE guideline is covered. Chapter 18 on the adjunctive role of radiographs in periodontal diagnosis reinforces the view that radiographs must be taken in accordance with principles of justification and optimisation, and referral criteria may help in deciding when to take radiographs and which views to use. Principles of periodontal diagnosis and treatment planning form the final chapter (19) in Part 3; essentially, the periodontal treatment plan follows a step-wise approach based on the European step 3 (S3)-level treatment guideline and the British Society of Periodontology and Implant Dentistry implementation of this for stage I–III periodontitis, as published in 2020–21.

16 Periodontal history, examination and diagnosis

Figure 16.1 Steps in taking a periodontal history, examination and diagnosis.

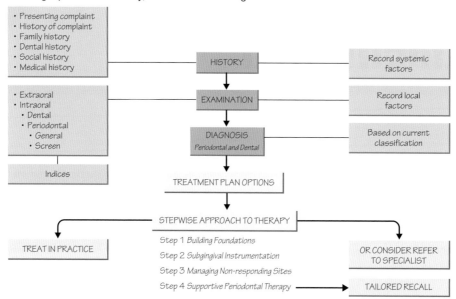

- Presenting complaint
- History of complaint
- Family history
- Dental history
- Social history
- Medical history

HISTORY → Record systemic factors

- Extraoral
- Intraoral
  - Dental
  - Periodontal
    - General
    - Screen

EXAMINATION → Record local factors

Indices

DIAGNOSIS
Periodontal and Dental → Based on current classification

TREATMENT PLAN OPTIONS

STEPWISE APPROACH TO THERAPY

TREAT IN PRACTICE

Step 1 *Building Foundations*
Step 2 *Subgingival Instrumentation*
Step 3 *Managing Non-responding Sites*
Step 4 *Supportive Periodontal Therapy*

OR CONSIDER REFER TO SPECIALIST

TAILORED RECALL

Figure 16.2 Points that a general description of a periodontal condition should cover.

- Qualitative assessment of oral hygiene and presence of supragingival calculus deposits
- Presence of obvious
  - gingival inflammation, swelling, loss of contour
  - gingival recession
  - suppuration
- Occlusal problems, drifting / tooth migration and related aesthetic problems
- Identification of local periodontal risk factors

Figure 16.3 A detailed examination of periodontal tissues and recording of periodontal indices.

Detailed examination of periodontal tissues and recording of periodontal indices:
1. Probing pocket depths in mm
   - From gingival margin to base of pocket
2. Clinical attachment levels in mm
   - From cemento-enamel junction to base of pocket
3. Bleeding on probing with a controlled force (~0.25 N)
4. Suppuration on gentle palpation of tissues or following probing
5. Furcation using codes 1,2,3
6. Recession in mm
   - From cemento-enamel junction to gingival margin
7. Mobility using codes I,II,III

Figure 16.4 Diagram of probing pocket depth, recession and clinical attachment loss.

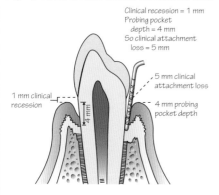

Clinical recession = 1 mm
Probing pocket depth = 4 mm
So clinical attachment loss = 5 mm

1 mm clinical recession

5 mm clinical attachment loss

4 mm probing pocket depth

Figure 16.5 Suppuration.

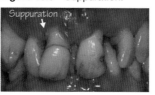

Suppuration

Figure 16.6 Classification of furcation involvement.

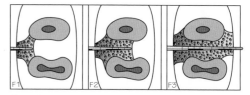

The probe is inserted between the roots of a multi-rooted tooth. A class 1 involvement (F1) is where a probe can be inserted less than 3 mm between the roots. A class 2 involvement (F2) penetrates more than 3 mm but not fully through the furcation, and a class 3 (F3) involvement extends completely between the roots.

Figure 16.7 Mobility.

Handles of two instruments placed on tooth and mobility graded according to movement in horizontal (buccolingual) and vertical direction:
- Grade I = 0.2–1 mm movement in horizontal direction
- Grade II = more than 1 mm movement in horizontal direction
- Grade III = more than 1 mm movement in horizontal direction + vertical movement

Figure 16.8 Radiographic assessment.

Features of periodontal significance to note:
- Degree and pattern of bone loss (horizontal or vertical)
- Progression of bone loss (serial radiographs)
- Subgingival calculus
- Overhanging restoration margins or deficiencies
- Furcation defects
- Endodontic-periodontal lesions
- Widened periodontal ligament space
- Root morphology

Features of dental significance to note:
- Teeth present
- Caries, recurrent caries
- Periapical radiolucencies
- Root fractures
- Root resorption
- Retained roots
- Impacted or unerupted teeth
- Cysts
- Other pathology affecting bone, TMJ, sinuses

Periodontology at a Glance, Second Edition. Valerie Clerehugh, Aradhna Tugnait, Michael R. Milward, and Iain L. C. Chapple.
© 2024 John Wiley & Sons Ltd. Published 2024 by John Wiley & Sons Ltd.

The history and examination should provide relevant information to enable the clinician to formulate a clinical diagnosis and treatment plan (Fig. 16.1).

Periodontal history

Eliciting a good history requires a structured approach, good communication skills and building up a rapport with the patient. The history for a patient presenting for a periodontal assessment should include details of the following.

1 *Presenting complaint.*
- If there is not a complaint, the reason for attendance should be noted.
- If there are other dental complaints these should also be noted.

2 *History of complaint/reason for attendance*: the onset, duration, severity and any triggers of the presenting complaint should be noted.

3 *Family history* of periodontal problems or early tooth loss.

4 *Previous dental history.*
- Past experience and the nature of dental work including restorative, prosthodontic and orthodontic treatment should be noted and the reason for any extractions should be sought.
- A record should be made of any previous periodontal treatment, whether plaque control advice has been given and what type.
- The patient should be asked about any adverse reaction or difficulties accepting local analgesia.
- The pattern of attendance for dental treatment (regular or irregular) should be noted, which may indicate compliance.

5 *Social history*: the social history should include a summary of any personal circumstances that may influence dental management or provision of treatment.
- Availability for treatment.
- How, and how often, tooth brushing is carried out and whether interdental aids are used.
- Tobacco smoking history (how many cigarettes smoked, for how many years, if tried to stop/interested in stopping); also smokeless tobacco habits.
- Alcohol consumption and number of units.
- Dietary factors relevant to caries risk, e.g. frequency of consuming sucrose-containing snacks or carbonated sucrose-containing drinks.

6 *Medical history.*
- A full medical history should be taken systematically, noting any relevant points. This permits the identification of patients who may:
  - be at risk from receiving a periodontal examination/treatment (e.g. on anticoagulants and needing INR (international normalised ratio) prior to treatment to avoid excessive bleeding)
  - pose an infection risk to the dental professional/other patients (e.g. carrier of blood-borne viruses human immunodeficiency virus, hepatitis B or C); universal cross-infection control is implicit
  - have systemic risk factors for periodontal diseases (e.g. poorly controlled diabetes).
- If there is uncertainty about any drugs in the UK, the *British National Formulary* (https://bnf.nice.org.uk) can be consulted.
- The medical history should be checked and updated every visit.

7 *Informed consent* needs to be obtained from the patient before proceeding with the subsequent periodontal management.

Periodontal examination

The dental examination begins with an extraoral examination followed by an intraoral examination of the soft and hard tissues, occlusion and any fixed or removable prostheses. The periodontal examination should be an integral component of the dental examination and can be considered in three parts.

1 General description of the periodontal condition (Fig. 16.2).
2 Periodontal screening using the Basic Periodontal Examination (UK, Europe) or Periodontal Screening and Recording (USA) (Chapter 17).
3 Detailed examination of the periodontal tissues and recording of periodontal indices (Fig. 16.3).
- Probing pocket depths, clinical attachment loss and recession (Fig. 16.4).
- Bleeding on probing with a controlled force (~0.25 N) (Chapple *et al.*, 2018).
- Suppuration (Fig. 16.5).
- Furcation (Fig. 16.6).
- Mobility (Fig. 16.7).

These indices are usually measured on six sites per tooth (mesiobuccal, buccal, distobuccal, mesiolingual, midlingual, distolingual) and recorded on a periodontal chart, such as published by the British Society of Periodontology and Implant Dentistry (2019), while acknowledging there is no universally accepted periodontal chart.

Special tests

In order to reach a diagnosis, additional information may be needed.
- Radiographs.
- Vitality tests.
- Other special tests.

Radiographs

Periapical radiographs, horizontal bitewings, vertical bitewings, panoramic views or combinations of these may be suitable for periodontal assessment but should only be taken when they are clinically justified and would change the management or prognosis of the patient (Chapter 18). The key findings of the radiographic examination must be concisely recorded in the notes (Fig. 16.8).

Vitality tests

Pulpal vitality can be tested by thermal (primarily cold) stimuli or electric pulp testers, and together with radiographic assessment may be useful in determining management options such as root canal therapy.

Other special tests

Other tests may include blood tests, e.g. full haematological screen, blood glucose levels, INR or microbiological plaque sampling.

Diagnosis

The diagnosis is dependent on the findings from the history and examination and should include the periodontal diagnosis, based on the current classification (see Chapters 2 and 19), and any dental condition that needs management. See Chapter 36 for details of Staging and Grading periodontitis, and Figure 36.2 for a clinical decision-making algorithm to guide practitioners on reaching a definitive diagnosis in the context of the 2018 classification system (Dietrich *et al.*, 2019).

Following the diagnosis, the treatment plan can be drawn up and agreed with the patient's consent.

Key points
- History taking requires a structured approach and good communication skills
- Periodontal examination is an integral part of the dental examination and comprises general assessment of the periodontium, periodontal screening and detailed periodontal indices
- Periodontal diagnosis is based on classification and may need special tests; other dental diagnoses should also be made

17 Periodontal screening

Figure 17.1 (a) Sextants and grid for recording BPE in adults. (b) Index teeth (highlighted in yellow) for recording sBPE in children/adolescents.

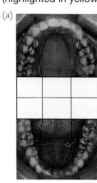

(a)

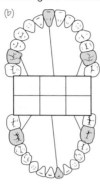

(b)

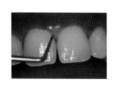

Figure 17.2 Features of probe used for periodontal screening using BPE/sBPE.

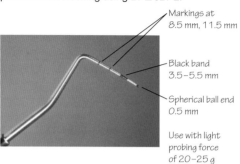

Markings at 8.5 mm, 11.5 mm

Black band 3.5–5.5 mm

Spherical ball end 0.5 mm

Use with light probing force of 20–25 g

Figure 17.3 BPE codes and criteria.

BPE Code	Criteria
0	Healthy periodontal tissues. Probing depths <3.5 mm. Black band entirely visible above gingival margin. No calculus/ no overhangs/ no other plaque retention factor. No bleeding on probing.
1	Bleeding on probing. Probing depths <3.5 mm. Black band entirely visible above gingival margin. No calculus/ no overhangs/ no other plaque retention factor.
2	Supragingival and/or subgingival calculus and/or overhangs and/or other plaque retention factor. Probing depths <3.5 mm. Black band entirely visible above gingival margin.
3	Probing depth(s) 3.5–5.5 mm. Black band partially visible above gingival margin indicating shallow pocket(s) of 4 mm or 5 mm.
4	Probing depth(s) >5.5 mm. Black band disappears in the pocket, indicating deep pocket(s) of 6 mm or more.
*	Furcation involvement

Figure 17.4 Diagrammatic use of probe and codes for BPE. (a) Code 0; (b) Code 1; (c) Code 2; (d) Code 3; (e) Code 4; (f) Code *.

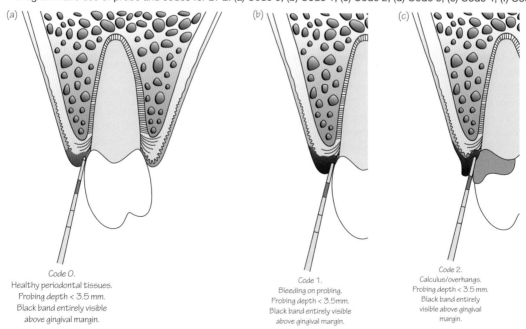

(a) Code 0.
Healthy periodontal tissues.
Probing depth < 3.5 mm.
Black band entirely visible above gingival margin.

(b) Code 1.
Bleeding on probing.
Probing depth < 3.5mm.
Black band entirely visible above gingival margin.

(c) Code 2.
Calculus/overhangs.
Probing depth < 3.5mm.
Black band entirely visible above gingival margin.

Periodontology at a Glance, Second Edition. Valerie Clerehugh, Aradhna Tugnait, Michael R. Milward, and Iain L. C. Chapple.
© 2024 John Wiley & Sons Ltd. Published 2024 by John Wiley & Sons Ltd.

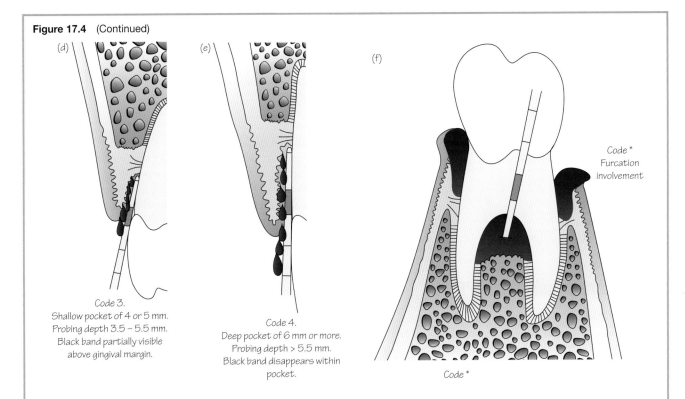

Figure 17.4 (Continued)

(d)

Code 3.
Shallow pocket of 4 or 5 mm.
Probing depth 3.5 – 5.5 mm.
Black band partially visible
above gingival margin.

(e)

Code 4.
Deep pocket of 6 mm or more.
Probing depth > 5.5 mm.
Black band disappears within
pocket.

(f)

Code *
Furcation
involvement

Code *

Figure 17.5 Use of radiographs in conjunction with BPE/sBPE.

1. BSP recommends that radiographs should be available for code 3 and 4 sextants:
   a. Type of radiograph is a matter for clinical judgement, but crestal bone should be visible.
   b. Many clinicians consider periapicals to be the gold standard for code 4 sextants i) to allow assessment of bone loss as % of root length and ii) to view periapical tissues.
2. Radiographs should only be considered following a thorough history and examination and be in accord with the principles of clinical justification and optimization (see Chapter 18)
3. Use selection criteria for dental radiography and periodontal patients to assist choice of radiographs (Faculty of General Dental Practitioners (UK), 2018)

Figure 17.6 BSP guidance on interpretation of BPE codes (see also Chapter 19 for BSP implementation of EFP S3-level clinical treatment guideline).

Code	BSP Guidance on Interpretation of BPE Codes (BSP, 2019)
0	No need for periodontal treatment
1	Oral Hygiene Instruction (OHI), including plaque and gingival bleeding scores
2	OHI Remove supragingival/subgingival calculus and other plaque retention factors
3	OHI. Risk factor control Initial therapy Post-initial therapy, do 6-point pocket chart in sextant(s) code 3
4	OHI. Risk factor control Full periodontal assessment including full mouth 6-point pocket chart Assess need for more complex treatment; referral to a Specialist may be indicated (see BSP Referral Policy and Parameters of Care, www.bsperio.org.uk)
*	Treat according to BPE code 0–4 and degree of furcation involvement Assess need for more complex treatment; referral to a Specialist may be indicated as above

Periodontal screening provides a quick and easy method of detecting periodontal disease so that appropriate treatment and patient education can be started at the earliest opportunity. In the UK, periodontal screening has been recommended for use in general dental practice by the British Society of Periodontology and Implant Dentistry (BSP) since 1986. The system initially employed was the Community Periodontal Index of Treatment Needs (CPITN) but this has since been reconfigured for use in individual patients as the Basic Periodontal Examination (BPE). It is also used in Europe. The UK implementation guidance of the 2018 Classification for Periodontal and Peri-implant Diseases and Conditions has been mapped to the BPE guideline (Dietrich *et al.*, 2019). The equivalent system in the USA is Periodontal Screening and Recording (PSR), which was introduced by the American Dental Association and the American Academy of Periodontology into general dental practice in 1992.

Why use periodontal screening?

- It is a simple, rapid and cost-effective method of assessing patients for periodontal diseases.
- It is comfortably tolerated.
- Periodontal screening summarises the necessary information with minimal documentation.
- It helps determine patients who would benefit from a more detailed periodontal examination and who may require more complex periodontal therapy.
- It helps avoid dento-legal problems when used as recommended for screening, recording and further evaluations.
- In children and adolescents, the simplified BPE (sBPE) is recommended following its adoption by the BSP and the British Society of Paediatric Dentistry in 2012; it was updated in 2021 (Clerehugh & Kindelan, 2021).

Limitations of periodontal screening

- It is not intended as a replacement for the full periodontal examination/periodontal indices.
- It cannot indicate the extent of periodontal involvement.
- It does not record plaque levels or details of clinical attachment loss (CAL)/recession.
- It is not suitable for monitoring periodontal status or response to treatment.
- It should not be used around implants, for which four- or six-point pocket charting should be used.

Who to screen

- All new patients.
- All recall patients as an integral part of a routine dental examination.

How to screen using the BPE

Sextants/index teeth

In adults, the mouth is divided into sextants (Fig. 17.1a). At least two teeth must be present in a sextant for it to be scored, otherwise the single tooth should be included in the score for the neighbouring sextant (www.bsperio.org.uk).

In teenagers and children, following full eruption of the teeth, periodontal screening can be undertaken on the index teeth (www.bsperio.org.uk): all four first permanent molars plus the maxillary right central incisor and mandibular left central incisor (Fig. 17.1b), (Clerehugh, 2008; Clerehugh & Kindelan, 2021) (see also Chapter 41).

Probe

To be suitable for periodontal screening, a number of features should be present, based on the WHO 621 probe (Fig. 17.2).

- A 0.5 mm spherical ball tip to aid detection of subgingival calculus deposits and limit penetration at the base of the pocket.
- A black band at 3.5–5.5 mm to delineate the normal sulci (<3.5 mm) and periodontal pockets (>3.5 mm).
- Sometimes additional marks at 8.5 and 11.5 mm are present on the 'C-type' probe version for clinical use.
- Lightweight.
- Recommended probing force of 20–25 g (0.20–0.25 N).

Recording BPE

The probe should be gently walked around all the teeth in each sextant in adults (except for third molars, unless first and/or second molars are missing), or around the index teeth in children/teenagers, covering six sites per tooth: distobuccal; midbuccal; mesiobuccal; distolingual/palatal; midlingual/palatal; mesiolingual/palatal.

This should take no more than 2–3 minutes in adults, and even less time in children and teenagers.

What to record for the BPE

The screening procedure assigns codes 0, 1, 2, 3, 4 or * according to the presence or absence of bleeding after gentle probing; supragingival or subgingival calculus, defective restoration margins or other plaque retention factors; shallow pockets (4 or 5 mm); deep pockets (6 mm or more); and furcation involvement (Figs 17.3, 17.4).

Adults

The worst finding in each sextant is recorded in a six-box grid (Fig. 17.1a). If code 4 is assigned, continue to examine all the sites in the sextant in order to gain full understanding of the sextant and to ensure furcations are not overlooked in posterior sextants.

Teenagers and children

The highest score around each index tooth is recorded in a six-box grid (Fig. 17.1b). Only codes 0, 1 or 2 should be determined up to the age of 11 years because of the likelihood of false pockets associated with newly erupting teeth. However, if the black band disappears into any unusually deep pockets, then further periodontal investigation is required, irrespective of age. In adolescents aged 12 years or over, the full range of codes can be used on the index teeth to facilitate early detection of periodontal pockets.

For all ages, both the number and the * should be recorded if furcation involvement is present.

How to use the screening information

- Guidance on use of radiographs is summarised in Fig. 17.5.
- BSP guidance on interpretation of BPE scores is shown in Fig. 17.6; the clinician's skill, knowledge and judgement should be used, taking into account individual patient factors. Deviation from the guideline may be appropriate in individual cases, for instance where there is lack of patient engagement. See Chapter 19 for details of the step-wise clinical treatment approach and the BSP implementation of the EFP S3-level clinical treatment guideline into clinical practice.
- BPE cannot be used for monitoring response to treatment. Pre- and posttreatment six-point pocket charts should be undertaken to assess response to periodontal therapy.
  - Where pocket charts are undertaken, only pockets of 4 mm or more should be recorded; bleeding on probing should always be recorded.
  - Once in the supportive phase of therapy, full-mouth probing depths should be recorded at least annually.

Key points

- Screening provides a simple, rapid method of assessing a patient's periodontal condition using:
  - Basic Periodontal Examination (BPE) in UK/Europe for adults; Simplified BPE (sBPE) for children/adolescents
  - Periodontal Screening and Recording (PSR) in the USA
- The mouth is divided into sextants in adults or index teeth if used in children/adolescents
- A probe based on the WHO 621 probe with a spherical ball tip and black band is gently walked around six sites per tooth
- The worst score is recorded for each sextant/index tooth in a six-box grid
- BPE/sBPE and PSR:
  - do not replace the need for a full periodontal examination
  - are not suitable for measuring response to treatment
- Information gathered helps the clinician determine:
  - the level of further examination needed
  - basic guidance on treatment needed
- BPE is not suitable for use around implants

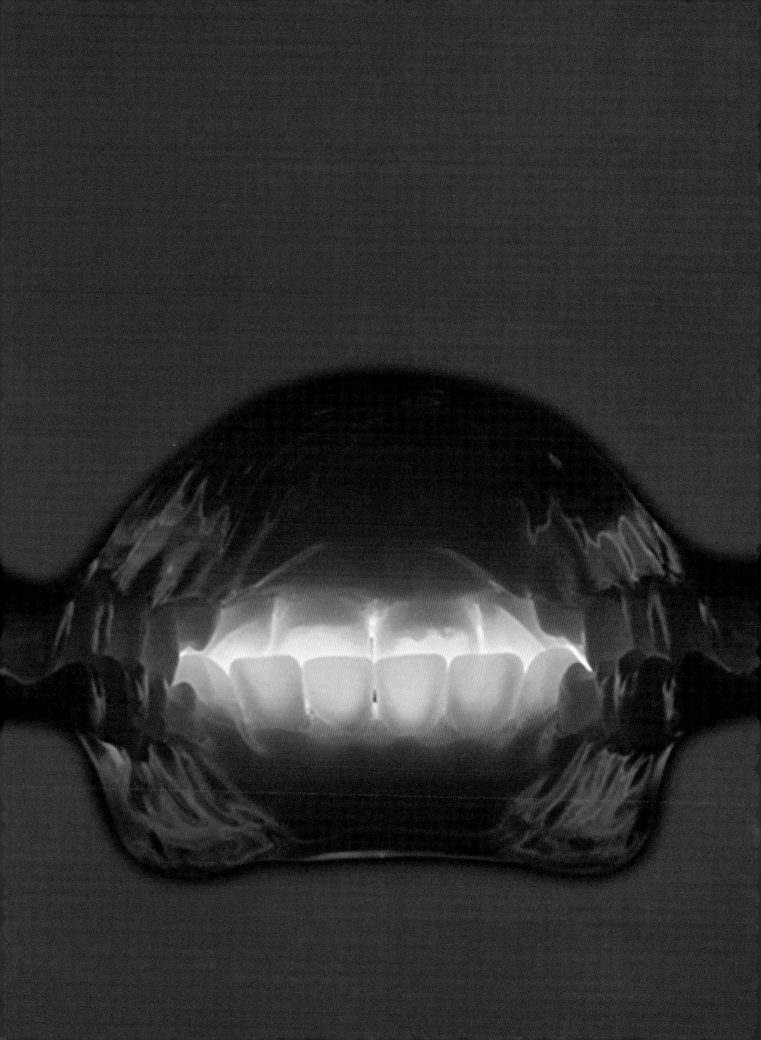

18 Role of radiographs in periodontal diagnosis

Figure 18.1 Ways of minimising radiation exposure when using radiographs.

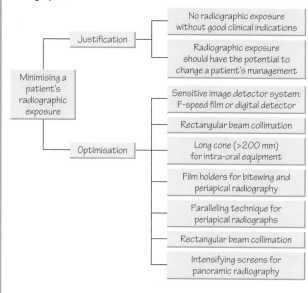

Figure 18.2 Key aspects of a radiographic periodontal assessment. CEJ, cement–enamel junction; TMJ, temporomandibular joint.

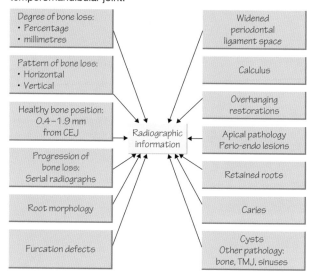

Figure 18.3 Panoramic radiograph showing bone loss.

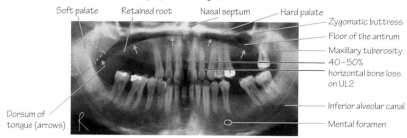

Panoramic radiograph showing some of the normal anatomical structures. A generalised horizontal pattern of bone loss is seen around the teeth. Percentage bone loss is estimated from an assessment of total root length relative to the degree of bone remaining, so for instance an estimate of 40–50% bone loss is seen around UL2.

Figure 18.4 Furcation defects.

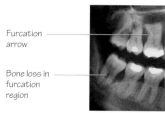

Part of a panoramic radiograph showing furcation defects with bone loss clearly evident between the roots of LR8. The furcation arrow indicates early furcation involvement in a three-rooted molar (UR6).

Figure 18.5 Calculus and deficient crown margin.

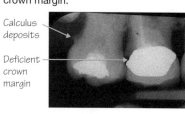

Figure 18.6 Plaque retention factors.
Source: Courtesy of Ms V. Yorke.

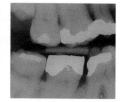

Horizontal bitewing radiograph showing multiple, heavily restored teeth, including poorly restored LR6 with distal open contact and deficient distal margin LR7.

Figure 18.7 Overhanging restoration margins.

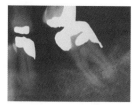

Part of a panoramic radiograph showing overhanging restorations distally on LL5 and particularly on LL7.

Periodontology at a Glance, Second Edition. Valerie Clerehugh, Aradhna Tugnait, Michael R. Milward, and Iain L. C. Chapple.
© 2024 John Wiley & Sons Ltd. Published 2024 by John Wiley & Sons Ltd.

Figure 18.8 Full-mouth periapical radiographs for a patient with advanced bone loss.

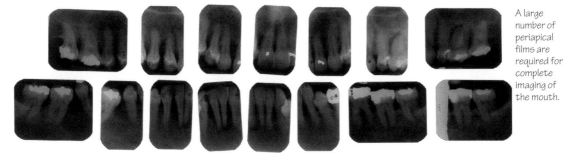

A large number of periapical films are required for complete imaging of the mouth.

Radiographs are used as an adjunct to a thorough clinical examination for diagnosing periodontal disease and planning treatment. The British Society of Periodontology and Implant Dentistry Flowchart (Appendix 3) provides guidance to the clinician on how to implement the 2018 classification to reach a diagnosis in clinical practice and the appropriate radiographs are integral to determining the staging and grading of a patient. There is some variation across different countries in the exact recommendations for radiographs but they are considered essential to assess the bony tissues supporting the teeth.

The details of regulations governing the use of radiographs also vary across countries, but in principle they all seek to protect the workforce and general public and limit the radiation dose to patients. Patients are protected by application of the principles of justification and optimisation (Fig. 18.1).

- *Justification* of a medical exposure is based on the practitioner's understanding of the hazards associated with taking a radiograph and the clinical information. A radiographic examination can be justified when it shows a potential net benefit to the patient, weighing the overall diagnostic gains against the possible disadvantages of the exposure.
- *Optimisation* is applied by employing a range of measures to minimise the radiation dose once it has been established that the radiograph should be taken.

Radiographic information

Radiographs can provide considerable information that may assist in the diagnosis and management of a patient's periodontal condition (Figs 18.2–18.7). The degree of bone loss can be expressed either as a percentage of the root length if the apex of the tooth can be visualised or in millimetres on a bitewing radiograph. The pattern of bone loss is not diagnostic but irregular bone loss can be suggestive of more rapid destruction than a horizontal pattern of loss. Angular or intra-bony defects have been considered to be associated with occlusal trauma but this is not diagnostic. The exact pattern of bone loss is often more dependent on the amount of separation between the roots.

Existing radiographs should be used as far as possible. Sequential radiographs can give information on disease progression; for instance, serial bitewing radiographs taken primarily for caries detection may provide information about bone levels over time. It is important that any radiographs taken solely to follow up periodontal disease are justified.

Radiographic views

The selection of views should be based on the diagnostic information required. Radiographs can be used alone or in combination as appropriate.

- Horizontal bitewing.
- Vertical bitewing.
- Periapical.
- Panoramic.

Horizontal bitewing

Horizontal bitewing radiographs are frequently prescribed primarily for caries detection. The alveolar crest can be visualised even if there have been several millimetres of bone loss. These radiographs provide a good image with consistent positioning and they may allow monitoring of bone changes if a series of these radiographs is available. Their disadvantage is that the apical structures cannot be visualised and the overall length of the root cannot be gauged.

Vertical bitewing

Vertical bitewing radiographs are taken by rotating the conventional bitewing through 90° so that more extensive bone loss can be seen while still imaging several teeth on one radiograph. This view has the same disadvantage as the horizontal bitewing in that the apical structures will not be available for assessment.

Periapical

Periapical radiographs are considered to be the most useful radiographs for assessment of periodontal structures. They image the full extent of the root so that the worst site of bone loss can be determined and subsequently used to determine the stage and grade of periodontitis. Periapical radiographs can be taken at selective sites or throughout the mouth to produce a full series (Fig. 18.8). The long cone paralleling technique enables a consistent image to be taken. Good clarity of the image is obtained by this technique and visualiation of the whole root although it can take time to obtain a full set of radiographs.

Panoramic

Panoramic radiographs enable all teeth to be seen on one image (Fig. 18.3). Newer machines generate images of good quality but detail is less fine compared to intraoral techniques. There is a tendency for overlap of teeth and reduced image quality in the anterior regions. Having reviewed the panoramic radiograph, selected periapical radiographs can be taken to supplement the information obtained if necessary.

Digital radiography

Digital radiography has become widely available, superseding film radiography so that many of the errors that were associated with wet film processing with chemicals are no longer a problem. Digital images are processed immediately. Images can be manipulated so, for instance, thin bone that could escape detection can be rendered visible by adjusting contrast and brightness and small bony changes can be detected on serial radiographs.

Cone beam computed tomography

Cone beam computed tomography (CBCT) produces high-resolution three-dimensional images leading to applications particularly in implant placement (see Fig. 28.6c,d) and orthodontics. CBCT may also offer superior imaging of bone defects and furcation lesions. The effective dose of CBCT is dependent on many factors but principally on the volume of tissue being irradiated. In general, the effective doses are larger than for conventional radiographs taken for periodontal use.

European evidence-based referral criteria have been produced to guide the clinical use of CBCT and have concluded that currently, CBCT is not indicated as a routine method of imaging periodontal bone support (SEDENTEXCT, 2012). CBCT is indicated for cross-sectional imaging prior to implant placement as an alternative to existing cross-sectional techniques where the radiation dose of CBCT is shown to be lower.

Selection of radiographs

Radiographic selection or referral criteria have been available for some years in the UK, Europe and the USA. The objectives for their use are to limit unnecessary radiation to the patient and increase the diagnostic value of the radiographs taken. They are used following completion of a thorough clinical assessment of the patient. The results of this clinical examination are then used to determine whether radiographs should be taken and to aid selection of views.

In compiling guideline, the convened bodies in the UK, Europe and the USA identified that there was limited evidence on which to base their recommendations and so the referral criteria available are derived largely from expert opinion and differ in specific detail. Having undertaken the radiographic examination, it is essential that all films are examined and the diagnostic findings should be reported in written form in the patient's notes, producing what is termed a radiographic report. This ensures that all valuable diagnostic information is extracted regardless of the primary reason for taking the radiographs.

Key points

- Radiographs are used with a thorough clinical examination to make a diagnosis and draw up a treatment plan
- Radiographs must be taken in accordance with the principles of justification and optimisation
- Radiographs can provide information on bone levels, local plaque retention factors and other features that can assist diagnosis and treatment planning of periodontal conditions
- Different radiographic views can provide different information, radiation exposure and image quality
- Referral criteria may help in deciding when to take radiographs and which views to use

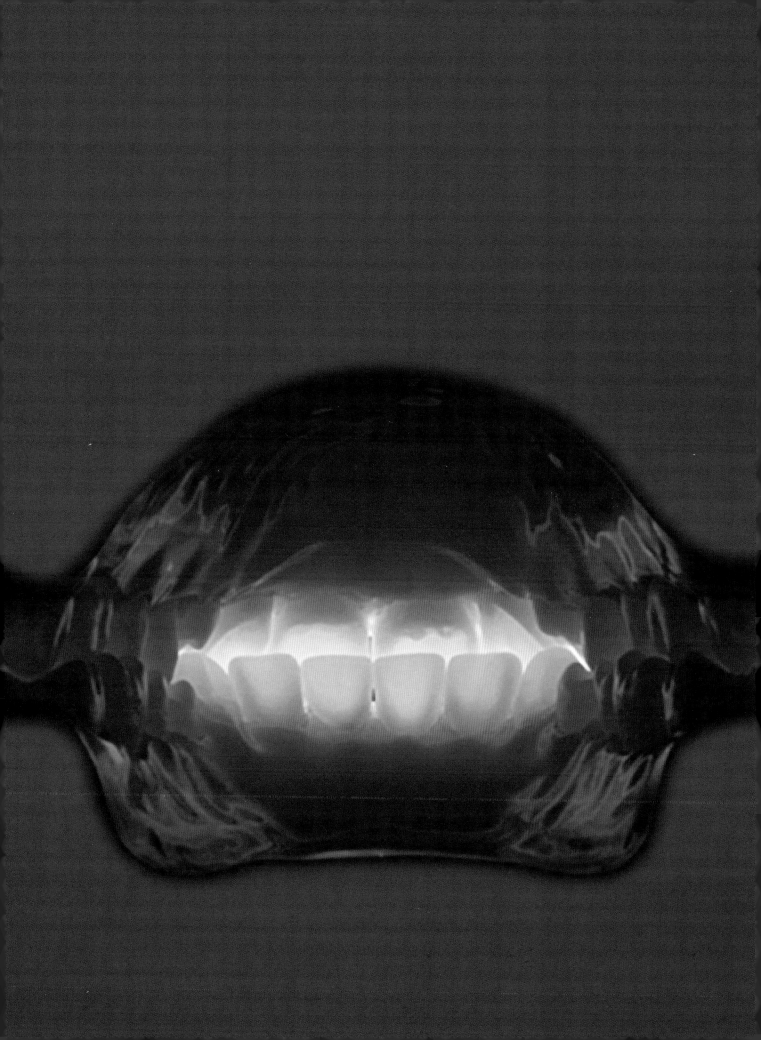

19 Principles of periodontal diagnosis and treatment planning

Figure 19.1 Stepwise approach to periodontal therapy.

```
                          HISTORY ────────── Record systemic factors,
                             │                    risk factors
Screening, radiographs,      ▼
  other special tests ───── EXAMINATION ────── Record local
                             │                    factors
Differential diagnosis       ▼
Diagnostic statement ────── DIAGNOSIS ──────── Based on current
                         Periodontal and Dental    classification
                             │
                             ▼
                  TREATMENT PLAN OPTIONS
                             │
                             ▼
              STEPWISE APPROACH TO THERAPY
        ┌────────────┬──────┴──────────┬──────────────┐
        ▼            │                 │              ▼
 TREAT IN PRACTICE   Step 1 Building Foundations    OR CONSIDER REFER
                     │                              TO SPECIALIST
                     Step 2 Subgingival Instrumentation
                     │
                     Step 3 Managing Non-responding Sites
                     │
                     ▼
                     Step 4 Supportive Periodontal Therapy ──▶ TAILORED RECALL
```

Figure 19.2 Dental examination of a patient.

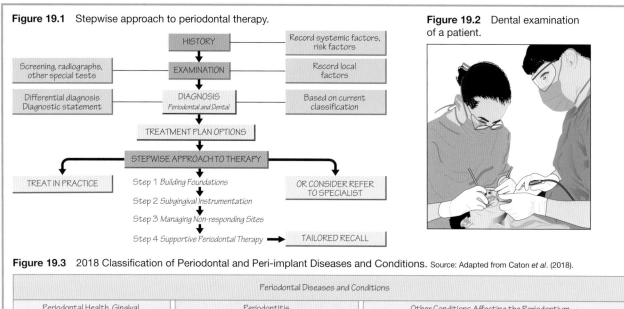

Figure 19.3 2018 Classification of Periodontal and Peri-implant Diseases and Conditions. Source: Adapted from Caton *et al.* (2018).

Periodontal Diseases and Conditions		
Periodontal Health, Gingival Diseases and Conditions Chapple et al., 2018 Trombelli et al., 2018	Periodontitis Papapanou et al., 2018 Jepsen et al., 2018 Tonetti et al., 2018	Other Conditions Affecting the Periodontium Jepsen et al., 2018 Papapanou et al., 2018

Periodontal Health and Gingival Health	Gingivitis Dental Plaque Biofilm-induced	Gingival Diseases Non-dental Plaque Biofilm-induced	Necrotising Periodontal Diseases	Periodontitis	Periodontitis as a Manifestation of Systemic Disease	Systemic Diseases or Conditions Affecting the Periodontal Supporting Tissues	Periodontal Abscesses and Endodontic-Periodontal Lesions	Mucogingival Deformities and Conditions	Traumatic Occlusal Forces	Tooth and Prosthesis Related Factors

Peri-implant Diseases and Conditions Berglundh et al., 2018			
Peri-implant Health	Peri-implant Mucositis	Peri-implantitis	Peri-implant Soft and Hard Tissue Deficiencies

Figure 19.4 Diagnostic statement for periodontitis.

Diagnostic Statement for Periodontitis				
Steps:				
Staging of Periodontitis	Stage I Early/Mild	Stage II Moderate	Stage III Severe	Stage IV Very Severe
Interdental Bone Loss *	< 15 % or < 2 mm**	Coronal third of root	Mid third of root	Apical third of root
* Maximum bone loss in % of root length ** Measurement in mm from CEJ if only bitewing radiograph available (bone loss) or no radiographs clinically justified (CAL)				
Extent	Localised (up to 30% of teeth) Generalised (more than 30% of teeth) Molar/incisor pattern			
Grading of Periodontitis	Grade A Slow	Grade B Moderate	Grade C Rapid	
% Bone Loss/Age	< 0.5	0.5–1.0	>1.0	
Risk Factor Assessment	eg Smoking (cigarettes/day, duration)		eg Diabetes Mellitus (if sub-optimal control)	
Assessment of Current Periodontal Status	Currently Stable BOP < 10% PPD ≤ 4 mm No BOP at 4 mm sites	Currently In Remission BOP ≥ 10% PPD ≤ 4 mm No BOP at 4 mm sites	Currently Unstable PPD ≥ 5 mm PPD ≥ 4 mm & BOP	
Formulation of brief periodontitis diagnostic statement: Extent; Stage; Grade; Current Status (Stability); Risk Factors Eg Diagnosis: generalised periodontitis, stage II, grade B, currently unstable. Risk factor – current smoker 10/day, 10 years				

Periodontology at a Glance, Second Edition. Valerie Clerehugh, Aradhna Tugnait, Michael R. Milward, and Iain L. C. Chapple.
© 2024 John Wiley & Sons Ltd. Published 2024 by John Wiley & Sons Ltd.

Figure 19.5 UK Clinical Practice Treatment Guideline for Periodontal Diseases.

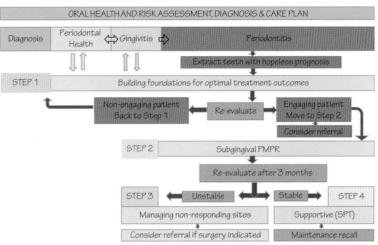

Figure 19.6 Step 1.

- Follows disease classification and diagnosis
- Aims to build foundations for optimal treatment outcomes
- Explain disease, local/systemic risk factors (RFs), treatment options
- Implement strategies for patient motivation and behaviour change to
  - achieve better self-performed oral hygiene (OH)
  - control RFs to reduce gingival inflammation
- Professional mechanical plaque removal (PMPR)
  - including removal of supragingival and subgingival calculus from crowns of teeth
- Eliminate local plaque retentive factors
- Other treatment based on clinical/radiograph exam

Figure 19.7 Engaging patient.

Favourable response to self-care advice:
- ≥ 50% improvement in plaque and marginal bleeding scores
OR
- Indicative plaque levels ≤ 20%
- Indicative bleeding levels ≤ 30%
AND
- Stated preference to achieve periodontal health

Figure 19.8 Non-engaging patient.

Unfavourable response to self-care advice:
- < 50% improvement in plaque and marginal bleeding scores
OR
- Indicative plaque levels >20%
- Indicative bleeding levels >30%
AND
- Stated preference to palliative care approach

Figure 19.9 Palliative periodontal care.

- Simple, pragmatic, cost-effective, non-judgemental maintenance protocol
  - Regular calculus removal
  - Re-motivation of non-engaging patients
  - Can be delivered by dental care professionals
- May improve length of tooth retention but less effective than full treatment protocol
  - Review if change from non-engaging to engaging patient

Figure 19.10 Step 2 for engaging patients.

- Follows evaluation of Step 1 after 3 months, including OH review, plaque score:
  - Non-engaging patient returns to Step 1 and repeats
  - Engaging patient moves to Step 2 OR consider referral if appropriate:
- Periodontal pocket depth (PPD) and bleeding charts
- Reinforce OH, RF control, behaviour change
- Subgingival PMPR (hand or powered)
  - Reduce plaque biofilm, calculus on root
- Use of adjunctive local/systemic antimicrobials when indicated by appropriately trained professionals

Figure 19.11 Step 3 for engaging patients.

- Follows re-evaluation 3 months after Step 2, including plaque score, PPD and bleeding charts
- Reinforce OH, RF control, behaviour change
- Manage non-responding sites (ie PPD ≥ 5mm, or PPD 4 mm with bleeding on probing (BOP))
- Re-perform subgingival PMPR on moderate (4–5 mm) residual pockets with BOP
- For deep residual sites (≥ 6 mm) with BOP, consider other causes eg intra-bony/furcation lesions and if referral indicated for access flap surgery or regenerative/resective surgery
  - If referral not possible, re-perform subgingival PMPR
- If all sites stable after Step 3, move to Step 4

Figure 19.12 Step 4 for engaging patients.

- Supportive periodontal therapy (SPT)
- Monitor periodontal status, PPD/BOP charts
- Repeat plaque score, reinforce OH, RF control, behaviour change
  - Re-motivate and re-educate patient
  - Repeat plaque control instruction
  - Re-treat disease using targeted PMPR to limit tooth loss
  - Arrange next recall
- Tailored recall at time interval appropriate to diagnosis

The periodontal diagnosis follows a thorough history and examination (Figs 19.1, 19.2; Chapter 16) and should be based on the current 2018 classification derived from the 2017 World Workshop for the Classification of Periodontal and Peri-implant Diseases and Conditions (Caton *et al.*, 2018) (Fig. 19.3; Chapter 2). If more than one periodontal disease/condition is present, more than one diagnosis should be made. If there is any uncertainty, a differential diagnosis can be made. For each periodontal condition diagnosed, a diagnostic statement would usefully include the type and extent of the periodontal disease and, in the case of periodontitis, its staging, grading, stability and risk factors (Dietrich *et al.*, 2019) (Fig. 19.4; Chapter 36; Appendix 3).

It is also important for other non-periodontal diagnoses to be made based on the extraoral and intraoral examination of soft and hard oral tissues, e.g. temporomandibular joint disorders, oral mucosal diseases, caries/root caries, deficient, fractured or overhanging restorations, apical pathology, retained roots, unerupted or impacted teeth, oral pathology such as cysts or tumours, and problems relating to fixed or removable prosthodontics.

The treatment plan is based on the periodontal and dental conditions diagnosed.

Periodontal treatment plan

European Federation of Periodontology (EFP) S3-level treatment guideline and BSP implementation for stages I–III periodontitis

The periodontal treatment plan follows a stepwise approach based on the EFP step 3 (S3)-level treatment guideline (Sanz *et al.*, 2020) and the BSP implementation of this (Kebschull & Chapple, 2020; West *et al.*, 2021) (Fig. 19.5; Appendix 4). S3 is the highest level of guideline development. It was based on 15 systematic reviews, assessment of available evidence and formulation of clinical recommendations (CRs) using a structured, moderated consensus process involving a guideline development group from 36 national periodontal societies within the EFP. The EFP used methodological guidance from the Association of Scientific Medical Societies in Germany and the Grading of Recommendations Assessment, Development and Evaluation (GRADE) Working Group.

The UK version was developed by a representative guideline group from the source guideline using a formal process called the GRADE ADOLOPMENT framework which allowed for the adoption (unmodified acceptance), adaptation (acceptance with modification) and *de novo* development of evidence and consensus-based CRs of direct clinical relevance to the UK dental community (West *et al.*, 2021). In total, 62 CRs were made for the various treatment modalities: nine for Step 1, 17 for Step 2, 16 for Step 3 and 20 for Step 4, with an expert consensus for each one for what is:

- recommended
- suggested
- undertaken on the judgement of the individual clinician.

Step 1 Building foundations for optimal treatment outcomes (Fig. 19.6)

Step 1 aims to successfully control the plaque biofilm and may lead to behaviour change/motivation. It includes tailored OHI; professional mechanical plaque removal (PMPR) to remove supragingival and subgingival plaque and calculus on the tooth crown; local and systemic risk factor (RF) control. CR 1.1 recommends that the same guidance on oral hygiene practices to control gingival inflammation is enforced throughout steps 1–4 of periodontal therapy, including supportive periodontal therapy (SPT). BSP advocates either full-mouth or, for speed in clinical practice, partial-mouth recording for plaque/bleeding scores on Ramfjord teeth: UR6, UR1, UL4, LL6, LR1, LR6. CRs 1.5–1.7 recommended RF control interventions, specifically smoking cessation or diabetes control by dentists or referral to appropriately trained professionals. On completion of Step 1, engaging patients as defined by NHS England (Fig. 19.7) can move to Step 2. Non-engaging patients (Fig. 19.8) should move back to Step 1 and repeat (Fig. 19.5) with the option for palliative care (Fig. 19.9).

Step 2 Subgingival biofilm and calculus control/removal (Fig. 19.10)

Step 2 is the cause-related phase of therapy and aims to control (reduce/eliminate) the subgingival plaque biofilm. It includes subgingival PMPR to remove subgingival plaque biofilm and subgingival calculus from the root surface and may also involve the use of adjunctive therapies for gingival inflammation (Chapter 23). On completion of Step 2, the outcome of therapy should be assessed to determine if the desired endpoints were reached.

Step 3 Management of non-responding sites (≥4 mm with BOP or ≥6 mm) (Fig. 19.11)

Step 3 is directed at treating non-responding sites (probing depth ≥4 mm with BOP or ≥6 mm). It aims to gain access to further subgingival instrumentation. This may involve repeated non-surgical subgingival PMPR for residual pockets of 4–5 mm with BOP or surgical interventions for PDs ≥6 mm; referral for appropriate surgical approaches by specialists or dentists with additional training may be indicated to achieve regeneration or resection in lesions (infra-bony or furcation) with increased complexity.

Step 4 Maintenance/supportive periodontal therapy (SPT) (Fig. 19.12)

Step 4 aims to maintain periodontal stability through SPT in all treated periodontitis patients, recognising that they are deemed 'periodontitis patients' for life. It combines preventive/therapeutic interventions from Steps 1–3 if needed.

The BSP was unable to make a clinical recommendation in respect of adjunctive use of antiseptics in dentifrices without further research (CR 4.12) but suggested consideration of adjunctive use of mouthwashes containing chlorhexidine, essential oils and cetyl pyridinium chloride in periodontitis patients undergoing SPT (CR 4.13). It is not known if other adjunctive agents such as probiotics, prebiotics, anti-inflammatory agents and antioxidant micronutrients are effective in controlling gingival inflammation during SPT (Figuero *et al.*, 2020; West *et al.*, 2021). Regular recall intervals are required, tailored to the patient's individual needs.

Recurrent disease should be managed in conjunction with an updated diagnosis and treatment plan. Compliance with OHI regimens and healthy lifestyle are integral along with any necessary PMPR and ongoing risk factor control.

For stage IV periodontitis, the focus shifts from treatment of the periodontitis to restoration of severe periodontitis cases using orthodontics, fixed and removable prosthodontics on teeth and/or implants, in conjunction with functional and occlusal considerations.

Key points

- Periodontal diagnosis:
  - follows a thorough history and examination
  - is based on the current 2018 classification
- The periodontal treatment plan for stages I–III periodontitis follows a stepwise approach based on the EFP S3-level treatment guideline and the BSP implementation of this:
  - Step 1: building foundations for optimal treatment outcomes
  - Step 2: subgingival biofilm and calculus control/removal (subgingival PMPR)
  - Step 3: management of non-responding sites
  - Step 4: maintenance/supportive periodontal therapy (SPT)
- Non-periodontal diagnoses should also be made and treatment arranged

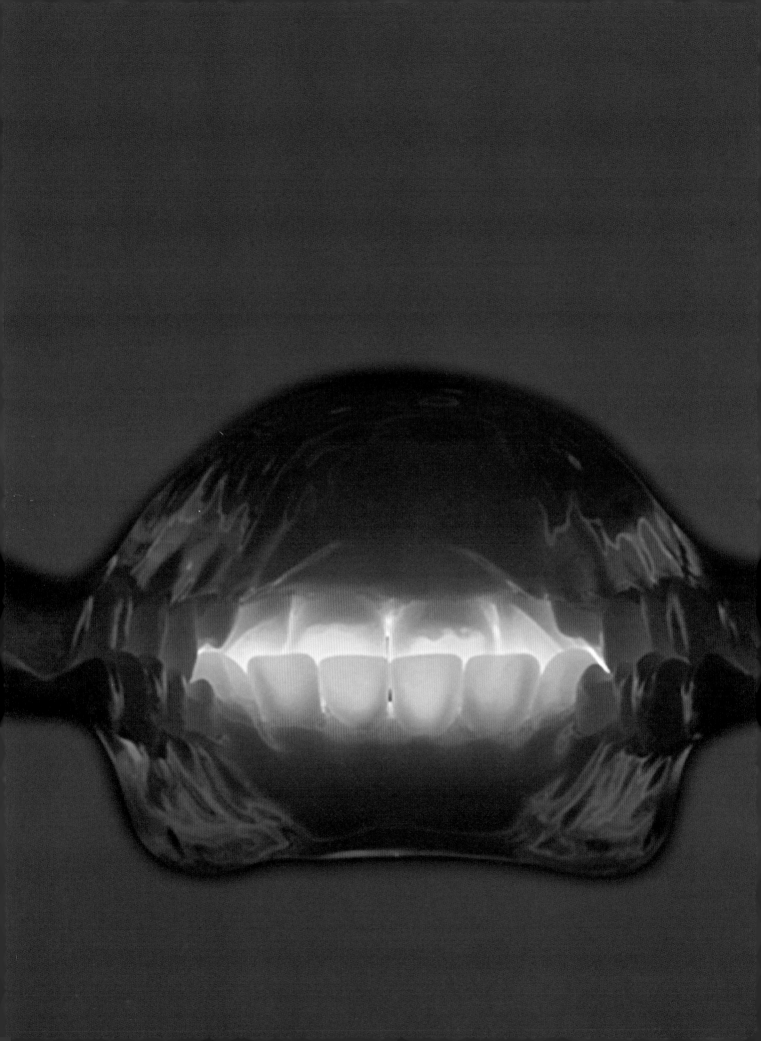

Fundamentals for periodontal patient care

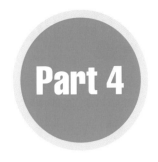

Part 4

Chapters

Overview

Part 4 addresses fundamentals for periodontal patient care, beginning with the crucially important topic of plaque control covered in the first chapter. A fundamental part of the management of periodontal diseases is the control of the supragingival plaque biofilm by the patient, commencing in the first step of therapy in accordance with the BSP implementation of the European S3-level guideline for stage I–III periodontitis, and being maintained throughout all four steps (Chapter 20). The next chapter (Chapter 21) covers non-surgical periodontal therapy, which is directed at removal of supragingival and subgingival plaque and calculus deposits and other local plaque retention factors; the chapter also includes updated terminology in this field. Professional mechanical plaque removal (PMPR) forms part of each of the four treatment steps in the BSP UK clinical practice guideline for the treatment of periodontal disease and forms the mainstay of professional periodontal management in general dental practice. The penultimate chapter describes the periodontal tissue response and healing following successful treatment, what happens if treatment fails, how to monitor the treatment response, and how to assign a periodontally stable or unstable outcome (Chapter 22). The final chapter (23) in Part 4 provides an updated consideration of the role of local and systemic antimicrobial therapy in the management of periodontal diseases and guidance on current controversies and usage.

20 Plaque control

Figure 20.1 (a) Manual brush *in situ*. (b) Powered brush *in situ*.

(a)

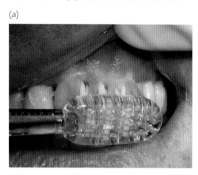

(b)

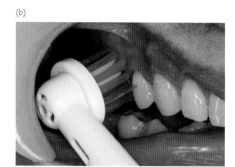

Manual Toothbrush
- Angle bristles at 45° to teeth and gingivae, vibrate the brush (modified Bass technique)
- Scrub technique appropriate for the child patient

Powered Toothbrush
Place alongside the tooth and gingivae
Brush action from:
- rotary head or
- sonic bristle vibration

Figure 20.2 Toothbrushing advice for patients.

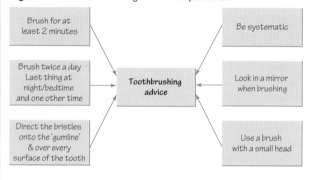

Brush for at least 2 minutes

Be systematic

Brush twice a day Last thing at night/bedtime and one other time

Toothbrushing advice

Look in a mirror when brushing

Direct the bristles onto the 'gumline' & over every surface of the tooth

Use a brush with a small head

Figure 20.3 Potential use of powered toothbrushes – points to consider.

- Patients with adequate oral hygiene skills should be instructed in the method they use rather than changed unnecessarily.
- Patients who seem unable to improve their cleaning with a manual brush may benefit from making a change and investing in a powered brush. Timer helps patient to brush for sufficient time.
- Powered toothbrushes can improve long-term compliance.
- Patients with reduced manual dexterity such as with arthritis may benefit from a powered toothbrush.
- Some disabled patients (e.g. with learning disabilities) or a carer may find a powered brush easier to use.
- Some patients especially children like using gadgets so may be more motivated to brush with a powered brush though the novelty may wear off.

Figure 20.4 (a) Interdental brushes. (b) Interdental brush *in situ*.

(a)

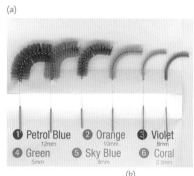

1. Petrol Blue 12mm
2. Orange 10mm
3. Violet 8mm
4. Green 5mm
5. Sky Blue 3mm
6. Coral 2.5mm

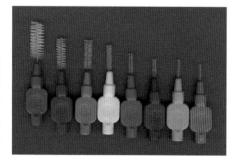

(b)

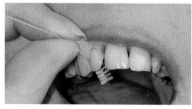

Periodontology at a Glance, Second Edition. Valerie Clerehugh, Aradhna Tugnait, Michael R. Milward, and Iain L. C. Chapple.
© 2024 John Wiley & Sons Ltd. Published 2024 by John Wiley & Sons Ltd.

Figure 20.5 Pharmacological plaque control agents.

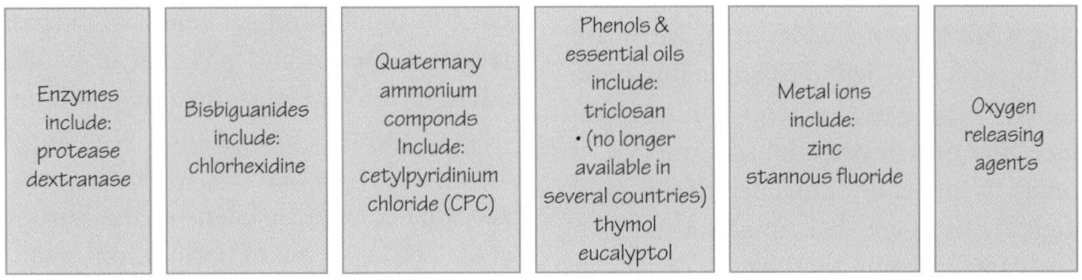

Enzymes include: protease dextranase	Bisbiguanides include: chlorhexidine	Quaternary ammonium componds Include: cetylpyridinium chloride (CPC)	Phenols & essential oils include: triclosan • (no longer available in several countries) thymol eucalyptol	Metal ions include: zinc stannous fluoride	Oxygen releasing agents

Figure 20.6 Use of chlorhexidine mouthwash.

Corsodyl® mouthwash
    Rinse with 10 ml of 0.2% for 1 minute twice daily
Peridex® mouthwash, PerioGard® mouthwash
    Rinse with 15 ml of 0.12% for 30 seconds twice daily

- When brushing is not possible for limited periods
- To help with acutely inflamed gingivae
- To relieve pain from ulcers or minor oral problems
- Specific cases of the medically compromised patient or patient with specific physical disability or learning disability
- Prior to ultrasonic scaling to reduce microbial load of aerosol spray
- Post-periodontal/oral surgery

Figure 20.7 Disclosed plaque.

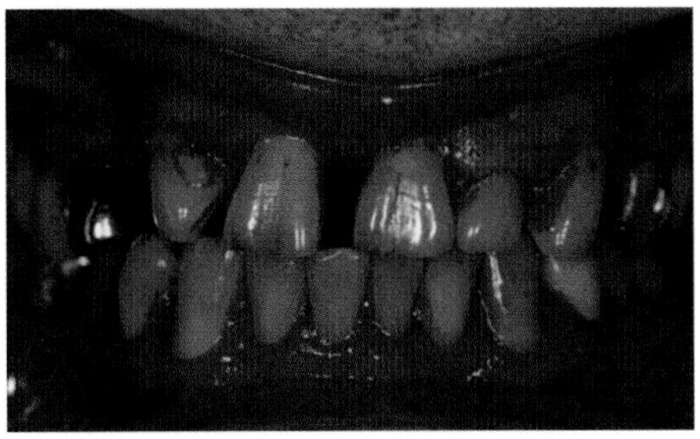

Figure 20.8 Tailor-made patient information.

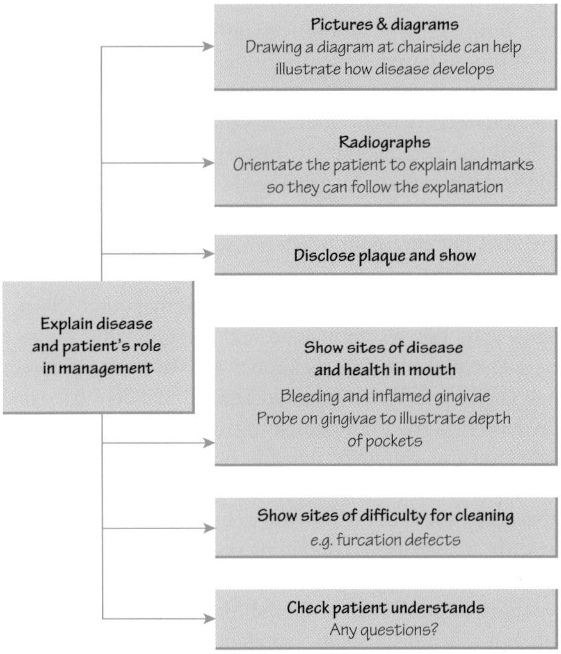

Explain disease and patient's role in management

- **Pictures & diagrams** Drawing a diagram at chairside can help illustrate how disease develops
- **Radiographs** Orientate the patient to explain landmarks so they can follow the explanation
- **Disclose plaque and show**
- **Show sites of disease and health in mouth** Bleeding and inflamed gingivae Probe on gingivae to illustrate depth of pockets
- **Show sites of difficulty for cleaning** e.g. furcation defects
- **Check patient understands** Any questions?

Supragingival dental biofilm, commonly known as plaque, is the primary aetiological factor in the periodontal diseases and there is substantial evidence to demonstrate the effectiveness of oral hygiene practices for gingivitis control (Chapple *et al.*, 2015; Van der Weijden & Slot, 2015). Therefore, a fundamental part of the management of periodontal diseases is the control of supragingival biofilm by the patient, undertaken as part of the first step of therapy in accordance with the BSP implementation of the European S3-level guideline for stage I-III periodontitis (West *et al.*, 2021). The patient needs information to understand why plaque removal is important in the treatment of their periodontal disease, education on the methods to use and motivation to maintain the recommended regime. Individually tailored oral health education can be effective in improving long-term compliance with oral hygiene practices.

Toothbrushing

A wide range of manual brushes of different designs are available. A recommended brush should have a small head, rounded nylon filaments and medium filaments. The modified Bass technique is commonly advised as it aims to clean into the gingival crevice without causing trauma (Fig. 20.1a).

Powered brushes are also widely used (Fig. 20.1b). A systematic review (Yaacob *et al.*, 2014) and meta-review (Van der Weijden & Slot, 2015) showed that powered toothbrushes reduce plaque and gingivitis more than manual toothbrushing in the short and long term, with another systematic review showing that oscillating, rotating, powered toothbrushes have improved efficacy (Robinson *et al.*, 2005).

Recommendation of which type of brush to use should be based on assessment of the individual patient (Figs 20.2, 20.3).

Interdental cleaning

An effective toothbrushing technique can only clean about 65% of the tooth surface and cannot remove interproximal plaque so interdental cleaning is also necessary. Interdental brushes, dental floss, tape and powered flossing devices are all available for interproximal use. Wood sticks have a triangular cross-section and although they can be used in open interdental embrasures, they can be damaging or break if used too aggressively and therefore have limited application. Dental floss and tape are advised when the interdental papillae completely fill the embrasures. Floss with a stiff end and expanded spongey part can be useful for threading under fixed prostheses and around tooth or implant abutments.

Where there is space for interdental brushes, these are recommended (Fig. 20.4), with interdental brushes being significantly more effective in cleaning than floss (Slot *et al.*, 2020). Structural equation modelling analysis showed that reductions in probing depths and bleeding on probing were mainly due to the greater efficiency of interdental brushes in removing interdental plaque rather than compression of the interdental papillae (Tu *et al.*, 2008).

Adjunctive pharmacological agents

Many agents have been incorporated into mouthwashes and toothpastes and key groups are shown in Fig. 20.5. Most are used to supplement brushing and interdental cleaning but some (e.g. chlorhexidine gluconate) can be used when toothbrushing is not possible, for instance after oral or periodontal surgery.

Chlorhexidine gluconate is generally considered the gold standard antiplaque/antigingivitis agent. It is mostly used as a mouthwash but is also available in some toothpastes or gels. It exhibits substantivity, i.e. the ability to adsorb to hard and soft tissues and subsequently adsorb in a biologically active form, and this prolongs the antibacterial activity following rinsing. Side-effects that limit its use include altered taste sensation, staining of teeth or tooth-coloured restorations, increased supragingival calculus formation and, rarely, mucositis. There is a very small risk of anaphylaxis, which although very rare means that the patient should be asked about any history of sensitivity to chlorhexidine and the medical history should be checked before it is prescribed or recommended. Prolonged usage is not generally recommended but the mouthwash is useful in specific clinical situations (Fig. 20.6).

A meta-analysis (Gunsolley, 2006) reported that other adjunctive agents with proven antiplaque and antigingivitis efficacy include (i) essential oils; (ii) triclosan 0.3% with a co-polymer (2.0% polyvinyl methyl ether and maleic acid) in a dentifrice formulation. However, triclosan-containing dentifrices are no longer available in several countries due to concerns over effects on hormone levels and potential long-term public health risks. If adjunctive antiseptic mouthrinses are to be considered, as well as chlorhexidine, formulations containing essential oils or cetylpyridinium chloride are suggested (West et al., 2021). Other agents that have more recently been proposed for delivery in dentifrices or mouthrinses include probiotics, prebiotics, anti-inflammatory agents and antioxidant micronutrients but evidence on their efficacy is lacking.

At present, there is no specific clinical recommendation for an adjunctive antiseptic dentifrice formulation without further research (West et al., 2021).

Disclosing plaque

An objective assessment of plaque removal can be achieved by using a disclosing solution or tablets which stain the plaque (Fig. 20.7). The tablet form can easily be used by the patient at home to assess their own cleaning and identify areas that they are missing. In the surgery, disclosing the plaque can initiate a discussion about the effectiveness of the patient's oral hygiene, allow targets to be set and progress to be charted. Personalising the advice given and engaging the patient in oral hygiene advice can help to improve compliance. Non-surgical therapy will be less successful if carried out when the oral hygiene is poor and in accordance with the steps of the European S-3 guideline (West et al., 2021), Step 2 of periodontal treatment delivering subgingival instrumentation should not be commenced in a non-engaging patient. The BSP UK Clinical Practice Guideline for the Treatment of Periodontal Disease flowchart defines an engaging patient as one with plaque levels of 20% or less and bleeding levels of 30% or less, or an improvement in plaque and marginal bleeding scores of 50% or more (BSP, 2021).

Changing behaviour

Oral health information and education can increase a patient's understanding and knowledge of their disease and give them the tools required to change their oral hygiene practices. However, tailored advice related to the patient's own mouth may be more effective for long-term compliance (Shou, 1998) (Fig. 20.8). Patients who believe that they have personal control over their health are more likely to respond to the advice they are given (Kiyak et al., 1998). The use of goal setting, self-monitoring and planning is effective in improving oral hygiene-related behaviour in patients with periodontal disease (Newton & Asimakopoulou, 2015). Motivational interviewing and other psychological methods may have potential to bring about behavioural change but there is not yet evidence of a significant impact on compliance with oral hygiene regimens (Carra et al., 2020; West et al., 2021).

Key points

- Both toothbrushing and interdental cleaning are necessary for optimal plaque control
- Pharmacological plaque control agents may be considered as part of an individual case; chlorhexidine is the most effective
- Disclosing plaque can be a useful tool for patient education and motivation
- Tailored oral hygiene advice is important in providing patient understanding and improved oral hygiene practices

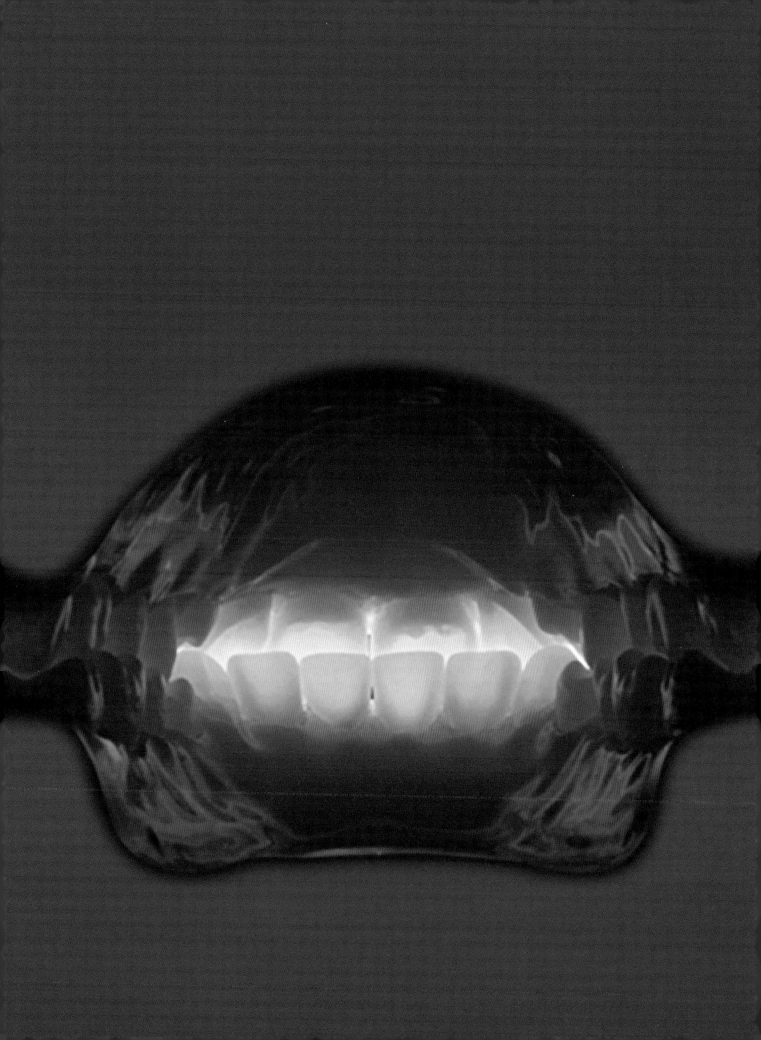

21 Non-surgical periodontal therapy

Figure 21.1 Terms relating to plaque and calculus removal.
Source: Adapted from BSP (2021).

Supragingival PMPR (Professional Mechanical Plaque Removal)	Removal of plaque, staining and supragingival calculus from the crown of a tooth or restoration	Replaces terms of scaling and polishing
Subgingival PMPR	Removal of subgingival plaque, calculus and endotoxin from the root surfaces	Replaces terms of subgingival scaling, subgingival debridement, subgingival instrumentation (though subgingival instrumentation used throughout European S3 Guideline) and root surface debridement
No modern equivalent: terms and concept are outdated	Removal of subgingival calculus and necrotic cementum	Root planing

Figure 21.3 Two classic studies demonstrating the effectiveness of plaque control.

Lovdal et al. (1961)	Badersten et al. (1984)
• 1500 subjects in Norway • Oral hygiene instruction and scaling and root planing repeated 2–4 times a year, over 5 years • Reduced gingivitis and tooth loss even in patients whose home-care was not substantially improved	• 16 subjects with moderate-advanced periodontitis • Oral hygiene instruction and root surface debridement of single rooted teeth • After 2 years elimination of gingivitis and pocket reduction even at very deep sites (> 9 mm)

Figure 21.2 Hand or ultrasonic instruments? (a) Hand instruments. (b) Ultrasonic instruments.

(a)

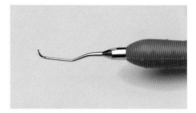

- Hand instrumentation allows the operator tactile sensitivity which is lost with ultrasonic instruments.
- Hand instruments are cheaper to buy and maintain than ultrasonics.
- Hand instruments are less likely to cause discomfort in sensitive teeth.
- No aerosol is generated (may impact on level of personal protective equipment required for use dependent on local rules).

(b)

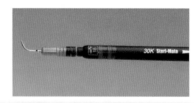

- Irrigation with water (or another coolant) in ultrasonic instruments clears the field of debris and blood but can in itself obscure vision.
- Magnetostrictive ultrasonics are contra-indicated in patients with some cardiac pacemakers.
- Piezoelectric and sonic instruments can be used in patients with cardiac pacemakers.
- Ultrasonic instruments can generate contaminated aerosols (additional personal protective equipment may be required in line with local rules).
- Ultrasonics can be useful to bring about quick removal of gross deposits (especially supragingivally).
- Ultrasonics can be less tiring for the operator.
- Ultrasonics can be used to remove overhanging margins on amalgam restorations.

Figure 21.4 Non-surgical periodontal therapy in a 46-year-old woman with deep pockets on UR3 and UR4, which bled on probing; she experienced occlusal trauma on UR4 following extraction of UL7 and LL7. (a) UR3 probing depth (PD) of >7 mm. (b) Angular vertical infra-bony defects UR3 and UR4. (c,d) Subgingival PMPR of UR3 using a hoe, following ultrasonic treatment. (e) Subgingival PMPR being finished on UR3 using a curette to create a clean smooth root surface; occlusal adjustment was undertaken on UR4 as part of the initial therapy. (f) PD at two years follow-up is less than 4 mm on UR3 (shown) and UR4. Bone level stability and corticated crest on UR3 at two years (g) and five years (h) follow-up.

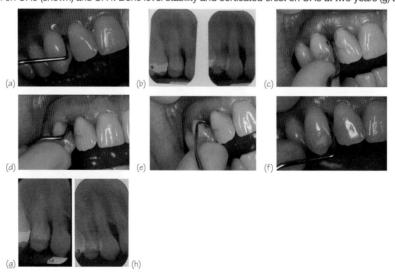

It is accepted that removal of the mechanical biofilm is required for successful periodontal treatment and a supportive care programme (Van Weijden & Slot, 2011; West *et al.*, 2021). Non-surgical professional mechanical plaque removal (PMPR) forms part of each of the four steps of treatment in the BSP UK clinical practice guideline for the treatment of periodontal disease (Chapter 19).

Non-surgical periodontal therapy is directed at removal of supragingival and subgingival plaque and calculus deposits which act as plaque retention factors. Removal of other local plaque retention factors is also part of this treatment and together these form the mainstay of periodontal management in general dental practice (Greenstein, 2000). Terms relating to the terminology of instrumentation past and present are shown in Fig. 21.1.

It was previously thought that endotoxin was firmly bound to cementum and that extensive cementum removal by scaling and root planing was required for treatment to be effective. However, studies have shown that endotoxin is weakly bound to the root surface and can readily be removed by powered or manual scalers and even by washing or polishing (Drisko *et al.*, 2000).

Periodontal instrumentation

The removal of deposits is technically demanding. Effectiveness is dependent on the depth of pocket, skill of the operator, root anatomy, time spent and instrument sharpness (for hand instruments). Supra- and subgingival PMPR is routinely carried out using hand instruments (Fig. 21.2a) (sickle scalers, curettes and hoes) and ultrasonic or sonic instruments (Fig. 21.2b) (Drisko *et al.*, 2000). The latter operate by tip vibration and a spraying/cavitation effect of the fluid coolant and therefore generate an aerosol as they are used. The vibrations of ultrasonic tips are generated by an electromagnetic field (magnetostrictive) or crystal transducer (piezoelectric); sonic tips are air driven with the vibrations generated mechanically. Ultrasonic and sonic instruments are generally less tiring for the operator and are reported as being time-saving compared to hand instruments (Drisko, 1993). Aerosol generation with the potential for air-borne spread of infectious agents, most notably COVID-19, can be a factor in determining choice of instrumentation.

Overhanging restoration margins are associated with greater bone loss (Chapter 14) and may be removed with burs and ultrasonic/sonic scalers, though sometimes a properly contoured replacement restoration is required.

Subgingival air polishing

Fine glycine particles are sprayed at the root surface to remove the biofilm. This cannot remove calculus but may have potential within the supportive phase of therapy after calculus removal has already been achieved.

Vector ultrasonic system

This produces less heat at the tip than other ultrasonic instruments and no aerosol. A review showed that it achieved similar levels of clinical improvement as other methods of periodontal treatment (Guentsch & Preshaw, 2008).

Effectiveness of plaque control and subgingival PMPR

Many studies have shown the effectiveness of plaque control and instrumentation in the treatment of periodontal diseases. Two classic papers are summarised in Fig. 21.3 (Lovdal *et al.*, 1961; Badersten *et al.*, 1984).

A number of studies have compared hand and ultrasonic or sonic instrumentation. Systematic reviews found no difference in outcomes although ultrasonic/sonic subgingival debridement required less time than hand instrumentation (Suvan *et al.*, 2020; Tunkel *et al.*, 2002). The decision on which instruments or which combinations of instruments to use is therefore based on other factors such as patient tolerance and operator preference.

Traditional therapy is delivered over a series of appointments and a successful outcome results in reduced probing depth, elimination of bleeding on probing, gain in attachment and stability of bone levels, even infill in some bony defects (Fig. 21.4). Periodontitis patients with a low proportion of residual periodontal pockets and little inflammation are more likely to have stability of clinical attachment levels and less tooth loss over time (Loos & Needleman, 2020). Full-mouth disinfection strategies have been proposed to minimise reinfection of treated pockets from areas with pathogens by completing treatment within 24 hours (Mongardini *et al.*, 1999). Some work suggested that this full-mouth treatment approach had superior clinical outcomes and microbiological effects than conventional therapy delivered by quadrant (Quirynen *et al.*, 2006). However, a systematic review reported that there was no clear evidence that the full-mouth scaling and root planing (now called subgingival PMPR; see Fig. 21.1) or full-mouth disinfection (with an adjunctive antiseptic) provided additional benefit compared to conventional scaling and root planing (Eberhard *et al.*, 2015), and full-mouth protocols are also associated with an acute systemic inflammatory response (Graziani *et al.*, 2015). The European S3 guideline suggesting that subgingival periodontal instrumentation can be performed with either traditional quadrant or full-mouth delivery within 24 hours was adopted by the British Society of Periodontology and Implant Dentistry (West et al., 2021).

Suvan et al. (2020) conclude that the decision on choice of treatment delivery can therefore be based on patient preferences and general considerations of medical status, tolerance of chair time or the need for repeated sessions of oral hygiene instruction. Where technical, local or systemic factors limit the success of non-surgical periodontal therapy alone, options such as adjunctive antimicrobials (Chapter 23) or surgical approaches (Chapters 24–26) may be indicated.

Use of local analgesia

Local analgesia is widely used when undertaking subgingival PMPR as it provides patient comfort and the vasoconstrictor can also provide a clearer field with less bleeding when deposited locally. A combination of blocks and infiltrations can be used. Anaesthesia of the soft tissues is the goal rather than pulpal anaesthesia. Some clinicians advocate treatment without local analgesia since some techniques may be acceptable to the patient without and allow larger areas of the mouth to be treated at one time. The decision for use of analgesia should be made on a patient-by-patient basis based on the instruments to be used, any dentine sensitivity and other considerations.

> **Key points**
> - Non-surgical therapy is aimed at the removal of supragingival and subgingival plaque deposits and plaque retention factors
> - Hand, ultrasonic and sonic instruments are equally effective for subgingival PMPR
> - The decision to use local analgesia for non-surgical therapy should be taken on a site and patient basis

22 Periodontal tissue response, healing and monitoring

Figure 22.1 Healing of the periodontal tissues. GCF, gingival crevicular fluid.

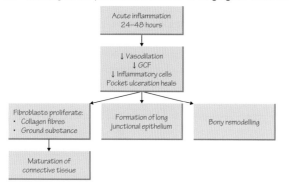

Figure 22.3 Indices for monitoring the response to periodontal therapy.

Response to oral hygiene instruction
- Plaque free score
- Marginal gingival bleeding score

Response to supragingival and subgingival PMPR
- Probing pocket depths
- Clinical attachment levels
- Bleeding on probing
- Suppuration
- Furcation defects
- Mobility
- Recession

Figure 22.2 (a) A periodontal lesion before treatment. (b) Early healing of a periodontal pocket. (c) Further healing of a periodontal pocket.

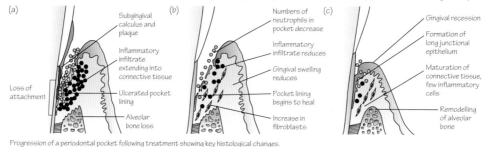

Progression of a periodontal pocket following treatment showing key histological changes.

Figure 22.4 Decision making following monitoring the response to periodontal therapy. Sites are re-evaluated according to the BSP treatment flow chart. Step 3 is undertaken to manage non-responding sites and includes further subgingival instrumentation or potential referral for surgical therapy depending on pocket depths and other considerations. Where a stable outcome has been achieved the patient can proceed to Step 4 and maintenance (supportive therapy). Extract from flow diagram of BSP UK Clinical Practice Guideline for the treatment of periodontal diseases, 2021. See Appendix 4 for complete diagram.

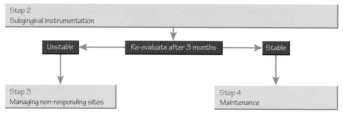

Following oral hygiene measures and supra- and subgingival PMPR, there are two potential outcomes: 1. The tissue may respond by healing or 2. The tissue may fail to heal.

Response to treatment

Following thorough supra- and subgingival PMPR and implementation of good oral hygiene, changes will occur in the microbial flora and periodontal tissues. After instrumentation, junctional epithelium re-establishes within two weeks but granulation tissue is still immature and not replaced by collagen fibres (Segelnick & Weinberg, 2006).

Repair of connective tissue continues for 4–8 weeks after instrumentation. Subgingival microbial recolonisation occurs within 4–8 weeks of supragingival and subgingival PMPR in the absence of improved plaque control, so maintenance of optimal oral hygiene is essential

Microbial flora

There is a reduction in the total numbers of micro-organisms in the periodontal pockets. The residual microbial flora shifts from predominantly Gram-negative anaerobic to one that is largely Gram-positive aerobic and associated with periodontal health, partly because of the reduction in plaque bulk allowing in higher oxygen concentrations within the plaque (Chapters 4 and 5). Since a subgingival microbiota with large numbers of spirochaetes and motile rods is re-established within 4–8 weeks of instrumentation in the absence of good plaque control (Magnusson et al., 1984), maintenance of optimal oral hygiene is essential to the healing process.

Periodontology at a Glance, Second Edition. Valerie Clerehugh, Aradhna Tugnait, Michael R. Milward, and Iain L. C. Chapple.
© 2024 John Wiley & Sons Ltd. Published 2024 by John Wiley & Sons Ltd.

Tissue response and healing

The response to supra- and subgingival PMPR is shown in Figures 22.1 and 22.2. As the periodontal tissue heals, there is a reduction in redness and swelling and the tissue becomes pink and firm. Clinically, the tissue feels more fibrous and the gingival cuff tightens. Bleeding on probing and suppuration subside.

A reduction in pocket depth results from a combination of events.
- Shrinkage of tissue following resolution of the inflammation.
- Potential development of gingival recession.
- Formation of a long junctional epithelium which attaches the gingiva to the cleaned root surface.
- Tightening of the gingival cuff as the gingival collagen fibre bundles reform.
- A small amount of gain in attachment may occur at the base of the pocket.

Healing can sometimes result in resolution of inflammation in the pocket with some reduction and leave a persistent pocket without bleeding. Such a site will be healthy but plaque may enter the deep residual pocket, making the site susceptible to recurrence of inflammation since stability is associated with the achievement of shallow pockets (Loos & Needleman, 2020). Such sites should be monitored closely and where there is any doubt about the need for advanced care to manage residual deep pockets, referral to a periodontal specialist is recommended (West et al., 2021).

Healing following conventional periodontal surgery is essentially the same and is discussed in Chapter 25. Healing following regenerative periodontal surgery is discussed in Chapter 26.

Studies have shown that:
- initially deeper sites show more recession than shallow sites
- initially deeper sites achieve more gain in clinical attachment.

Failure of treatment

Failure to heal will result in persistence of inflammation with the following signs: bleeding on probing, redness, swelling, persistent deep pockets or increasing depths, suppuration, increasing mobility. The most common reasons for failure to respond are:
- Inadequate patient plaque control due to lack of compliance or dexterity.
- Residual subgingival calculus deposits harbouring subgingival plaque, deep pockets, furcation lesions, concavities and root grooves or an inexperienced operator.

It can be hard to tell by probing if a root surface has been cleaned of subgingival calculus. Studies examining extracted teeth following debridement show that achieving a completely calculus-free root surface is very difficult. Only 20–30% of sites that bleed on probing will go on to demonstrate further attachment loss. Nonetheless, bleeding on probing from the base of the pocket suggests a site which is not responding, particularly if the bleeding persists at the same site with sequential monitoring.

Systemic risk factors (e.g. continued smoking, poorly controlled diabetes) may also contribute to treatment failure. Where rate of disease progression is high with the presence of pathogens such as Aggregatibacter actinomycetemcomitans, failure to eradicate these pathogens may impact on healing, and the patient's individual host response will also determine treatment outcome.

The algorithm for clinical periodontal assessment (Dietrich et al., 2019; Fig. 36.2; Appendix 3) implementing the 2018 classification describes periodontal status as currently unstable when there are PPD ≥5 mm sites or BOP at 4 mm sites. Should pockets of this type remain following therapy then healing has not occurred at all sites in the mouth and treatment has not been completely successful. Further treatment will then be required in accordance with Step 3 of the EFP S3 guideline (Sanz et al., 2020) and the BSP implementation of them (West et al., 2021) as discussed in Chapters 24–27.

Monitoring

To assess a patient's response to the therapy that has been undertaken, the periodontal condition needs to be monitored. This is achieved by repeating the indices taken at baseline (Fig. 22.3). The findings are then compared.

Healing will be indicated by a reduction in pocketing and bleeding indices. Evidence shows that achieving shallow periodontal pockets (≤4 mm) that do not bleed on probing in patients with full-mouth bleeding scores <30% will result in the best chance of stability of periodontal health and the lowest risk of tooth loss (Loos & Needleman, 2020). The BSP UK flow diagram for clinical practice guideline for the treatment of periodontal diseases (Appendix 4) defines the unstable case with non-responding sites as having moderate residual pocketing (4–5 mm) or deep residual pockets (≥6 mm) (Fig. 22.4; see also Fig. 19.5). The algorithm for implementation of the 2018 classification (Dietrich et al., 2019; Appendix 3) defines a stable case as one with:
- BOP <10%.
- PPD ≤4 mm.
- No BOP at 4 mm sites.

Satisfactory healing has occurred after treatment when these outcomes are met and the patient's periodontal status can be considered stable. Implementation of supportive care is then important to maintain the patient in accordance with Step 4 of the EFP S3 guideline (Sanz et al., 2020) and the BSP UK Clinical Practice Guideline for the Treatment of Periodontal Diseases (West et al., 2021; Appendix 4) as discussed in Chapter 19.

The patient's ability to implement plaque removal at home is assessed by repeating the plaque score.

Furcation and mobility indices are also repeated. Although these may improve following treatment, successful healing may in many cases not be associated with a significant change in these indicators. Mobility can occur in the presence of a healthy but reduced periodontal support (Chapter 15). Recession may well increase with healing. Furcation defect management in association with increased PPD and BOP is described in Chapter 27.

Probing should be avoided in the first few weeks following treatment to allow early healing and tissue maturation. The indices are therefore recommended to be carried out at 8–12 weeks (minimum of six weeks) after treatment to assess response. Bony changes will take significantly longer to become apparent and routine radiographic techniques will not detect early bony changes and indications of healing. Any decision to take radiographs to monitor bone levels must be based on the principles discussed in Chapter 18, and radiographs should not be taken unless they can be clinically justified.

When the response to treatment has been monitored, the clinician can decide whether the periodontal outcome is unstable or stable and the patient moves to Step 3 or 4 in accordance with current guideline (Fig. 22.4).

Key points
- Following successful treatment:
  - the microbial flora shifts from one that is principally Gram negative and anaerobic to Gram positive and aerobic
  - pocket depths and bleeding are reduced
  - the gingivae become more pink and fibrous
- Treatment failure may result from poor plaque control, residual calculus or other local and systemic factors
- Monitoring 8–12 weeks after treatment identifies responsive and non-responsive sites and enables subsequent treatment decisions to be made in accordance with EPF S3 clinical guideline and BSP clinical practice guideline

23 Role of antimicrobial therapy in periodontal diseases

Figure 23.1 Advantages and disadvantages of using antimicrobials for periodontal diseases.

a) Systemic Antimicrobials

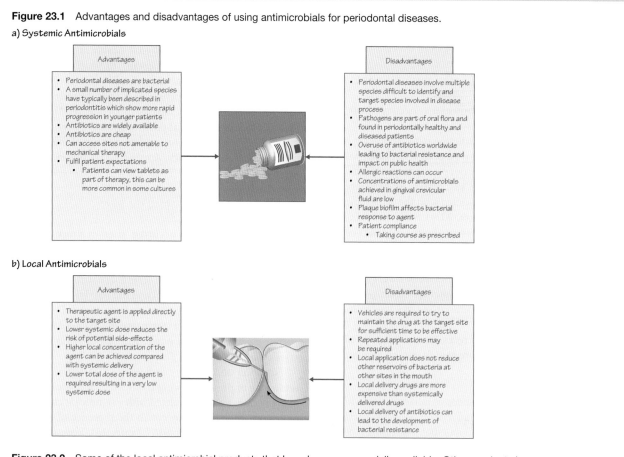

Advantages
- Periodontal diseases are bacterial
- A small number of implicated species have typically been described in periodontitis which show more rapid progression in younger patients
- Antibiotics are widely available
- Antibiotics are cheap
- Can access sites not amenable to mechanical therapy
- Fulfil patient expectations
  - Patients can view tablets as part of therapy, this can be more common in some cultures

Disadvantages
- Periodontal diseases involve multiple species difficult to identify and target species involved in disease process
- Pathogens are part of oral flora and found in periodontally healthy and diseased patients
- Overuse of antibiotics worldwide leading to bacterial resistance and impact on public health
- Allergic reactions can occur
- Concentrations of antimicrobials achieved in gingival crevicular fluid are low
- Plaque biofilm affects bacterial response to agent
- Patient compliance
  - Taking course as prescribed

b) Local Antimicrobials

Advantages
- Therapeutic agent is applied directly to the target site
- Lower systemic dose reduces the risk of potential side-effects
- Higher local concentration of the agent can be achieved compared with systemic delivery
- Lower total dose of the agent is required resulting in a very low systemic dose

Disadvantages
- Vehicles are required to try to maintain the drug at the target site for sufficient time to be effective
- Repeated applications may be required
- Local application does not reduce other reservoirs of bacteria at other sites in the mouth
- Local delivery drugs are more expensive than systemically delivered drugs
- Local delivery of antibiotics can lead to the development of bacterial resistance

Figure 23.2 Some of the local antimicrobial products that have been commercially available. Other products have come on and off the market and not all products mentioned are available in all countries worldwide.

Agent	Product
Actisite® (Alza Corporation, USA)	EVA fibre containing 25% tetracycline HCl - needs removing
Arestin™ (OraPharma Inc., USA)	Minocycline HCl (1 mg) encapsulated microspheres
Atridox™ (Atrix Laboratories Inc., USA)	Doxycycline hyclate (8.8%) resorbable gel
Dentomycin® (Blackwell Supplies, UK)	Minocyline 2% lipid gel
Elyzol® (Colgate-Palmolive, UK)	Metronidazole 25% in a mono/triglyceride gel
Periochip® (Dexcel Pharma, UK)	Chlorhexidine (2.5 mg) in hydrolysed gelatine

Periodontal disease has a bacterial aetiology and therefore much work has been done to investigate the potential role of antimicrobial therapy in the management of periodontal diseases (Fig. 23.1). Mechanical therapy cannot always remove the subgingival biofilm deposits, for instance because of deep pockets or a furcation defect, or reach bacteria that may have invaded soft tissue or dentinal tubules. Also, treated sites can be recolonised by pathogens from non-dental sites. Antimicrobial therapy can be delivered by systemic or local routes.

Systemic antimicrobial therapy
Systemic antimicrobial agents have a role in periodontal therapy in a few specific clinical situations.

Periodontology at a Glance, Second Edition. Valerie Clerehugh, Aradhna Tugnait, Michael R. Milward, and Iain L. C. Chapple.
© 2024 John Wiley & Sons Ltd. Published 2024 by John Wiley & Sons Ltd.

- Periodontitis grade C in younger adults with a high rate of progression.
- Necrotising periodontal diseases (such as necrotising gingivitis).
- Periodontal abscess.

Periodontitis

Following the 2017 World Workshop on the Classification of Periodontal and Peri-implant Diseases and Conditions (Caton *et al.*, 2018), the term 'aggressive periodontitis' was dropped as it had been recognised that periodontitis is a spectrum of disease. At the severe end of the spectrum, cases are seen where there is significant bone and attachment loss for the age of the patient with an indication of rapid progression and such cases are likely to be classified as grade C. It is important to remove the plaque biofilm for antimicrobials to be most effective. Although PMPR in these cases can improve the clinical condition, a number of studies have shown that this alone can fail to eliminate certain periodontal pathogens (Mombelli *et al.*, 2000) The use of systemic antimicrobials can be effective in reducing pathogenic species such as *Aggregatibacter actinomycetemcomitans*. The effectiveness of treatment may be enhanced if debridement can be completed in a short time while the drug is being taken.

Historically, studies have described the use of different antibiotics to treat periodontitis categorised as aggressive, including tetracycline, doxycycline, metronidazole, amoxicillin and azithromycin. Different combinations of drugs, dosages and durations of therapies have been used. Systematic reviews (Sgolastra *et al.*, 2012; Rabelo *et al.*, 2015) support the effectiveness of metronidazole alone and metronidazole in combination with amoxicillin when used as an adjunct to non-surgical therapy. Azithromycin, a macrolide antibiotic similar to erythromycin, has been shown to be improve clinical attachment levels and can be used in patients who are allergic to penicillins (Haas *et al.*, 2008).

Antibiotics can also be used in combination with surgery in cases of periodontitis showing rapid progression. The prescription of systemic adjunctive antimicrobials as an adjunct to subgingival PMPR should be undertaken by specialist periodontists or equivalently trained practitioners as part of the management of complex cases of disease (West *et al.*, 2021).

Controversies in systemic antimicrobial therapy for periodontitis

Systemic antibiotics have been prescribed by some clinicians following periodontal surgery, such as post guided tissue regenerative surgery. There is limited evidence to indicate the efficacy of use in these situations.

Research by Lopez *et al.* (2006) reported the use of antibiotics alone (without subgingival instrumentation) as a treatment of periodontitis that was equally as effective as subgingival instrumentation. The authors highlighted that many patients in undeveloped and developing regions did not have access to conventional periodontal therapy and that systemic antibiotics could be evaluated as a cost-effective treatment of periodontal disease in populations where access to dental care was limited. This is hugely controversial since all medical evidence recommends limiting unnecessary antibiotic usage to reduce antibiotic resistance and hypersensitivity reactions in the wider global population.

European S3-level treatment guideline and the BSP implementation of the guideline (West *et al.*, 2021) do not recommend the routine use of systemic antibiotics as an adjunct to subgingival instrumentation in patients with periodontitis because of the issues around patient and public health.

Necrotising periodontal diseases

Necrotising periodontal diseases can occur in gingivitis and periodontitis patients who are temporarily or moderately compromised.

In gingivitis patients, necrotising gingivitis (NG) is an endogenous infection by mainly anaerobic bacteria (Chapter 39). Where there is lymph node involvement, it is effectively treated with metronidazole in conjunction with non-surgical debridement (400 mg three times daily for three days) (Scottish Dental Clinical Effectiveness Programme, 2021). A mouthrinse such as chlorhexidine should also be used to control the plaque until the painful infection subsides.

In periodontitis patients, necrotising periodontitis (NP) is a more destructive condition and antimicrobials are indicated as part of the overall management.

Periodontal abscess

A periodontal abscess can occur as an acute exacerbation or after treatment in a patient with a pre-existing pocket. A periodontal abscess may also occur in a non-periodontitis patient, for instance as a result of impaction of a foreign body. Antibiotics may be used in treatment where adequate drainage cannot be achieved and there are signs of a spreading infection such as lymph node enlargement (Chapter 40).

Low-dose systemic antimicrobial therapy

Tetracyclines have a number of non-antibiotic properties that can have therapeutic benefit. They can inhibit:
- host collagenases and metalloproteinases
- collagenases from other sources such as neutrophils, macrophages, osteoblasts and osteoclasts
- bone resorption.

Subantimicrobial doxycycline (SDD) up to 40 mg daily has been formulated as an adjunct to subgingival instrumentation seeking to utilise these non-antimicrobial properties at a dose lower than would affect the microbial flora. A systematic review showed improvements in pocket depths with use of SDD (Donos *et al.*, 2019). However, European S3-level treatment guideline and the BSP implementation of the guideline suggest that SDD should not be used as an adjunct to subgingival instrumentation based on considerations around antibiotic stewardship (West *et al.*, 2021).

Local antimicrobial therapy

These agents have been developed for the treatment of periodontitis in adults, aiming to release the agent over a sustained period into the periodontal pocket. Clinical trials have used local delivery agents either as the sole treatment or in conjunction with subgingival PMPR. The reported levels of additional gain in clinical attachment and pocket depth reduction are modest, ranging from studies showing no additional benefit to an additional mean gain of attachment in the order of 1 mm.

Several commercial local delivery antimicrobial agents have been developed. These have included the products in Fig. 23.2 (though not all these systems have been continuously available in the marketplace since their original launch). Five of the products contain an antibiotic (metronidazole, minocycline, tetracycline or doxycycline). The last one uses the antimicrobial agent chlorhexidine, which is available in mouthwashes. Chlorhexidine products have not shown the development of bacterial resistance but there have been some rare reports of severe anaphylactic reactions. Tetracycline products have shown greater improvements in pocket probing depths than chlorhexidine-containing systems (Matesanz-Perez *et al.*, 2013).

European S3-level treatment guideline and the BSP implementation of the guideline state that locally administered sustained-release antibiotic agents and chlorhexidine may be considered as an adjunct to subgingival instrumentation in periodontitis patients (West *et al.*, 2021). West *et al.* note that the cost of such products, which is generally borne by the patient, impacts on cost-effectiveness. Typically, products can be used for patients who have isolated active pockets that are unresponsive to non-surgical therapy. They may be considered in cases where surgery is not considered appropriate, for example in a smoker, where there are other systemic contraindications to surgery or where patient tolerance of a surgical procedure is in doubt.

Although the average potential clinical improvement anticipated from the use of local delivery agents may be small, in an individual site or patient this may be enough to change a progressive situation into a manageable one.

Lasers and adjunctive photodynamic therapy

Lasers

Depending on the wavelength and how they are used, there is evidence for subgingival calculus removal and some antimicrobial effect although the level of impact is not clear. The European S3-level treatment guideline suggested that lasers should not be used as adjuncts to conventional therapy and this guideline has been adopted by the British Society of Periodontology and Implant Dentistry (West *et al.*, 2021).

Antimicrobial photodynamic therapy (aPDT)

This is a laser-based system which combines a non-thermal laser light with a photosensitising dye which attaches to the outer cell membrane of Gram-negative bacteria. Light activation of the solution leads to the formation of toxic reactive oxygen species which can kill periodontal pathogens, potentially reaching those that would remain after conventional instrumentation. A systematic review (Salvi *et al.*, 2020) found insufficient evidence of efficacy and the European S-3 guideline suggested that adjunctive antimicrobial photodynamic therapy at specific wavelengths should not be used in patients with periodontitis and this recommendation was adapted by the BSP.

Key points

- Despite the bacterial aetiology of periodontal disease, the involvement of indigenous species restricts the use of antibiotics in their management
- Systemic antimicrobials can have an adjunctive role in the management of:
  - periodontitis grade C in younger adults with a high rate of progression
  - necrotising periodontal diseases (such as necrotising gingivitis).
  - periodontal abscess with systemic involvement
- Local antimicrobials can be applied directly to the target site
- Local antimicrobials have shown only modest gains in clinical attachment
- Lasers and aPDT use are currently not recommended in patients with periodontitis

Advanced periodontal patient care: periodontal surgery, dental implants, periodontal-orthodontic interface

Part 5

Chapters

Overview

Part 5 covers topics on more advanced periodontal patient care. The first chapter introduces the topic of periodontal surgery, where it fits within the stepwise approach to periodontal treatment (see Part 3, Chapter 19), what periodontal surgery might be used for and various contraindications. The second chapter outlines the different types of periodontal surgery (Chapter 25), with a further chapter devoted to regenerative periodontal therapy and the range of surgical procedures that can be used, their uses, and potential outcomes from the different regenerative surgical techniques (Chapter 26). Bone defects and furcation lesions are described and illustrated in the next chapter, with therapeutic options and outcomes discussed for non-surgical versus surgical access for debridement, cross-referring to the relevant previous chapters (Chapter 27). The chapter introducing dental implants follows (Chapter 28), and a new chapter has been included on the topic of peri-implant mucositis and peri-implantitis, reflecting their inclusion for the first time in the 2018 classification following the World Workshop on the Classification of Periodontal and Peri-Implant Diseases and Conditions (see Chapter 29). The final chapter in Part 5 (Chapter 30) explores the dynamic two-way relationship between periodontal diseases and orthodontics: there may be periodontal sequelae following orthodontic treatment or there may be periodontal drifting as a result of periodontitis requiring orthodontic intervention; the patient should be in step 4 of therapy before any periodontal-orthodontic interventions are considered.

24 Periodontal surgery

Figure 24.1 Advantages and disadvantages of non-surgical periodontal therapy.

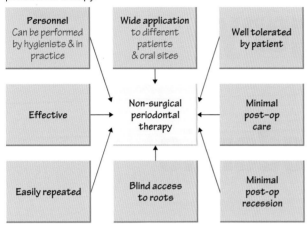

Figure 24.2 Advantages and disadvantages of surgical periodontal therapy.

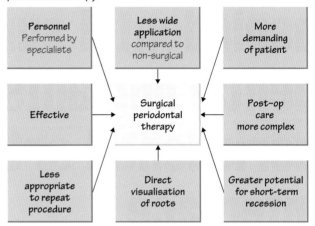

Figure 24.3 Clinical outcomes of surgical therapy.

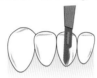

- Postoperative oral hygiene is critical to outcome of surgical therapy
- Pocket elimination, attachment gain and resolution of bleeding can be achieved by surgical therapy
- Bony infill can occur in 2 and 3 wall intrabony defects following resective surgical therapy
- Regenerative surgery is effective at treating intrabony defects of 3 mm of more
- Residual pockets associated with class II and III furcation involvement in maxillary and mandibular molars may be managed by regenerative surgery

Figure 24.4 Postoperative instructions to patients.

In the first 24 hours:
- Take care till local analgesia wears off
- Avoid vigorous rinsing of the mouth
- Avoid vigorous exercise
- Avoid alcohol
- Do not pull on lip or cheek to 'look'
- Pain relief can be gained by paracetomol 500 mg – 1 g or ibuprofen 400–600 mg and repeated 6 hours later if required. Do not exceed doses as recommended on the packet. Avoid aspirin
- Some oozing of the surgical site is not unusual
- Bleeding can be controlled by application of pressure with a clean handkerchief or pack placed on the site for 20 minutes. Seek help if bleeding continues
- Eat a soft diet initially and over the first few days

After 24 hours:
- Rinse around site with chlorhexidine mouthwash twice daily (for 1 to 2 weeks as advised) (Chapter 20)
- Clean other teeth as normal as close to the surgical site as is reasonable but avoid the site itself (for 1–2 weeks as advised)
- Some swelling can occur but should subside within a few days
- Seek advice if any concerns

As described in Chapter 19, steps 1 and 2 of the BSP implementation of the S3-level treatment guideline (West *et al.*, 2021) aim to control the supragingival and subgingival plaque biofilm. These steps include tailored OHI, professional mechanical plaque removal (PMPR), local and systemic risk factor control and may also involve the use of adjunctive therapies for gingival inflammation (Chapter 23). The steps are effective in controlling periodontal disease in many situations. However, there are limitations as to what can be achieved and in specific circumstances, surgical techniques have a role to play in disease management (Figs 24.1, 24.2). The European S3-level guideline and BSP implementation of the guideline suggest that in the presence of deep residual pockets (≥6 mm) in patients with periodontitis Stage III after the first and second steps of periodontal therapy access flap surgery is performed (West *et al.*, 2021). Non-surgical techniques are generally most effective in shallow and moderate pockets and less so in deep pockets. However, there is no absolute cut-off depth of pocket at which non-surgical debridement is ineffective. Non-surgical therapy may be unable to achieve thorough root debridement if there is reduced access to a pocket or if there is complex anatomy such as furcation defects, root concavities or infra-bony pockets.

The patient's response to the second step of therapy should be reviewed and the outcomes evaluated to determine if treatment has been successful (Chapter 21). If a successful outcome to therapy has not been achieved then consideration may be given to using the third step of periodontal therapy, that of surgical therapy. Surgical therapy would rarely be considered following a

Periodontology at a Glance, Second Edition. Valerie Clerehugh, Aradhna Tugnait, Michael R. Milward, and Iain L. C. Chapple.
© 2024 John Wiley & Sons Ltd. Published 2024 by John Wiley & Sons Ltd.

single round of non-surgical therapy and so a further course of non-surgical therapy would generally be advocated before determining whether surgical options should be considered.

Periodontal surgery will only benefit some patients for whom the endpoints of periodontal therapy have not been achieved so the decision to use surgery will need to be made weighing up all the factors (Fig. 24.3). Patients who are not engaging with home-care are unlikely to benefit from periodontal surgery so it is not recommended in such patients (West *et al.*, 2021). There is also evidence that sites of 5–6 mm probing pocket depths which are followed up and do not bleed on repeated assessment are likely to be stable. These sites can be monitored to ensure that there is no additional loss of attachment and surgery may have only limited benefit in such cases (Fig. 24.4). A pragmatic approach to advocating surgery is required even where there are sites which are unresponsive since patient factors play a large role in determining if surgery has a role in management; non-surgical management and monitoring is the most conservative approach and is acceptable to the widest group of patients and situations.

Uses of periodontal surgery

Periodontal surgery can be used to:
- provide access to a site for debridement by the operator
- make a site accessible to the patient for cleaning
- correct gross gingival morphology
- regenerate tissues
- improve aesthetics.

Access to a site for debridement

Non-surgical debridement is a blind procedure and direct visualisation of the root surfaces and residual deposits can improve the effectiveness of deposit removal in deep pockets. Direct access may be useful where there is a furcation defect or suspected root groove.

Access to a site for cleaning

Following periodontal destruction, the patient may be left with tissue contours that are hard to maintain, e.g. thickened flaps after recurrent episodes of necrotising gingivitis or partial access to a furcation area. The periodontal tissues can be recontoured using periodontal surgery for optimal plaque removal by the patient.

Correction of gross gingival morphology

Excess tissue removal may be required subsequent to gingival enlargement though management may be more appropriately achieved by working with the patient's medical team to review and potentially change the drug therapy (Chapter 34).

Regeneration of periodontal tissues

Regenerative techniques can enable new supporting structures to develop. These techniques are only appropriate in specific clinical situations (Chapter 26).

Improve aesthetics

Aesthetics may be improved by root coverage following gingival recession using a variety of mucogingival surgical techniques (Chapter 33).

Contraindications to periodontal surgery

- If patient plaque control is not of a high standard.
- In patients with systemic diseases such as severe cardiovascular disease, malignancy, kidney and liver disease, bleeding disorders and uncontrolled diabetes. Consultation with the general medical practitioner and specialists is essential.
- Pregnancy: surgery is best delayed until after childbirth.
- Smoking is known to adversely affect healing. Smokers have shown a poorer short- and long-term response to surgical treatment than non-smokers. Many clinicians do not perform periodontal surgery on smokers.
- Where the long-term prognosis and value of the tooth to the dentition is questionable.

Surgical flaps

Many of the surgical procedures require the raising of tissue flaps which allows access to the underlying root and bony defects. The soft tissue can then be manipulated in such a way that the flap is either replaced approximately back to the original position or moved to an adjacent site.

Traditional flap designs have lateral incisions which allow greater access and visibility of the root surfaces but impair the blood supply and decrease the stability of the flap. Conservative flap designs aim to access the roots with less impact on the hard and soft tissues using intrasulcular incisions. Papilla preservation flaps are designed to maintain the papillary architecture. Flap designs with the maximum preservation of interdental soft tissue are recommended and, in some situations, limiting the flap elevation is also recommended to improve wound stability (West *et al.*, 2021). Surgery should only be provided by appropriately trained clinicians and the choice of technique will ultimately depend on the clinician's experience and skill.

A full-thickness flap is one comprising all the soft tissue, which is lifted from the underlying bone using a periosteal elevator. This flap is used commonly. A split-thickness flap is one that is dissected so that the gingiva is separated from the mucoperiosteum which remains on the bone. This flap is used in some of the surgical procedures described in Chapter 33.

Good wound healing depends on early formation of a blood clot and stability of the wound. Even minimal tensile forces on the early blood clot can change its morphology and the more stretched the fibrin in the clot, the harder it is for the capillaries to permeate the blot clot (Varju *et al.*, 2011). Flap adaptation and stability is achieved by careful suturing and will also impact on healing. Thinner suture materials and magnification are generally advocated.

Postoperative care

Information regarding the surgical procedure is given to the patient prior to undertaking surgery and as part of gaining the patient's consent, explaining the likely discomfort, pain management and potential complications. The microbial environment of the oral cavity means that any surgical procedure in the mouth risks wound infection so optimal oral hygiene is imperative. The patient should be given verbal and written instructions on how to care for the mouth in the postoperative period (Fig. 24.4) and arrangements should be made for a follow-up visit. The patient should be provided with contact details in case they have any concerns following the treatment.

Key points
- Periodontal surgery can be used to:
  - provide access to a site for debridement by the operator
  - make a site accessible to the patient for cleaning
  - correct gross gingival morphology
  - regenerate periodontal tissues
  - improve aesthetics
- Postoperative oral hygiene is decisive for the outcome of surgical therapy
- Clear postoperative instructions should be provided to the patient

25 Types of periodontal surgery

Figure 25.1 Types of periodontal surgery.

Surgery to eliminate disease and produce conditions to minimise recurrence (Chapter 25)	Surgery to eliminate disease and regenerate lost periodontal structures (Chapter 26)	Surgery for root coverage (mucogingival surgery) (Chapter 33)
Pocket elimination or reduction • Gingivectomy (Fig 25.2) • Apically repositioned flap (Fig 25.3)	Guided tissue regeneration.	Pedicle grafts • Rotational flaps • Advanced flaps: coronally advanced flap. Often used with enamel matrix derivatives, connective tissue graft or acellular dermal matrix allograft material.
Accessing root for cleaning • Replaced flaps (modified Widman flap, Fig 25.4) • Open flap with intra-sulcular incisions • Papilla preservation flap	Enamel matrix derivative (Emdogain®, Biora).	Guided tissue regeneration. Used with or without enamel matrix derivatives.
Distal wedge excision and tuberosity reduction (Fig. 25.5).	Bone grafts (Chapter 27).	Free grafts • epithelialised gingival grafts • subepithelial connective tissue graft
	Other growth factors and emerging therapies	Allografts

Figure 25.2 Gingivectomy.

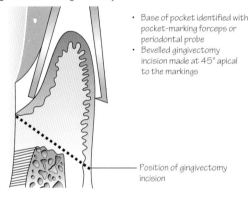

• Base of pocket identified with pocket-marking forceps or periodontal probe
• Bevelled gingivectomy incision made at 45° apical to the markings

Position of gingivectomy incision

Figure 25.3 Apically repositioned flap. (a) Inverse bevel incision to alveolar crest (dashed line). (b) Flap moved apically (arrow). (c) Flap sutured just above the alveolar crest.

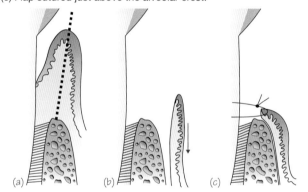

(a) (b) (c)

Figure 25.4 Modified Widman flap. (a) Inverse bevel incision to alveolar crest (dashed line). (b) Following removal of inner lining of pocket, the root surface can be accessed for cleaning. (c) Flap is replaced at or close to its presurgical position.

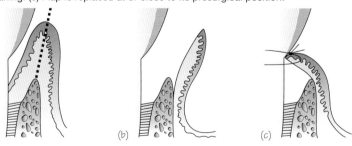

(a) (b) (c)

Periodontology at a Glance, Second Edition. Valerie Clerehugh, Aradhna Tugnait, Michael R. Milward, and Iain L. C. Chapple.
© 2024 John Wiley & Sons Ltd. Published 2024 by John Wiley & Sons Ltd.

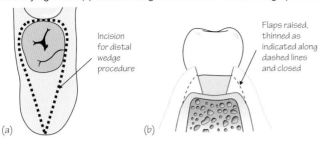
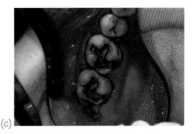

Figure 25.5 Distal wedge procedure. (a) Occlusal view. The incision is made around the last standing molar and the wedge of tissue is removed. (b) Vertical section. The tissue wedge is removed and the flaps thinned and approximated over the underlying bone. (c) Clinical image. Incisions for distal wedge procedure. Source: Courtesy of Mr P.J. Nixon.

Gingivectomy

This can be used for:

- persistent gingival enlargement such as drug-induced gingival enlargements (Chapter 34)
- exposing a furcation involvement with a wide zone of attached gingiva for access to oral hygiene measures
- persistent active sites with supra-bony pockets of >5 mm, where adequate attached gingiva would be left following surgery.

The techniques used for periodontal surgery can be divided as shown in Figure 25.1. This technique reduces the width of the attached gingiva so should not be used where this zone is limited. Gingivectomy for pocket elimination not associated with gingival deformity or overgrowth has largely been replaced by flap surgery.

Procedure

- The base of the pocket is identified with pocket marking forceps or a periodontal probe (Fig. 25.2).
- A bevelled gingivectomy incision is made at 45° apical to the markings both buccally and lingually/palatally. It is made as a continuous not scalloped incision.
- Tissue is removed with curettes.
- The exposed root surfaces are debrided.
- The dressing is placed.

Healing

The connective tissue becomes covered with blood clot. There is transient acute inflammation with reorganisation of the blood clot. The open wound epithelialises, covering the site in 7–14 days and keratinising in 2–3 weeks.

Apically repositioned flap

This procedure eliminates pockets by displacing the flap apically and the flap is sutured just coronal to the alveolar crest. This technique preserves the zone of attached gingiva. The roots are left exposed so aesthetics and postoperative sensitivity are poorer than with the more widely used replaced flaps.

Procedure

- Two vertical, parallel, relieving incisions are made to the bone at either end of the flap. These are carried out buccally and lingually. Care is required lingually with the distal relieving incision to prevent damage to the lingual nerve.
- An inverse bevel incision is made along the gingival margin, and scalloped around the necks of the teeth to separate the pocket lining and inflamed connective tissue from the flap (Fig. 25.3).
- The flaps are raised, leaving the separated pocket lining *in situ*.
- The separated pocket lining and connective tissue are removed from the roots with curettes.
- The roots are debrided.
- The buccal and lingual flaps are displaced apically and sutured. The palatal flap cannot be displaced so it is treated by inverse bevel incision alone.
- A dressing is placed to help maintain apical displacement.

Healing

There is transient acute inflammation with reorganisation of the blood clot between the tooth and flap into granulation tissue (one week).

There is replacement of granulation tissue by connective tissue (2–5 weeks). The epithelial migration commences from the margin of the flap and gives rise to new junctional epithelium (approximately four weeks).

There is some resorption of the alveolar bone margin resulting from raising a flap. This is minimised by a careful surgical technique. Long term, the gingival margin may shift coronally by about 1 mm.

Replaced flaps

Flaps with paramarginal incisions

The modified Widman flap (MWF) technique has been widely used and was designed to access the roots for cleaning and to remove the inflamed pocket epithelium.

Procedure

- An inverse bevel incision is made up to 1 mm from the gingival margin buccally and palatally/lingually to separate the pocket epithelium and inflamed connective tissue from the flap (Fig. 25.4).
- The separated tissue can be removed either directly by a curette or after two further incisions:
  - an incision from the base of the pocket to the bone crest
  - a horizontal incision after the flap is reflected from the crest of the bone to the tooth surface.
- Reflection of the flap (note there are no relieving incisions in this technique).
- Debridement of the root surfaces.
- The flap is replaced at the original level and is sutured, aiming to gain complete interdental coverage to avoid root exposure.
- A dressing is placed if it is considered necessary.

Healing

There is transient acute inflammation with reorganisation of the blood clot between the tooth and flap into granulation tissue (one week) which is replaced by connective tissue (2–5 weeks).

The epithelial migration commences from the margin of the flap and gives rise to new long junctional epithelium. This occurs over several weeks and is easily disrupted by premature probing. Pocket reduction is achieved by long junctional epithelial attachment to the cleaned root surface. Long term, the gingival margin may shift coronally by about 1 mm.

Open flap instrumentation with intrasulcular incisions (OFD)

This flap allows access to root surfaces while conserving soft tissue.

Procedure

- Intrasulcular incisions are made to allow sufficient access to root surfaces without exerting tension on the flaps. Relieving incisions are avoided where possible. Conservation of soft tissue is prioritised.
- Full-thickness flaps are raised buccally and lingually/palatally.
- Granulation tissue is removed and the root surfaces instrumented.
- Flaps are replaced to their original position and sutured in place.

Healing

Healing occurs as with the MWF. Gingival recession is generally less than with the MWF.

Papilla preservation flaps

Flaps are designed to preserve the interdental papillae (Cortellini et al., 1995). These flaps combined with the use of microsurgical techniques can lead to better aesthetics by minimising postoperative recession.

Distal wedge excision

Excess flabby tissue of the tuberosity distal to the last standing tooth can be excised to reduce a pocket and enable instrumentation of the root surface. Flaps are raised and a wedge of tissue is removed (Fig. 25.5). The flaps are thinned and approximated to the underlying bone.

Key points

- The categories of periodontal surgery are:
  - surgery to eliminate disease and produce conditions to minimise its recurrence
  - surgery to eliminate disease and regenerate lost periodontal structures
  - surgery for root coverage
- Gingivectomy is used to excise excess tissue and reduce pockets
- An apically repositioned flap is used to eliminate pockets
- A replaced flap is used to gain access to roots without achieving immediate postoperative pocket reduction
- Pocket reduction occurs following healing with the formation of long junctional epithelium

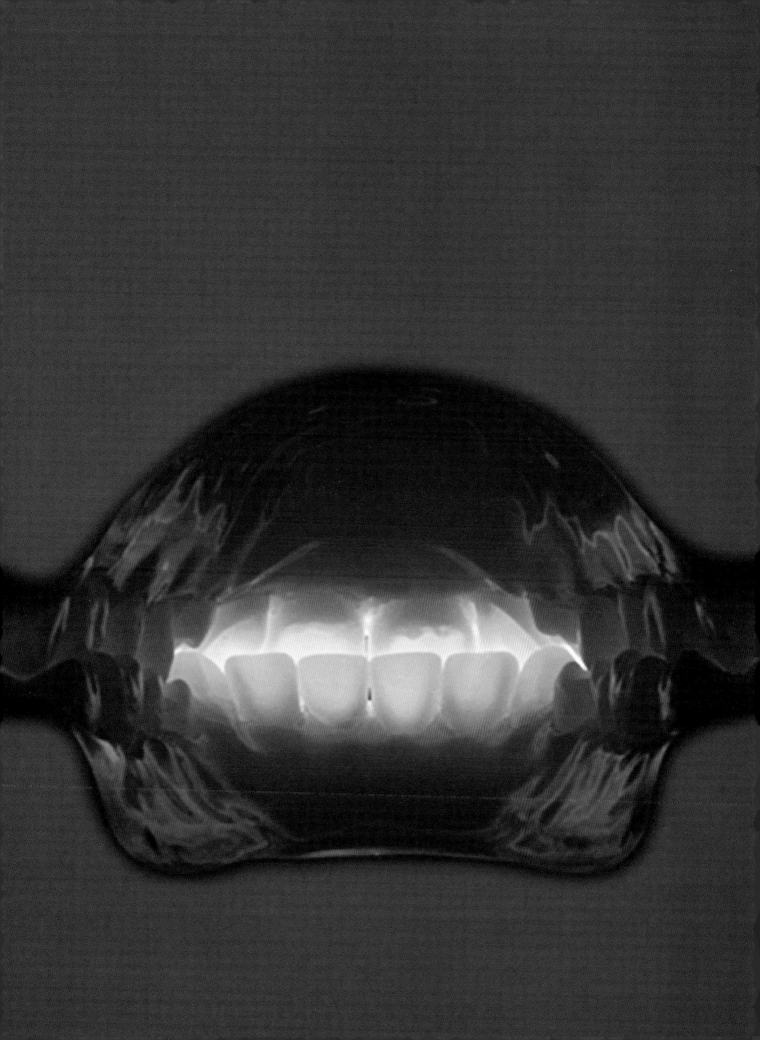

26 Regenerative periodontal therapy

Figure 26.1 Guided tissue regeneration.

Epithelium of replaced flap

Membrane preventing epithelium and connective tissue from contacting root surface

Cell migration

Periodontal ligament

Figure 26.2 Types of membrane for guided tissue regeneration.

Non-resorbable
• Flexible Teflon® (ePTFE): Gore-tex®

Resorbable
• Lactide/glcolide co-polymer: Resolut®
• Polylactic acid + citric acid ester: Guidor®
• Polylactic acid (made at chairside for custom fit): Atrisorb®
• Collagen: Bio-Gide®, Conform®
• Allogeneic: AlloDerm®

Figure 26.3 Guided tissue regeneration: membrane placement.

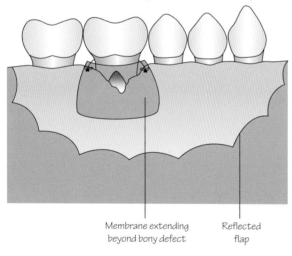

Membrane extending beyond bony defect

Reflected flap

Figure 26.4 Procedure for use of Emdogain.

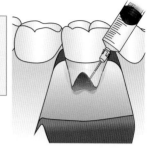

• After gaining surgical access to the site the cleaned root surfaces are conditioned with an EDTA (ethylene diamine tetra acetate) gel to remove the smear layer.
• The Emdogain gel is syringed directly onto the washed roots and the flap replaced.

Figure 26.5 A case treated by the use of Emdogain and PerioGlas. (a) Preoperative radiograph of the surgical site. (b) Reflection of the buccal flap. (c) Application of Emdogain following the use of ethylene diamine tetra-acetate (EDTA) conditioner. (d) Flaps replaced and secured with sutures. (e) Radiograph taken 18 months postoperatively. Source: Courtesy of Mr P.J. Nixon.

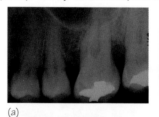 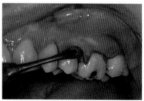
(a) (b)
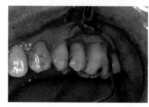 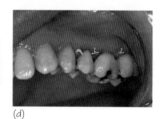
(c) (d)
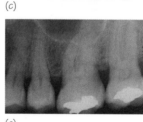
(e)

Figure 26.6 Potential growth factors for periodontal regeneration. Growth factors are known to affect osteogenic cells and are being actively investigated for a potential role in periodontal regeneration.

• Platelet-derived growth factor (PDGF)
• Insulin-like growth factor (IGF)
• Fibroblast growth factor (FGF)
• Transforming growth factor-β (TGF-β)
  – Including bone morphogenetic proteins

Periodontology at a Glance, Second Edition. Valerie Clerehugh, Aradhna Tugnait, Michael R. Milward, and Iain L. C. Chapple.
© 2024 John Wiley & Sons Ltd. Published 2024 by John Wiley & Sons Ltd.

Regenerative periodontal therapy encompasses a number of surgical procedures that aim specifically at gaining healing of periodontal destruction by developing new periodontium rather than by repair with a long junctional epithelial attachment. These techniques include:

- guided tissue regeneration
- enamel matrix derivative (Straumann® Emdogain®, Straumann, Crawley, UK)
- bone grafts (Chapter 27)
- growth factors.

Guided tissue regeneration

Following conventional flap surgery, healing occurs by proliferation of epithelial cells and formation of a long junctional epithelium which attaches onto the cleaned root surface. This repaired structure does not mimic the original periodontal attachment.

Guided tissue regeneration (GTR) has been described as a reordering of the migration of cells into the surgical site so that cells from the periodontal ligament are able to proliferate and migrate into the healing site. The outcome is then a re-established periodontium rather than a repaired periodontium (Fig. 26.1).

The technique consists of placement of a membrane that acts as a barrier and excludes the migrating epithelium and connective tissue, creating a space around the cleaned root surface. This is repopulated by cells that can then mature to form new periodontal ligament fibres, which insert into bone.

Types of membrane

There are two types of membrane (Fig. 26.2).

Non-resorbable

The first membranes to be developed were non-resorbable. Titanium reinforcement was added to create and maintain the space between the flap and root more effectively. A disadvantage of this type of membrane is that a second surgical procedure is required to remove it.

Resorbable

These were devised to avoid the second surgical procedure for removal of the membrane. Polylactic membranes are degraded by enzymes in the Krebs cycle. Collagen membranes are broken down by collagenases and subsequently by other proteinases. Collagen membranes are made from animal collagen and have to be produced in a way that ensures they are antigen free.

Use of GTR

- Treatment of two- or three-walled intra-bony defects (Chapter 27).
- Treatment of furcation defects (Chapter 27): most predictable in class II lesions of mandibular molars.
- Treatment of recession defects (Chapter 33).
- For alveolar ridge defects and limited generation of new bone for implant placement.

Procedure

- Intracrevicular incisions are used and the flaps are raised at the site of the defect. This is in order to achieve the following:
  - to preserve as much of the keratinised attached gingiva as possible
  - to separate the pocket epithelium.
- The root surfaces are cleaned.
- The membrane is cut to fit the area so that it covers the defect and extends slightly beyond it (Fig. 26.3).

- Most membranes are then sutured into place.
- Flaps are replaced so that none of the membrane is exposed to the oral cavity.
- Non-resorbable membranes are removed 4–6 weeks after placement. The healing tissue appears as a red gelatinous material, which needs to be carefully separated from the membrane to allow the membrane to be removed.
- The resorbable membranes break down over time.

GTR can be used alone or with enamel matrix derivatives or bone grafts.

Enamel matrix derivative

Enamel matrix derivative is a mixed peptide combination derived from immature enamel which have been found to induce cementum formation and periodontal regeneration. These peptides have been used to formulate the commercial product Straumann Emdogain. The surgical technique is much simpler than for GTR (Fig. 26.4).

Straumann Emdogain can also be used in conjunction with bone graft materials (Chapter 27) such as Bio-Oss® (Geistlich Pharma AG), PerioGlas® (Nova Bone) or Straumann BoneCeramic 400–700® that act as scaffolds for bone deposition (Fig. 26.5). Straumann Emdogain can also be used with the technique of GTR.

Outcomes

Although studies have shown significant gains in bone levels and clinical attachment with GTR, there is variability in the gains reported. Complete resolution of intra-bony defects is rarely found. GTR has shown attachment gains in class II furcation defects, particularly at lower molar sites, but results are less predictable in class III defects (Chapter 27). Factors that may influence the outcome include plaque levels, the morphology of the site and factors relating to the surgical technique. Membrane stability is very important in achieving success, and exposure of the membrane with subsequent bacterial contamination is associated with reduced attachment gains.

Recent studies have shown similar results from non-resorbable and resorbable membranes and that there are improved clinical outcomes compared with open flap debridement, showing a mean adjunctive benefit of 1.34 mm in CAL and 1.2 mm in pocket depth reduction. Although there is inevitably an increase in cost associated with regenerative surgery, this can be offset by a lower cost of managing disease recurrence when looked at over a 20-year period (Cortellini et al., 2017).

The use of barrier membranes or enamel matrix derivative materials with or without the addition of bone grafts is recommended (West et al., 2021). The EFP S3-level guideline recommends periodontal regenerative surgery to treat teeth with residual pockets associated with intra-bony defects 3+ mm or class II furcations on mandibular molars and suggest that class II furcations in maxillary molars be treated with regenerative techniques. The guideline has also been adopted by the BSP (West et al., 2021).

Other growth factors and emerging therapies

Growth factors and cell mediators regulate cellular activities such as migration and proliferation (Fig. 26.6). They function in low concentrations and act locally. They bind to high-affinity cell membrane receptors and activate cellular mechanisms.

Bone morphogenetic proteins (BMP) are a group of proteins belonging to the transforming growth factor (TGF)-β group. These factors are able to stimulate bone and cartilage and cementogenesis. In the periodontal site, they may be able to stimulate cells not only from the remaining periodontal ligament but also from other tissue such as the flaps.

A systematic review on the use of growth factors (Darby & Morris, 2013) concluded that use of recombinant human platelet-derived growth factor-BB led to greater clinical attachment level gain, bone fill and rate of bone growth compared to an osteoconductive control (β-tricalcium phosphate).

Cell-based therapies are also being investigated, including using cells to act as carriers for growth factors or providing stem cells which can then differentiate into other cell types. Scaffolds are often used to provide space for regeneration to occur.

Developments in these materials can lead to scaffolds that regulate cell ingrowth and organise the developing tissue.

Gene therapy offers the possibility of altering the host response by inserting genes into cells but is in the earliest stages of investigation.

Key points

- Guided tissue regeneration involves placement of a membrane to create a space for the migration of cells from the periodontal ligament
- Enamel matrix derivative is available as Straumann Emdogain which induces cementum and periodontal regeneration
- Growth factors may have the potential to regenerate the periodontium

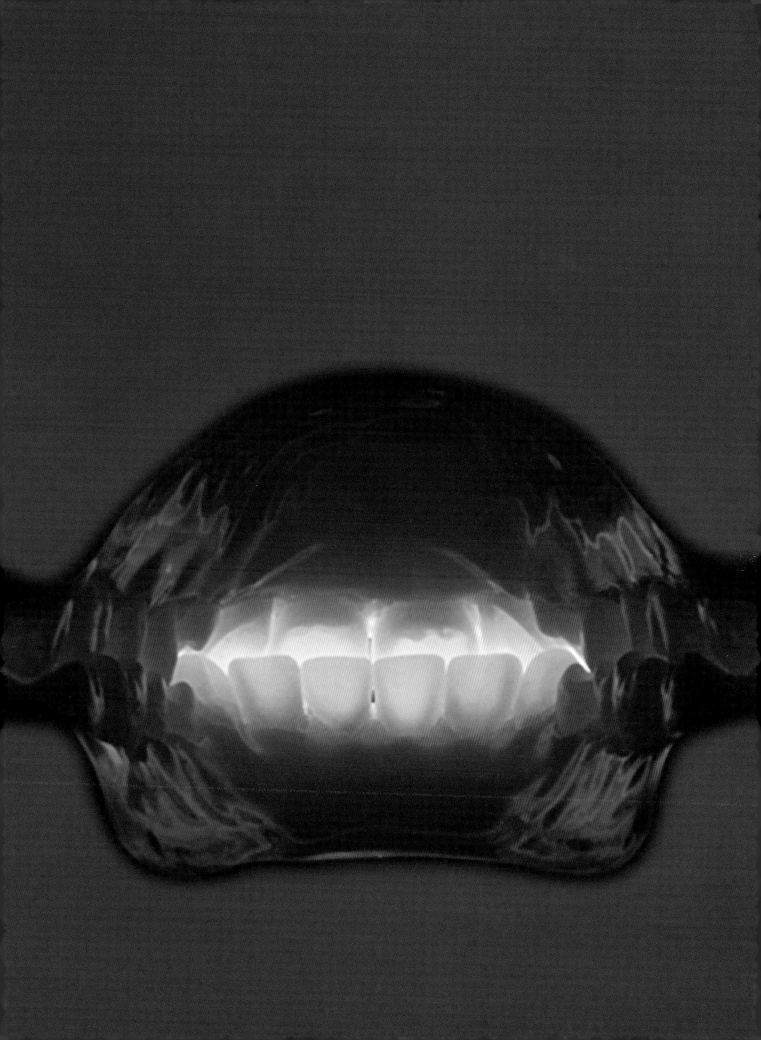

27 Bone defects and furcation lesions

Figure 27.1 Anatomy of bone defects.

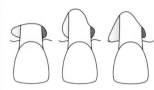

Three-walled bone defects   Two-walled defect   One-walled defect

Bony defects are often described according to the number of supporting bone walls that surround the tooth: one-, two- or three-walled defects. A three-walled defect is bounded by one tooth surface and three osseous surfaces. Clinical and radiographic investigations can aid the diagnosis of a bone defect but the actual anatomy can only fully be assessed if a surgical flap is raised.

Figure 27.2 Treatment of bone defects.

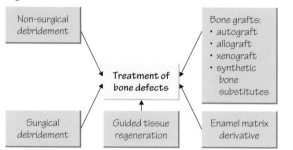

Figure 27.3 Use of synthetic bone graft (PerioGlas®). (a) Synthetic bone graft material on an instrument prior to placement. (b) Placement of the synthetic bone graft material. Source: Courtesy of Mr P.J. Nixon.

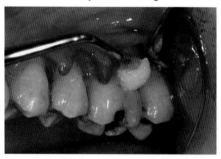

(a)

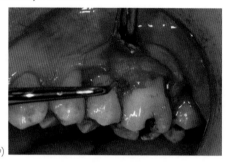

(b)

This case was treated using Emdogain® and PerioGlas®. The placement of Emdogain® and the subsequent healing following the use of both materials is shown in Fig. 26.5.

Figure 27.4 Classification of furcation involvement.

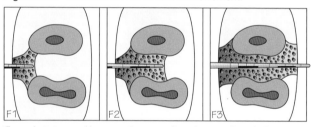

F1   F2   F3

The probe is inserted between the roots of a multi-rooted tooth. A class 1 involvement (F1) is one where a probe can be inserted less than 3 mm between the roots. A class 2 involvement (F2) penetrates more than 3 mm but not fully through the furcation, and a class 3 (F3) involvement extends completely between the roots.

Figure 27.5 Treatment of furcation lesions.

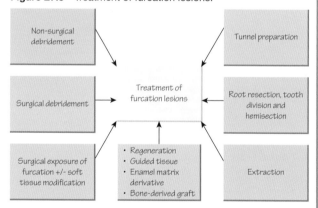

Figure 27.6 Root resection.

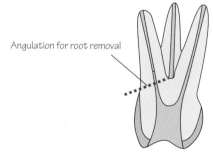

Angulation for root removal

Endodontic treatment is required. Flaps are raised and the root to be removed is sectioned along the line indicated. The root is elevated. The remaining tooth is contoured to give access to cleaning and the flaps are replaced leaving the tooth supported on the two remaining roots. A permanent restoration is placed to seal the cut root canal. Careful oral hygiene measures are needed to clean under the crown at the amputation site.

Periodontology at a Glance, Second Edition. Valerie Clerehugh, Aradhna Tugnait, Michael R. Milward, and Iain L. C. Chapple.
© 2024 John Wiley & Sons Ltd. Published 2024 by John Wiley & Sons Ltd.

Bone defects

Alveolar bone resorption leads to the creation of bony defects (infra-bony or intra-bony), which differ in anatomy from one tooth site to another (Fig. 27.1).

Treatment of bone defects

The different types of treatment that have been used are depicted in Fig. 27.2.

Non-surgical debridement

- Bone defects can be treated as at any other site by non-surgical debridement.
- Healing is with a long junctional epithelium and potentially some bony infill, particularly where there are several walls to the defect.

Surgical access for debridement

- Raising a surgical flap can improve access to the site and enable thorough removal of the inflammatory tissue.
- Healing is as for non-surgical debridement.
- The bony defect can be reshaped during the procedure. This may result in further bone loss so use with caution to create an architecture that allows better flap adaptation.
- Bone fill may be obtained in two- and three-walled defects but great variability in the degree of fill has been found.

Simple debridement of the defect (either indirectly or directly) is most successful if the defect is not too large and there are several bone walls.

Bone grafts

Bone grafts can be used with a surgical technique to access the bony defect. The graft may be derived from a number of sources.

- *Autografts* (from same individual) taken from other oral sites or the iliac crest (an invasive procedure). Fresh marrow often leads to ankylosis and tooth resorption so it is frozen before use. Bony infill can be gained but the site generally heals with a long junctional epithelial attachment.
- *Allografts* (from same species) have included freeze-dried bone allograft (FDBA) and freeze-dried demineralised bone allograft (FDDBA). Studies have shown bony infill and some regeneration of new bone, periodontal ligament and cementum. The possibility of disease transfer is a potential problem though probably a very low risk. The graft is likely to act as a scaffold which is replaced by new tissue.
- *Xenografts* (from different species) have been commercially produced from the mineral component of bovine bone (Bio-Oss®, Geistlich Pharma AG). There is potentially a risk of transmission of infective agents. However, this material has been used widely and appears to have osteogenic potential in periodontal intra-bony defects.
- *Synthetic bone substitutes* include hydroxyapatite, ceramics and bioactive glasses (e.g. PerioGlas®, NovaBone) (Fig. 27.3). The bioactive materials show formation of new cementum and bone and periodontal ligament, while hydroxyapatite tends to result in bony infill with a long junctional epithelial attachment.

Enamel matrix derivative and guided tissue regeneration

See Chapter 26.

Treatment of intrabony defects

The European S3-level treatment guideline and the BSP implementation of this (West *et al.*, 2021) recommend the treatment of teeth with residual deep pockets associated with an intra-bony defect of 3 mm or more with periodontal regenerative surgery since these techniques show better outcomes compared to open flap debridement. Either barrier membranes or enamel matrix derivative, with or without the addition of bone-derived grafts, are recommended in these clinical situations. Although regenerative techniques are more expensive in the short term, Cortellini *et al.* (2017) found that the cost was lower than that of managing disease recurrence over a 20-year period. Clinicians need to continually re-evaluate the different regenerative biomaterials available to make the appropriate choice for each patient.

Furcation lesions

Bone loss around multi-rooted teeth can expose part of or the entire furcation region where the roots divide. This complicates the anatomy of the bony defect, creating a site that is potentially hard for the patient and operator to clean. Furcation lesions can be diagnosed clinically by careful probing or radiographically. They are usually classified according to the degree of horizontal involvement (Fig. 27.4) although the vertical extent of the lesion should also be assessed.

Treatment of furcation lesions

The different methods of treatment are depicted in Fig. 27.5.

Non-surgical and surgical access for debridement

- Class 1 and 2 defects can be managed by Professional Mechanical Plaque Removal (PMPR) and supportive therapy.
- Access to a furcation defect may be improved by raising a flap for thorough subgingival PMPR of the site.

Surgical exposure (± soft tissue modification)

A gingivectomy or apically repositioned flap can be used to uncover a furcation defect to produce a site accessible to plaque control by the patient.

Regeneration

Regeneration and regenerative techniques are discussed in Chapter 26.

- Guided tissue regeneration (GTR) can be used to treat class 2 furcation involvement and also used with other graft materials.
- GTR has been used to treat class 3 defects but with less predictable results.
- Enamel matrix proteins have been used to treat class 2 defects. Regenerative surgery is recommended for the treatment of class 2 furcation defects in mandibular molars and suggested for treating maxillary molars with class 2 defects (West *et al.*, 2021). The use of enamel matrix derivative alone or bone-derived grafts with or without a resorbable membrane is recommended (West *et al.*, 2021).

Tunnel preparation

Can be used in the lower molars to produce a furcation accessible from buccal to lingual for cleaning.

- The buccal and lingual flaps are raised and displaced apically.
- The furcation defect may be recontoured for a brush to pass through easily.
- A periodontal pack in the furcation maintains the site during healing.

Root resection, tooth division and hemisection

These surgical techniques are used where there is advanced bone loss around one of the roots and the remaining roots will have enough support to allow the tooth to function. The value of the tooth to the patient should be assessed. Endodontic treatment is undertaken so unfavourable canal morphology can be a contraindication.

• *Root resection* is used generally for the three-rooted upper molars with a loss of the mesiobuccal or distobuccal root (Fig. 27.6).
• *Tooth division* is used infrequently in lower molars where bone loss is severe in the furcation region but roots individually have reasonable bone support. The tooth is divided and each part is subsequently prepared for a single tooth crown.
• *Hemisection* is used in lower molars with advanced bone loss around one root. Following division of the tooth, one root is retained and the other elevated. The remaining root can then be used as a bridge retainer to support a pontic replacing the missing portion or as a premolar-sized crown.

Extraction

Extraction may be the appropriate management of a tooth with advanced furcation involvement where the tooth is compromised and not considered a key tooth in the dentition. Nonetheless, furcation involvement alone is not a reason for extraction and it is recommended that molars with class 2 and 3 furcation involvement receive periodontal therapy (West *et al.*, 2021).

Key points

• Bone defects can be managed by non-surgical and surgical therapy aimed at debridement of the defect
• Regeneration in intrabony defects may be achieved by the use of bone grafts, guided tissue regeneration and enamel matrix derivative
• Regeneration in intra-bony pockets of 3 mm or more is recommended
• Furcation defects can be managed by non-surgical and surgical therapy aimed at debridement of the defect
• Regeneration in furcation lesions may be achieved using bone grafts, guided tissue regeneration and enamel matrix derivative
• Periodontal regenerative therapy is recommended or suggested for the management of class 2 furcation involvements
• Advanced or complex furcation defects may be managed by tunnel preparation or resection of part of the tooth
• Furcation involvement alone is not a reason for extraction

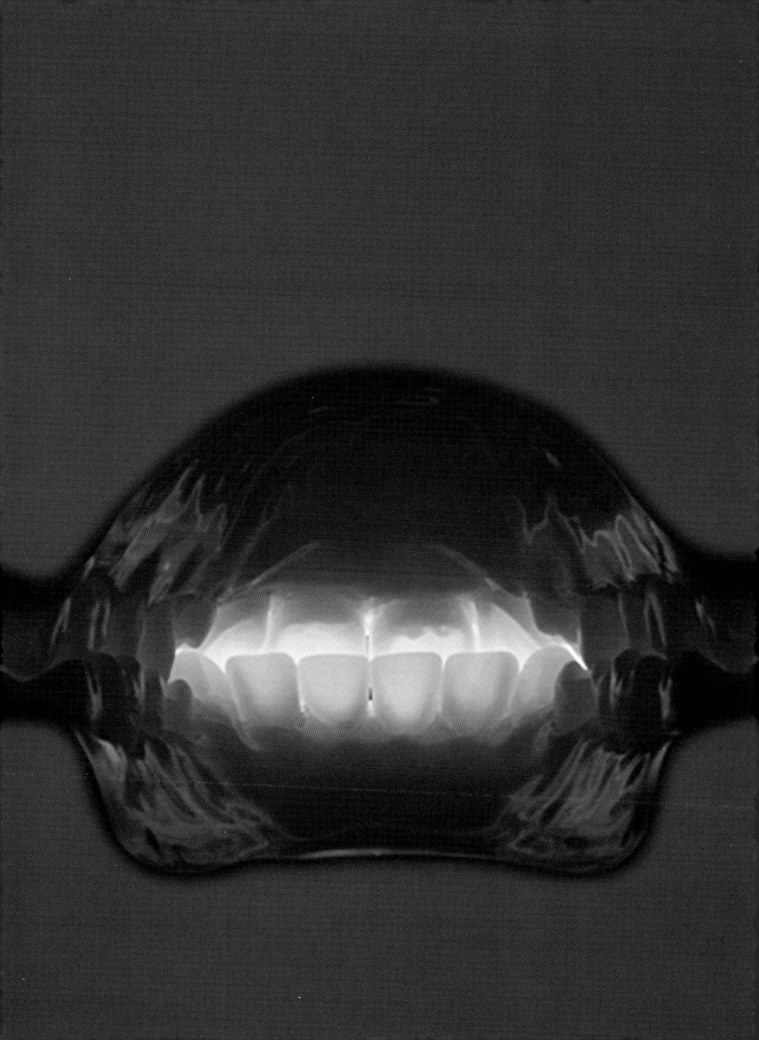

28 Dental implants

Figure 28.1 Factors to consider prior to implants.

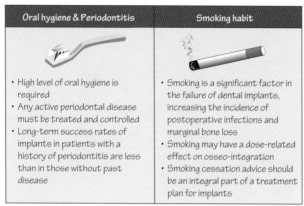

Oral hygiene & Periodontitis	Smoking habit
• High level of oral hygiene is required • Any active periodontal disease must be treated and controlled • Long-term success rates of implants in patients with a history of periodontitis are less than in those without past disease	• Smoking is a significant factor in the failure of dental implants, increasing the incidence of postoperative infections and marginal bone loss • Smoking may have a dose-related effect on osseo-integration • Smoking cessation advice should be an integral part of a treatment plan for implants

Figure 28.3 Implant replacing an upper left lateral incisor. (a) Implant at UL2 with impression coping *in situ*. (b) Final restoration of UL2. (c) Radiograph showing the healthy implant with final restoration at year year post placement. Source: Courtesy of Mr P.J. Nixon.

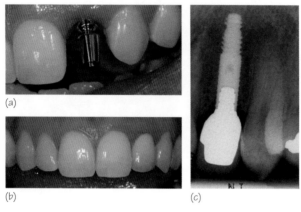

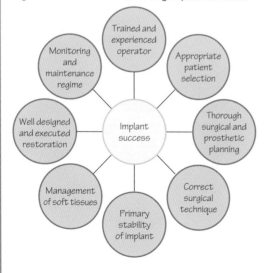

(a)

(b)

(c)

Figure 28.5 Factors in achieving implant success.

Implant success
- Trained and experienced operator
- Appropriate patient selection
- Thorough surgical and prosthetic planning
- Correct surgical technique
- Primary stability of implant
- Management of soft tissues
- Well designed and executed restoration
- Monitoring and maintenance regime

Figure 28.2 Implant with coronal restoration.

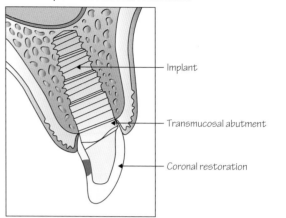

- Implant
- Transmucosal abutment
- Coronal restoration

Figure 28.4 Clinical considerations for implant therapy.

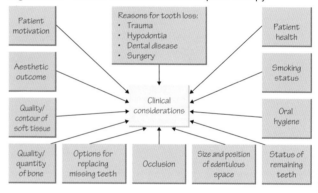

Clinical considerations
- Patient motivation
- Aesthetic outcome
- Quality/ contour of soft tissue
- Quality/ quantity of bone
- Options for replacing missing teeth
- Occlusion
- Size and position of edentulous space
- Status of remaining teeth
- Oral hygiene
- Smoking status
- Patient health

Reasons for tooth loss:
- Trauma
- Hypodontia
- Dental disease
- Surgery

Figure 28.6 Implant and peri-implant tissues.

The barrier epithelium is about 2 mm long with an underlying zone of connective tissue of about 1.5 mm. The epithelium is attached to the implant via hemidesmosomes. The fibres in the connective tissue run parallel to the implant surface with no attachment to its surface.

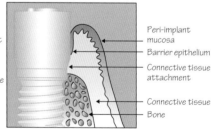

- Peri-implant mucosa
- Barrier epithelium
- Connective tissue attachment
- Connective tissue
- Bone

Figure 28.7 Implant planning. (a) UR1 implant crown wax-up. This is used to plan the crown and construct stents. (b) Stent with marker for location used when taking radiographs and during surgery. (c) Cone beam CT image to show maxillary bone in area of implant (UR1 site). Software allows the proposed implant to be positioned and shows that there is a deficiency of labial bone in the region, indicating that some form of bone regeneration or grafting may be required. (d) Cone beam CT used to generate a 3D image of the maxillary teeth and surrounding bone with the planned dental implant in UR1 site. Source: Courtesy of Dr A Al-Taie.

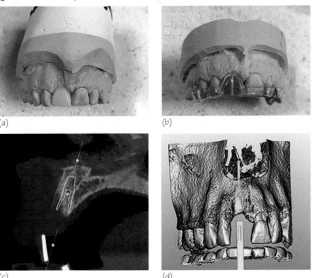

Figure 28.8 Implant placement. (a) Surgical stent in place for placement of implant to replace missing UL1. (b) Preparation of implant site. The site is prepared with low-speed drills to produce a hole matched to the selected implant. (c) Dental implant in place with a cover screw over the implant. Source: Courtesy of Dr A Al-Taie.

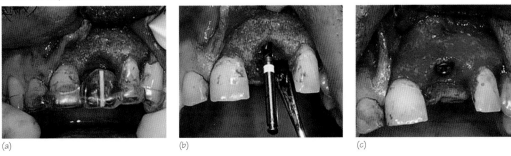

Dental implants give the clinician and patient a valuable option for restoring edentulous spaces. Implants may be used to replace single or multiple teeth and to replace teeth that have been lost because of periodontal disease. A number of factors need to be considered when determining the suitability of a patient for implants.

Treatment outcomes are improved in patients with good oral hygiene, periodontal health and in non-smokers and these factors may need addressing prior to the placement of implants (Fig. 28.1). A systematic review by Chrcanovic *et al.* (2015) has shown that smoking significantly affects failure rates, the risk of postoperative infections and marginal bone loss. Final restoration of implants may be with single crowns (Figs 28.2, 28.3), bridges or overdentures. Implants are retained in the mouth by osseointegration, the name given to the tight connection that develops as bone forms in close approximation to the implant surface.

The key parts of the implant-retained restoration are:
- an implant placed into bone
- a component connected to the implant that projects through the mucosa into the mouth (transmucosal abutment)
- a coronal restoration.

A large number of implant systems are available, each with differing characteristics such as implant shape, lengths and widths, type of fixation of components and surface characteristics. Within each system, there are components to aid planning before surgery, provide guidance at the time of placement and enable fabrication of temporary and final restorations. The risk of future peri-implant mucositis does not seem to be related to the implant system.

Implants may be placed in a healed ridge but may also be placed immediately following extraction using an atraumatic extraction technique to preserve the tissues.

Osseointegration

Dental implants are made of titanium, a highly reactive and biocompatible metal, which forms a non-corrosive surface oxide layer in contact with the tissues. A large implant–bone interface is achieved by surface modifications, screw threads, grooves or perforations that allow forces to be transmitted over a wide area. Studies have shown that osteoblasts require a porous and rough surface in order to synthesise and lay down bone against the implant. A roughened implant surface is produced either by coatings (titanium-plasma spray coating or hydroxyapatite) or by grit blasting and etching. Osseointegration occurs around and within all these features. The attachment of tissues around an implant is shown in Fig. 28.4. In the healthy peri-implant unit, the peri-implant mucosa is about 3–4 mm high and comprises a core of connective tissue covered by either keratinised or non-keratinised mucosa. Keratinised tissue (often considered optimal if it is ≥2 mm) is preferable for peri-implant tissue health (Kungsadalpipob *et al.*, 2020).

Implant planning

There are various clinical considerations to be taken into account before providing implants, with many factors that influence their success (Figs 28.5, 28.6), so careful planning is essential (Fig. 28.7). The patient's aesthetic and functional needs should be assessed and the tissues examined clinically. Articulated study models and a diagnostic set-up are needed to identify the optimum sites for surgical placement that will enable favourable restorative reconstruction. The diagnostic set-up can be used to make stents as a guide for interpreting radiographs and for the surgical placement of the implants. Radiographs are required to assess bone and visualise anatomical structures. Specialist radiographs such as cone beam computed tomography provide 3D imaging of the bone which is especially valuable in more complex cases. The clinician needs sufficient information to plan the number of implants required, the width, length and positioning of the implants and whether additional grafting is required in advance or at placement. It is important that the restorative work is planned and designed to create a favourable morphology for oral hygiene as well as to address the aesthetic and functional needs of the patient.

Implant placement

Following the planning process, a hole which is matched to the selected implant is prepared with precision low-speed drills and irrigated to avoid damage to the bone. Drills are used in sequence to gradually widen a pilot hole and prepare it to the correct depth. Care is taken to ensure that the diameter and length of implant are appropriate to avoid damage to adjacent structures. The implant is placed in the prepared hole and screwed into its final position with a handpiece or driver. A good fit of the implant provides primary stability which will promote osseointegration (Fig. 28.8).

A one- or two-stage technique can be used.

- The *one-stage method* leaves the implant exposed with placement of a gingival former (healing abutment) or temporary restoration to allow soft tissue adaptation. Often, the implant is not loaded during the osseointegration period. Techniques have been described for early loading of the implant.
- The *two-stage method* involves placement of the implant and cover screw and coverage with the mucosal tissues while osseointegration occurs. This generally takes between three and six months depending on the implant location. The implant is then exposed, a gingival former (healing abutment) is placed to contour the soft tissues during healing, and the restoration is subsequently constructed.

Guided tissue regeneration and bone grafts

Providing that primary stability is achieved, bony defects around the implant can be treated with guided tissue regenerative techniques. Where significant increases in bone width or height are required, more extensive surgical procedures such as block bone grafts or sinus lifts are needed. These require a high level of skill and an additional healing period prior to implant placement.

Key points

- Dental implants are retained by osseointegration
- A soft tissue cuff similar to gingivae develops around the implant
- Successful implants that can be maintained long term will depend on appropriate patient selection and good planning of the surgical and restorative work
- Additional techniques such as guided tissue regeneration and bone grafting can augment bone at the implant site

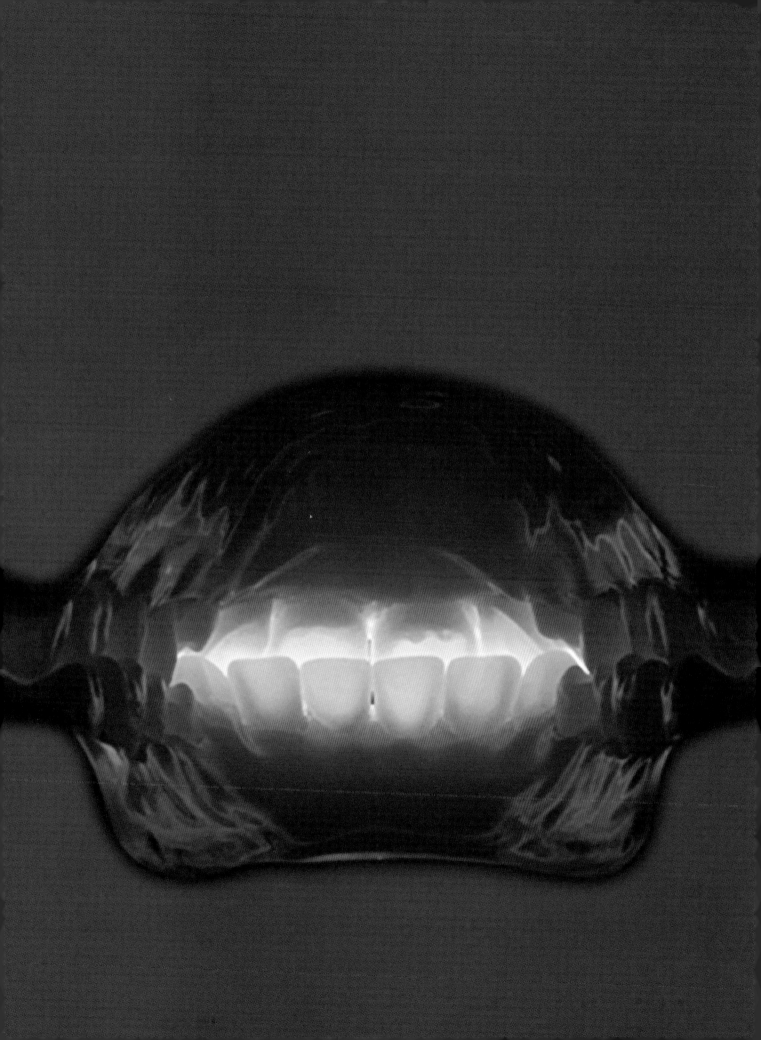

29 Peri-implant mucositis and peri-implantitis

Figure 29.1 (a) Diagnosis of peri-implant mucositis. (b) Diagnosis of peri-implantitis.

(a)

Diagnosis requires:

- Presence of bleeding and/or suppuration on gentle probing with or without increased probing depth compared to previous examinations.
- Absence of bone loss beyond crestal bone level changes resulting from initial bone remodelling.

(b)

Diagnosis requires:

- Presence of bleeding and/or suppuration on gentle probing.
- Increased probing depth compared to previous examinations.
- Presence of bone loss beyond crestal bone level changes resulting from initial bone remodelling.

In the absence of previous examination data diagnosis of peri-implantitis can be based on the combination of:

- Presence of bleeding and/or suppuration on gentle probing.
- Probing depths of ≥6 mm.
- Bone levels ≥3 mm apical of the most coronal portion of the intraosseous part of the implant.
- Note that recession of the gingival margin should be considered in the probing depth evaluation.

Figure 29.2 Radiograph of a failing implant. Radiograph taken 12 years post placement of implants showing bony craters on the mesial and distal aspects of the implant on the right. The bone levels are substantially better on the implant on the left.
Source: Courtesy of Mr P.J. Nixon.

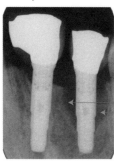

Extensive mesial and distal bone resorption

Figure 29.3 (a) Radiograph of UR3 implant shows limited loss of bone consistent with peri-implant mucositis in association with clinical findings of soft tissue inflammation. (b) Radiograph of UR1 shows bone loss particularly on the mesial aspect of the implant. (c) Clinical photograph of the two implants following removal of suprastructure. Implant at site of UR3 has reddened mucosa and bleeding on probing. Implant at site of UR1 shows suppuration from around the implant and deep pockets were identified. Non-surgical therapy was implemented. The UR3 implant responded to treatment and healed. The UR1 implant developed further bone loss and mobility and was removed.
Source: Courtesy of Mr J. Patel.

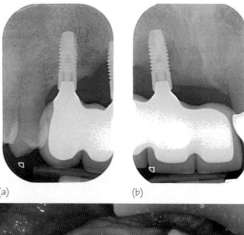

(a)   (b)

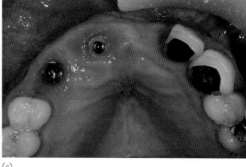

(c)

Figure 29.4 Treatment modalities used for peri-implantitis.
Source: Heitz-Mayfield & Mombelli (2014).

Non-surgical	Surgical
• Mechanical debridement • Laser debridement • Air-abrasive device • Subgingival chlorhexidine irrigation • Local antibiotics • Systemic antibiotics	• Removal of exposed implant threads to achieve a smoother surface • Resective surgery • Bone regeneration techniques such as GBR or bone grafts

Figure 29.5 Prevention and management of peri-implant diseases. Source: Adapted from Heitz-Mayfield & Mombelli (2014).

Pre-treatment phase:
- Oral hygiene instruction and smoking cessation counselling
- Design and assessment of prosthesis for access for plaque control
- Prosthesis removal and adjustment as required

Surgical access (if resolution of peri-implantitis not achieved non-surgically)
- Full-thickness mucoperiosteal flap for thorough cleaning of contaminated implant (may include adjustment of implant surface)
- Stabilisation of intraosseous peri-implant defect with bone substitute/bone graft/bioactive substance +/- resorbable barrier membrane

Postoperative anti-infective protocol:
- Peri- or postoperative systemic antibiotics
- Chlorhexidine rinses during healing period

Maintenance care:
- 3 to 6 month maintenance including oral hygiene instruction and supramucosal biofilm removal

Figure 29.6 (a) Preoperatively the labial tissue shows inflammation and bleeding adjacent to the UR1 implant and suprastructure. (b) Labial flap raised showing the loss of the labial bone plate and presence of granulation tissue at the UR1 implant. (c) Bone loss due to peri-implantitis has led to exposed implant threads. (d) Implant threads smoothed to facilitate healing. Source: Courtesy of Mr J. Chesterman.

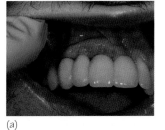
(a)

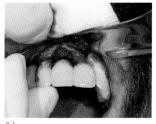
(b)

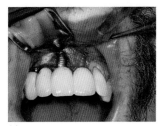
(c)

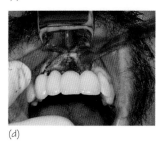
(d)

Bacterial plaque can form on implants and plaque retention can lead to inflammation of the peri-implant tissues.

When the inflammation is limited to the soft tissues around a dental implant and there is an absence of bone loss beyond the changes associated with the initial bone remodelling related to the implant placement, then the disease is termed peri-implant mucositis. The criteria to define peri-implant mucositis are shown in Fig. 29.1a. The clinical features of inflammation are bleeding on gentle probing, redness and swelling. Suppuration may be present. An increase in probing depth may be seen associated with swelling of the tissue or reduced resistance to probing but without bone loss. Peri-implant mucositis is characterised by a well-defined inflammatory lesion with blood vessels, plasma cells and lymphocytes.

Peri-implant mucositis has been reported as present in up to 48% of implants followed up from nine to 14 years (Roos-Jansåker et al., 2006) or in about 80% of subjects restored with implants (Lindhe & Meyle, 2008). Smoking, diabetes mellitus and radiation therapy are also associated with peri-implant mucositis, as is a history of periodontitis. Although peri-implant mucositis may be present for extensive periods without progression, sites of peri-implant mucositis may be considered an increased risk for the development of peri-implantitis.

Peri-implantitis is a plaque-associated pathological condition occurring in tissues around dental implants, characterised by inflammation in the peri-implant mucosa and subsequent progressive loss of supporting bone. The criteria to define peri-implantitis are shown in Fig. 29.1b. Peri-implantitis may affect a significant number of implants and patients, occurring in between 28% and 56% of subjects (12–40% of sites) in one study (Lindhe & Meyle, 2008). There has been a large variation in reported prevalence because of different thresholds of bone loss and pocket depths used to define peri-implantitis. The establishment of clear criteria to define the disease should enable reporting to be more consistent in future studies.

The peri-implantitis lesion tends to be less encapsulated than those around a tooth. Although plasma cells and lymphocytes dominate at both sites of peri-implantitis and periodontitis, more macrophages and neutrophils are found in peri-implantitis with signs of acute inflammation and large numbers of osteoclasts along the surface of the crestal bone. The inflammatory lesion is also often larger at peri-implantitis sites compared with periodontitis sites.

In the presence of inflammation around an implant, the tip of the probe can pass beyond the apical cells into the connective tissue and almost to the bone crest. The onset of peri-implantitis may occur early in the lifetime of the implant (Berglundh et al., 2018). There appears to be an increased susceptibility for bone loss around implants. This may be because there are no inserting collagen fibres as there would be around a tooth. Bone defects in peri-implantitis often appear crater-like (Fig. 29.2). Progression of peri-implantitis appears to be faster than that of periodontitis (Berglundh et al., 2018). The implants may be stable but can show mobility when bone loss becomes severe. Ultimately, the progression of peri-implantitis can lead to failure with loss of the implant and associated restoration(s) (Fig. 29.3).

Periodontal maintenance of implants

An effective oral hygiene maintenance programme is key to preventing the development of inflammation around implants and work has shown that patients on a maintenance programme involving mechanical debridement and oral hygiene instruction have less peri-implant mucositis than those without follow-up care (Costa et al., 2012).

A baseline radiograph should be obtained at the time of suprastructure placement against which future radiographs can be assessed for bone loss. Patients with implants should be regularly monitored for any indication of inflammatory changes. Implants should be monitored regularly by probing with a light probing force and with follow-up radiographs. Regular supportive therapy of professionally administered plaque control is required to reinforce and assist plaque removal around implants. Since the titanium surface of implants is easily damaged, plastic, carbon fibre or titanium instruments have been proposed for calculus removal although others advocate traditional stainless steel instruments to be more effective for calculus removal.

Treatment of peri-mucositis and peri-implantitis

Although resolution of peri-implant mucositis is possible, not all data indicate that resolution is achieved in all patients. Early detection of peri-implant mucositis allows non-surgical debridement with effective oral hygiene to be implemented (Salvi & Ramseier, 2014). Though some have also advocated the adjunctive use of chlorhexidine (De Siena et al., 2013) or other adjuncts, the efficacy of these has not yet been demonstrated (Heitz-Mayfield et al., 2011; Salvi & Ramseier, 2014; Schwartz et al., 2014).

Many different treatments have been advocated for peri-implantitis but no gold standard has yet been identified (Esposito et al., 2012). A review by Renvert et al. (2008) showed only minimal effects on the clinical parameters of peri-implantitis from non-surgical submucosal debridement alone. A systematic review of the treatment of peri-implantitis found a wide range of treatment regimes in use (Heitz-Mayfield & Mombelli, 2014) (Fig. 29.4). Historically, studies have shown considerable variation in inclusion criteria and definitions of peri-implantitis and many report short follow-up periods. Javed et al. (2013) reviewed the literature on clinical efficacy of antibiotics in the treatment of peri-implantitis. They concluded that there was no clear advantage to antibiotic therapy for the treatment of peri-implantitis. Heitz-Mayfield and Mombelli (2014) found favourable short-term treatment outcomes reported in the majority of patients. However, lack of response to treatment, progression of disease and disease recurrence with implant loss were also reported.

High-quality randomised clinical trials are required to determine the optimum management of peri-implantitis. Although evidence is lacking for specific recommendations for treatment, some aspects seem to be of benefit (Heitz-Mayfield & Mombelli, 2014) (Figs 29.5, 29.6).

Key points

- Peri-implant diseases are common and can result in loss of the implant
- Peri-implant mucositis is a mucosal condition that can be well managed by effective oral hygiene, with or without non-surgical debridement
- Peri-implantitis is similar to the periodontitis lesion but there may be more susceptibility to bone loss.
- Regular supportive therapy is required to prevent plaque retention around implants that can lead to peri-implant mucositis and peri-implantitis
- No single treatment regime has been identified for treatment of peri-implantitis

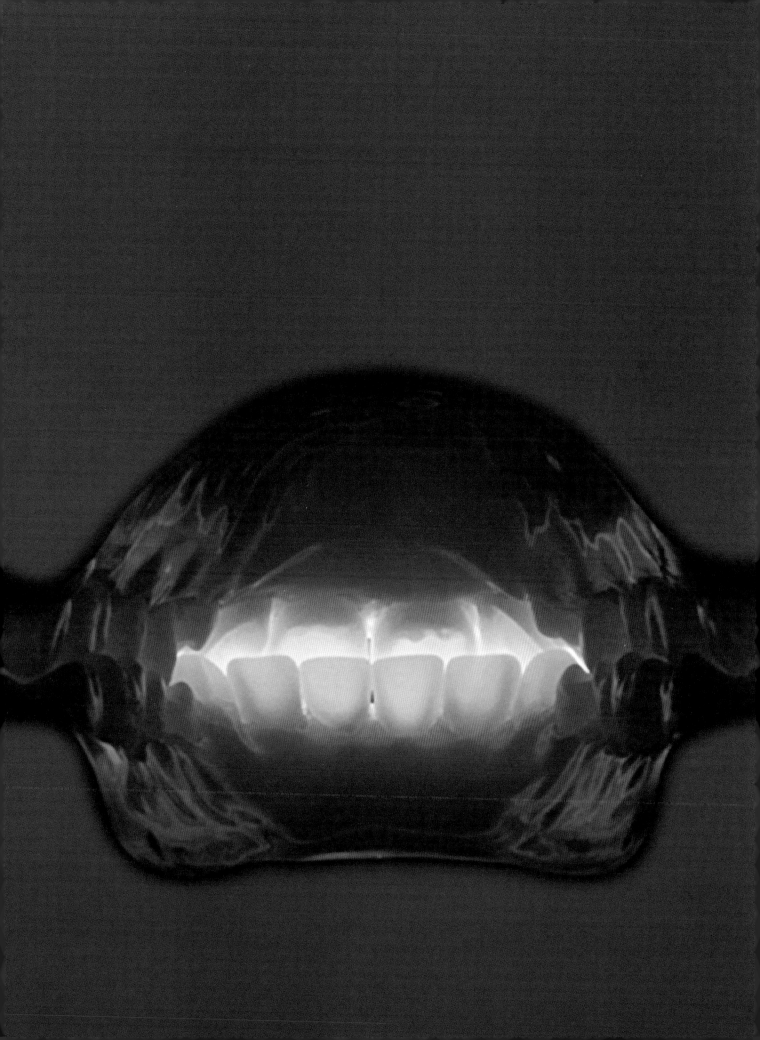

30 Periodontal–orthodontic interface

Figure 30.1 Hawley retainer.

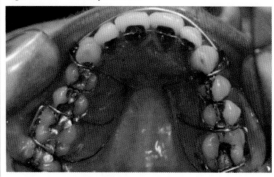

Figure 30.2 (a–c) Fixed orthodontic appliances in a 15-year-old Asian girl. Note the poor plaque control, gingival inflammation and swelling anteriorly and posteriorly.

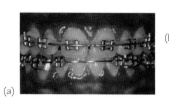
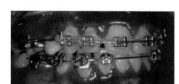
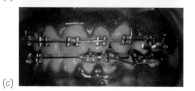

Figure 30.3 (a,b) Interspace brush. Single tufted brush for cleaning around fixed appliance brackets, arch wires and elastics.

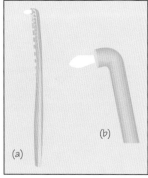

Figure 30.4 (a–c) A 28-year-old female patient (non-smoker) with a history of localised Stage IV Grade C periodontitis, prior to periodontal therapy. Note inflammation around the lateral incisors, upper left central incisor and instanding lower left lateral incisor. Also note the position of the upper left central incisor which has drifted and dropped out of line of the arch and is rotated and tilted.

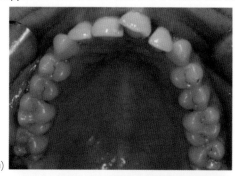
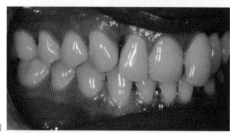
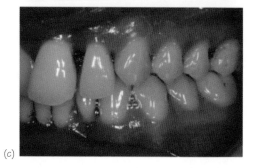

Figure 30.5 (a–f) Radiographs of patient in Fig. 30.4. (a,d) Vertical bitewing radiographs showing subgingival calculus and bone loss on the distal of the upper first molars and lower left second molar. (b,c,e,f) Periapical radiographs showing subgingival calculus and bone loss on the upper right lateral incisor, upper left central and lateral incisors and lower left lateral incisor.

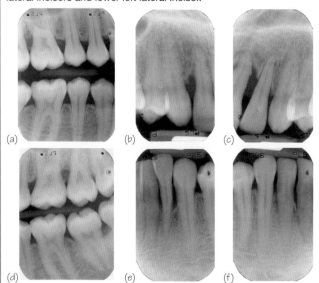

Periodontology at a Glance, Second Edition. Valerie Clerehugh, Aradhna Tugnait, Michael R. Milward, and Iain L. C. Chapple.
© 2024 John Wiley & Sons Ltd. Published 2024 by John Wiley & Sons Ltd.

Figure 30.6 Adult orthodontics in periodontally compromised patients.

Adult orthodontics in periodontally compromised patients
• Adults who elect to have orthodontic treatment usually have the motivation to complete orthodontic treatment; increased compliance
• Medical, social and dental history can complicate orthodontics
• Lack of facial growth may inhibit orthodontic movements
• Less cellular activity, therefore takes longer before tooth movement occurs
• May experience more pain following arch wire adjustments, therefore lighter orthodontic forces needed

• Lack of periodontal support:
  • reduces resistance to unwanted tooth movement, creating anchorage problems – light forces are needed to avoid tipping or extrusion
  • increases risk of root resorption due to reduced available root surface area and decreased vascularity

• Reduced adaptation of periodontal fibres leads to requirement for stricter retention regime – permanent retention advocated

Figure 30.7 (a,b) The patient in Fig. 30.4 after periodontal therapy. The patient disliked the appearance and position of her upper left central incisor but wanted to retain the tooth if at all possible. Lip trapping occurs and localised recession.

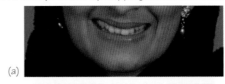
(a)

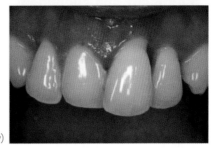
(b)

Figure 30.8 Stages of orthodontic treatment for the patient in Fig. 30.7: (a) fixed upper appliance; (b) bonded palatal upper retainer; (c) fixed lower appliance; and (d) aligned (permanently retained) upper anterior teeth and fixed lower appliance. There is improved aesthetics and spontaneous improvement in recession on the upper left central incisor following orthodontic tooth movement.

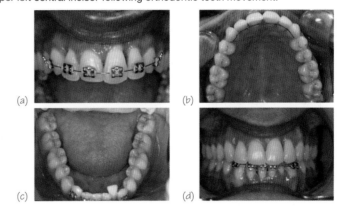
(a) (b) (c) (d)

Figure 30.9 (a) Pre-periodontal and orthodontic treatment of drifted upper central incisors in a female adult patient with periodontitis. (b) After treatment. (c) Bonded orthodontic retainer.

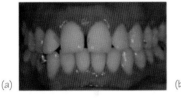
(a)

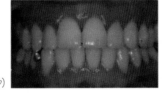
(b)

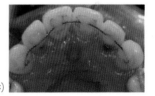
(c)

Figure 30.10 (a–c) Pre-periodontal treatment of a 33-year-old female patient with Stage IV Grade C periodontitis that led to drifting and proclination of the upper left central incisor, which had suffered recurrent periodontal abscesses. The prognosis of the tooth was deemed poor but it responded to periodontal therapy, at the patient's request, and orthodontic treatment was instigated with an upper removable appliance.

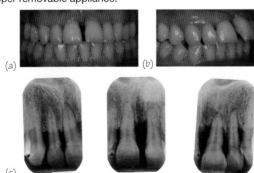
(a) (b)
(c)

Figure 30.11 Following orthodontic therapy of the patient in Fig. 30.10, the diastema closed (a) and a bonded retainer was placed (b). A six-year follow-up showed periodontal and orthodontic stability.

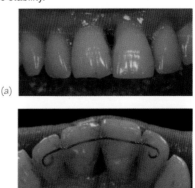
(a)

(b)

A dynamic two-way relationship exists between periodontal diseases and orthodontics: (i) some patients undergoing orthodontic treatment experience secondary periodontal sequelae which can adversely affect their periodontal health unless appropriately managed; (ii) periodontal diseases can lead to incisor drifting, and aesthetic concerns that might subsequently be addressed by orthodontic treatment.

Orthodontic treatment and secondary periodontal sequelae

Orthodontic appliances can act as plaque retention factors, therefore optimum oral hygiene is essential during treatment. Traditionally, provision of orthodontic treatment has been deemed the domain of children, but the uptake of adult orthodontics has increased dramatically in recent years. The use of fixed appliances outweighs that of removable appliances nowadays.

Removable orthodontic appliances

The Adams clasps of the upper removable appliance (URA), whether active or passive (as a retainer), engage the undercut – usually of the maxillary first molar teeth (Fig. 30.1) – and impinge directly on the marginal interdental papilla and buccal gingivae. This can create local plaque retention problems leading to gingival inflammation and eventually, if unchecked, loss of attachment and alveolar bone loss.

Fixed orthodontic appliances

Plaque accumulation is a particular problem around fixed orthodontic appliances, which are renowned for:
- a hyperplastic gingival response to the plaque biofilm (Fig. 30.2)
- the potential for enamel demineralisation around the brackets and bonded attachments for the arch wires.

Plaque control

Exemplary oral hygiene is essential throughout treatment. For patients with fixed appliances, this can be achieved by small-headed manual brushes, interdental brushes, single tufted interspace brushes to get underneath the arch wires and around the brackets (Fig. 30.3), or powered brushes with orthodontic heads. The URA should be removed for toothbrushing, kept clean itself and then replaced.

The danger of inadequate plaque control is gingivitis which, although reversible with adequate plaque control, can, if unchecked, progress to irreversible periodontitis.

Fluoride and diet

To prevent enamel demineralisation around the brackets and bonded attachments, in addition to optimum oral hygiene the patient should be provided with:
- topical fluorides, especially fluoride mouthwash
- dietary advice to limit cariogenic intakes/acidic sweetened beverages.

Periodontal screening prior to orthodontic treatment

In view of the risks of periodontal disease from undergoing orthodontic treatment, it is critical to screen patients for periodontal diseases *prior* to commencing orthodontic treatment using the Basic Periodontal Examination (or Periodontal Screening and Recording) (Chapter 17) and to ensure periodontal review and supportive therapy are provided during treatment.

Other risks

- *Recession.* Providing teeth are orthodontically moved within the alveolar bone, there is little risk of gingival recession. If excessive proclination is anticipated, then connective tissue grafting can be undertaken to create keratinised gingiva prior to tooth movement.
- *Root resorption.* There is a risk of root resorption of 1–2 mm during orthodontic tooth movement, which leads to a shortened root length. Around 15% of patients may experience resorption of 2.5 mm or more which would have implications in a periodontally compromised patient.

Periodontal drifting

Periodontal drifting is a pathological migration of teeth that have reduced bone support and have lost clinical attachment as a consequence of periodontitis. Patients will usually complain of spacing appearing between their front teeth, incisor(s) dropping out of the line of the arch, and tipping or rotation (Figs 30.4, 30.5). It can occur relatively slowly, for instance in Grade A periodontitis, but more rapidly as in Grade B or C periodontitis especially when periodontal risk factors are present (Chapter 36). Occlusal factors are thought to play a role (Chapter 15).

Usually, the age group most affected will be adults, so prior to considering orthodontics, patients must be carefully assessed, counselled as to treatment options, the risks (see above) and benefits explained, and informed consent gained. Several differences exist between adults and children seeking orthodontic treatment (Fig. 30.6).

Periodontal–orthodontic management

Periodontal–orthodontic management involves a number of steps for a successful outcome (Figs 30.7–30.11).
- Step 1 and 2, and if necessary step 3 of periodontal treatment should be undertaken and completed and the periodontal condition should be stable. The patients should be in the supportive phase of therapy (step 4). There should be no active pockets or residual inflammation (Fig. 30.7) (Chapter 19).
- Oral hygiene must be optimum.
- There should be assessment on an individual basis to check:
  - that there is adequate bone through which to move the drifted teeth and sufficient bone for postorthodontic retention

- that there are sufficient teeth and bone and periodontal support for the fixed or removable orthodontic appliance to be functional.
- The patient should be aware of how long they will need to wear the orthodontic appliance(s), and the frequency of visits.
- The patient should be instructed how to care for their appliance(s).
- Appropriate fluoride supplements and diet advice should be provided to prevent demineralisation around the appliance(s) as recommended by Public Health England (2021).
- A periodontal maintenance programme (step 4) should be in place during the orthodontic treatment (Fig. 30.8).
- The periodontally compromised patient should be aware of the need for permanent orthodontic retention following the completion of orthodontic treatment (Figs 30.8b, 30.9c, 30.11b).

Key points

- To prevent periodontal sequelae due to orthodontic treatment:
  - periodontal screening should precede orthodontic treatment
  - oral hygiene must be optimum during treatment
  - fluoride supplements/diet advice are needed to prevent demineralisation
- Periodontal drifting may lead patients to seek orthodontic treatment
- There are differences between orthodontics in adults and children
- Risk/benefit should be advised and informed consent gained
- Periodontal–orthodontic management involves a number of steps for a successful outcome

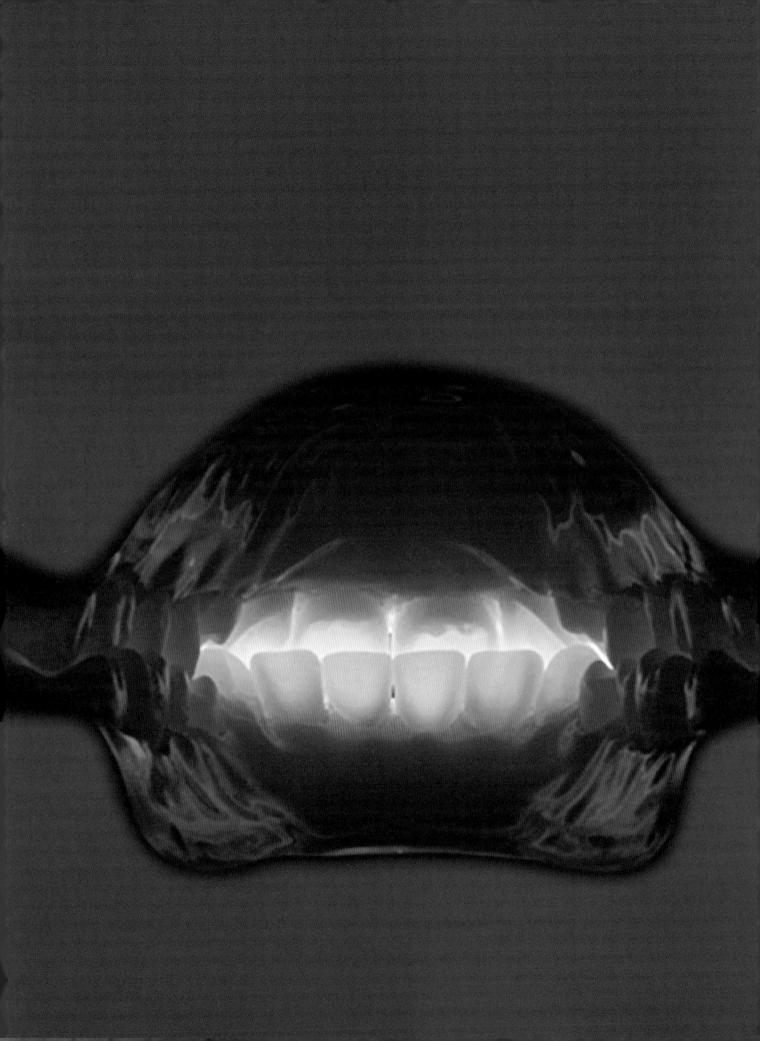

Periodontal diseases and periodontal management

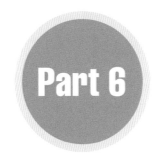

Part 6

Chapters

Overview

Part 6 contains chapters on various periodontal diseases and conditions integral to the 2018 classification, and their management, including plaque biofilm-induced gingivitis (Chapter 31), non-plaque-induced gingival conditions and lesions (Chapter 32), gingival recession and gingival enlargement (Chapters 33 and 34), periodontitis (Chapter 35), necrotising periodontal diseases (Chapter 39) and, periodontal abscesses and endodontic-periodontal lesions (Chapter 40). Periodontal diseases in children and adolescents and in older adults are considered in separate chapters (Chapters 41 and 42). Specific chapters are devoted to the periodontal management of patients who smoke and patients with diabetes (Chapters 37 and 38), recognising the importance of these two conditions as risk factors for periodontitis, as covered in Part 2. Staging and grading of periodontitis has been included as a new chapter, having been introduced for the first time in the 2017 World Workshop, and the chapter also presents a pragmatic, workable framework by the BSP for its implementation into clinical practice in the UK (Chapter 36). The final chapter covers delivery of periodontal care, including the value of the dental team approach, the referral process and what to include, and emphasises that good diagnosis, communication and record keeping are imperative (Chapter 43).

31 Plaque biofilm-induced gingivitis

Figure 31.1 Dental plaque biofilm-induced gingivitis.

> A. **Associated with dental plaque biofilm alone**
> B. **Mediated by local or systemic risk factors**
>   i) **Local risk factors (predisposing factors)**
>   a) **Dental plaque biofilm retention factors**
>   1) Supragingival or subgingival calculus
>   2) Subgingival restoration margins
>   3) Tooth anatomical factors e.g. root groove, enamel pearl, furcation
>   4) Malocclusion/crowding
>   5) Fixed and removable prosthodontic or orthodontic appliances
>   b) **Oral dryness/Lack of saliva e.g. in relation to lack of lip seal/mouthbreathing**
>   ii) **Systemic risk factors (modifying factors)**
>   1) Sex steroid hormones – puberty; pregnancy; NB little effect in relation to menstrual cycle or most modern low-dose oral contraceptives
>   2) Diabetes mellitus (hyperglycaemia)
>   3) Smoking
>   4) Blood dyscrasias - leukaemia
>   5) Nutritional – vitamin C deficiency
>   6) Pharmacological agents – e.g. related to hyposalivation or gingival enlargement; high-dose contraceptive pill
> C. **Drug-influenced gingival enlargement**
>   1) Anti-epileptic drugs e.g. phenytoin; sodium valproate
>   2) Calcium channel blockers e.g. nifedipine, amlodipine, felodipine, diltiazem, verapamil
>   3) Immuno-suppressants e.g. ciclosporin
>   4) High-dose contraceptives

Figure 31.3 Section through a tooth with established, clinically evident plaque-induced gingivitis.

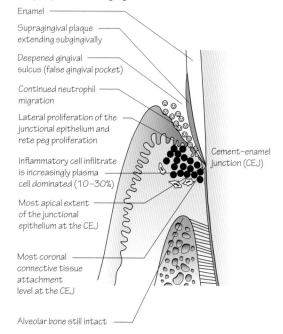

Figure 31.2 Definitions of dental plaque biofilm-induced gingivitis.

> **Site level (see also Figure 31.3):**
> Inflammatory lesion resulting from interactions between the dental plaque biofilm and host's immune-inflammatory response which remains contained within the gingiva and does not extend to the periodontal attachment (cementum, periodontal ligament and alveolar bone) or the mucogingival junction.
>   – Reversible by reducing levels of dental plaque at/apical to gingival margin
>
> **Patient case level:**
> Gingivitis on an intact periodontium and gingivitis on a reduced periodontium is defined as ≥ 10% bleeding sites with probing depths ≤ 3mm:
>   – Localised gingivitis: 10–30% bleeding sites.
>   – Generalised gingivitis: >30% bleeding sites.
>
> **Note:** a periodontitis case cannot simultaneously be defined as a gingivitis case, therefore a patient with a history of periodontitis with gingival inflammation is still a periodontitis case.

Figure 31.4 Plaque-induced gingivitis: plaque visible at the gingival margin, blunted papillae and red, swollen gingiva.

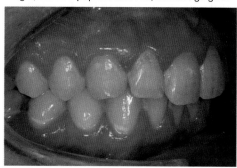

Figure 31.5 A false gingival pocket.

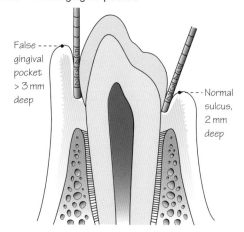

Periodontology at a Glance, Second Edition. Valerie Clerehugh, Aradhna Tugnait, Michael R. Milward, and Iain L. C. Chapple.
© 2024 John Wiley & Sons Ltd. Published 2024 by John Wiley & Sons Ltd.

Figure 31.6 (a) Pretreatment: a false gingival pocket associated with a subgingival cavity (arrow) and plaque retention on the mesial UL2. The papilla is swollen and red. (b) Post treatment for gingivitis: the inflammation is diminished. The cavity on UL2 is now supragingival and accessible for restoration.

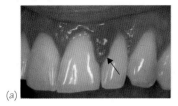 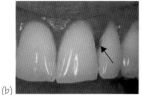

(a) (b)

Figure 31.7 Plaque accumulation around a fixed orthodontic appliance in a 17-year-old female. There is gingival inflammation and a hyperplastic response to plaque.

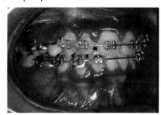

Figure 31.8 A 13-year-old boy with pronounced gingivitis anteriorly which is associated with poor plaque control and lack of saliva there due to incompetent lips, a high lip line and being a mouth breather in relation to nasal blockages.

High lip line and incompetent lips;
(a) mouthbreathes   (b)   Oral dryness, lack of saliva exacerbates plaque-induced gingivitis anteriorly

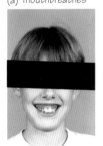 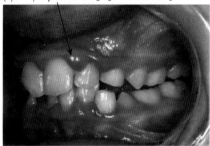

Figure 31.9 Pregnancy-associated gingivitis. (a) A 21-year-old pregnant patient with inflamed, swollen lower anterior gingivae which bleed on gentle probing. (b) A different pregnant patient with an even more marked response to plaque and severe gingival overgrowth (epulis), especially on the lower incisors.

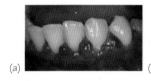 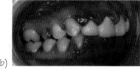

(a) (b)

Figure 31.10 Drug-induced gingival overgrowth in an adult male patient with inadequate plaque control who was taking ciclosporin and a calcium channel blocker (nifedipine) following a renal transplant.

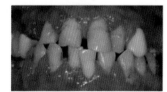

Figure 31.11 Diagnostic look-up table for clinical practice. Health versus gingivitis. Source: Modified from Chapple et al. (2018), Table 1.

Diagnostic Look Up Table for Clinical Practice	Health	Gingivitis
Intact periodontium		
Clinical Attachment Loss (CAL)	No	No
Probing Pocket Depths (PD) (assumes no false pockets)	≤ 3 mm	≤3 mm
Bleeding on Probing (BOP)	< 10%	Yes (≥ 10%)
Bone Loss (Radiological)	No	No
Reduced periodontium. Non-periodontitis patient		
Clinical Attachment Loss	Yes	Yes
Probing Pocket Depths (all sites & assumes no false pockets)	≤ 3 mm	≤3 mm
Bleeding on Probing	< 10%	Yes (≥ 10%)
Bone Loss (Radiological)	Possible	Possible
Successfully treated, stable periodontitis patient		
Clinical Attachment Loss	Yes	Yes
Probing Pocket Depths (all sites & assumes no false pockets)	≤ 4 mm [1,2,3]	≤ 3 mm [3]
Bleeding on Probing	< 10%	Yes (≥ 10%)
Bone Loss (Radiological)	Yes	Yes

Footnotes: [1] No site ≥ 4 mm with BOP; [2] if PD ≥ 4 mm with BOP, this is no longer a closed pocket; [3] higher risk of disease recurrence in successfully treated case so PD threshold set higher for health than gingivitis;

There is considerable variation between subjects in susceptibility to the development of gingival inflammation. It is currently thought that dental plaque biofilm-induced gingivitis and periodontitis are a continuum of the same disease; however, the interface is complex (Chapters 8, 9).

Classification and definitions

The World Workshop on the Classification of Periodontal and Peri-Implant Diseases and Conditions held in 2017 classified dental plaque biofilm-induced gingivitis into various types (Fig. 31.1) and defined it at the site level/patient case level (Fig. 31.2) (Chapple et al., 2018). A correct diagnosis is reached after considering the findings of the history and examination and relies on knowledge of the current 2018 classification.

Features of plaque biofilm-induced gingivitis

Histopathological features are shown in Fig. 31.3. Clinical signs (Fig. 31.4) include:

- redness/change in colour of the gingiva.
- swelling/loss of knife edge of marginal gingiva.
- false gingival pockets may be present in an intact periodontium in which the most apical extent of the junctional epithelium is still at the CEJ but the sulcus is deepened to >3 mm due to gingival swelling (Figs 31.5, 31.6).
- loss of contour (blunting) of the interdental papilla.
- bleeding on gentle probing.
- discomfort on gentle probing may occur.

Clinical symptoms the patient may complain of include:

- bleeding gums, metallic/altered taste.
- halitosis.
- appearance (swollen red gums).
- pain/soreness possible but not usually key feature, unlike necrotising gingiviits (Chapter 39).
- difficulty eating.
- reduced oral health-related quality of life.

Plaque-induced gingivitis on a reduced periodontium

The features of gingivitis as above may occur on a periodontium with reduced periodontal support in: (i) a non-periodontitis patient (e.g. recession, crown lengthening); (ii) a successfully treated periodontitis patient in whom loss of attachment and loss of alveolar bone are present but not progressing.

Predisposing/modifying factors

Rate of progression, severity and extent of gingivitis may be influenced by the following.

Local risk factors (predisposing factors)

- Supragingival or subgingival calculus.
- Subgingival restoration margins, overhangs or cavities (Fig. 31.6).
- Tooth anatomical factors, e.g. root groove or enamel pearl.
- Malocclusion or crowding.
- Fixed and removable prosthodontic or orthodontic appliances (Fig. 31.7).

- Oral dryness/lack of saliva, e.g. incompetent lips/lack of lip seal, which compromise the protective benefits of saliva (Fig. 31.8).

Systemic risk factors (modifying factors)

- Sex steroid hormones.
  - Puberty: increased inflammatory response of the gingiva to plaque and hormones during the circumpubertal period.
  - Menstrual cycle: a small cohort of women experience a marked inflammatory response of the gingiva immediately prior to ovulation, but for most, this is clinically undetectable.
  - Pregnancy: there can be a pronounced inflammatory response of the gingiva to plaque and hormones during the second and third trimesters (Fig. 31.9a); pregnancy epulis is an exaggerated inflammatory response that typically presents interdentally as a mushroom-like mass with a pedunculated base from the gingival margin but can be more extensive (Fig. 31.9b).
- Diabetes mellitus: inflammatory response of the gingiva to plaque which is aggravated by poorly controlled blood glucose levels and hyperglycaemia.
- Smoking is a major risk factor for periodontitis but also affects the microvasculature of the gingival tissues which can mask clinical signs of gingivitis such as bleeding on probing.
- Blood dyscrasias: gingivitis associated with abnormal function or number of blood cells (e.g. leukaemia, a malignant condition that can manifest with increased bleeding and purple-red, enlarged, spongy gingiva).
- Vitamin C deficiency (scurvy) is uncommon in developed countries but in some parts of the world can lead to bright red, swollen, ulcerated gingivae which tend to bleed readily.
- Medications may be associated with:
  - drug-influenced gingival enlargement, e.g. phenytoin (for epilepsy), ciclosporin (an immunosuppressant) or calcium channel blockers (commonly used for hypertension or heart problems) (Fig. 31.10; Chapter 34).
  - drug-influenced gingivitis, e.g. contraceptive pill.
  - drug-related reduced salivary flow, e.g. antidepressants, antihistamines, antihypertensives.

Management

Effective management of plaque-induced gingivitis requires the correct diagnosis (Chapple et al., 2018; Dietrich et al., 2019) (Fig. 31.11) and any local or systemic factors to be identified (Chapters 11, 14). The suspicion of leukaemia requires urgent medical referral. Initial Step 1 therapy is generally amenable to primary dental care and involves the disruption and removal of the plaque biofilm, with measures put in place to control the biofilm and prevent recurrence of the gingivitis (Chapter 19; Appendix 4).

- Plaque and bleeding on probing indices.
- Oral hygiene instruction:
  - toothbrushing advice – manual or powered brush.
  - interdental cleaning advice – floss/tape or interdental brushes.
  - advice on toothpastes and mouthwashes.
- Smoking cessation advice.
- Manage modifiable systemic risk factors, e.g. liaise with diabetes care team to help improve diabetes control.
- Eliminate predisposing local plaque retention risk factors.

- Supragingival PMPR by dental professional to remove supragingival plaque, staining and calculus on tooth crown and subgingival plaque and calculus from gingival crevice which is subgingival.
- Arrange caries management, endodontic treatment, extractions and immediate/transitional prosthodontic treatment.
- Review and monitor response to Step 1.
- If there is inadequate plaque control and residual disease is present in a non-engaging patient, then repeat Step 1.
- If there is adequate plaque control and resolution of disease in an engaging patient, then arrange supportive therapy and an appropriate tailored recall to prevent disease recurrence (Step 4).

Key points

- There are different types of dental plaque biofilm-induced gingivitis
- Diagnosis:
  - follows history and examination
  - is aided by knowledge of the current classification
- Management:
  - relies on control/disruption of the plaque biofilm and the elimination of predisposing local/modifiable systemic risk factors
  - can generally be provided in the primary dental care setting

32 Non-plaque-induced gingival conditions and lesions

Table 32.1 Classification of gingival diseases: non-dental plaque induced (Chapple *et al*., 2018).

A. Genetic/developmental disorders
  i. *Hereditary gingival fibromatosis*

B. Specific infections
  i. *Bacterial origin*
    (a) *Neisseria gonorrhoeae*
    (b) *Treponema pallidum*
    (c) *Mycobacterium tuberculosis*
    (d) Streptococcal gingivitis
  ii. *Viral origin*
    (a) Coxsackie virus (hand-foot-and-mouth disease)
    (b) Herpes simplex I & II (primary or recurrent)
    (c) Varicella zoster (chicken pox & shingles – V nerve)
    (d) Molluscum contagiosum
    (e) Human papilloma virus (squamous cell papilloma; condyloma acuminatum; verruca vulgaris; focal epithelial hyperplasia)
  iii. *Fungal origin*
    (a) Candidosis
    (b) Other mycoses, e.g. histoplasmosis, aspergillosis

C. Inflammatory and immune conditions
  i. *Hypersensitivity reactions*
    (a) Contact allergy
    (b) Plasma cell gingivitis
    (c) Erythema multiforme
  ii. *Autoimmune diseases of skin and mucous membranes*
    (a) Pemphigus vulgaris
    (b) Pemphigoid
    (c) Lichen planus
    (d) Lupus erythematosus
       Systemic lupus erythematosus
       Discoid lupus erythematosus
  iii. *Granulomatous inflammatory lesions (orofacial granulomatoses)*
    (a) Crohn's disease
    (b) Sarcoidosis

D. Reactive processes
  i. *Epulides*
    (a) Fibrous epulis
    (b) Calcifying fibroblastic granuloma
    (c) Vascular epulis (pyogenic granuloma)
    (d) Peripheral giant cell granuloma

E. Neoplasms
  i. *Premalignancy*
    (a) Leukoplakia
    (b) Erythroplakia
  ii. *Malignancy*
    (a) Squamous cell carcinoma
    (b) Leukaemic cell infiltration
    (c) Lymphoma
       Hodgkin's
       Non-Hodgkin's
    (d) Chondrosarcoma

F. Endocrine, nutritional & metabolic diseases
  i. *Vitamin deficiencies*
    (a) Vitamin C deficiency (scurvy)

G. Traumatic lesions
  i. *Physical/mechanical trauma*
    (a) Frictional keratosis
    (b) Mechanically induced gingival ulceration
    (c) Factitious injury (self-harm)
  ii. *Chemical (toxic) burn*
  iii. *Thermal insults*
    (a) Burns to gingiva

H. Gingival pigmentation
  i. *Melanoplakia*
  ii. *Smoker's melanosis*
  iii. *Drug-induced pigmentation (antimalarials, minocycline)*
  iv. *Amalgam tattoo*

Figure 32.1 The surgical sieve: arriving at a correct differential diagnosis.

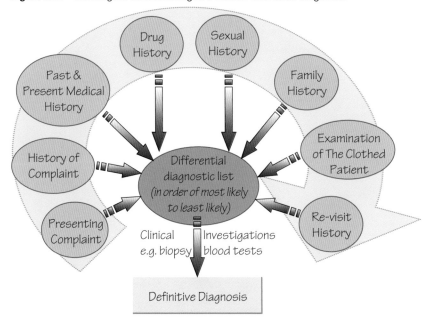

Periodontology at a Glance, Second Edition. Valerie Clerehugh, Aradhna Tugnait, Michael R. Milward, and Iain L. C. Chapple.
© 2024 John Wiley & Sons Ltd. Published 2024 by John Wiley & Sons Ltd.

Figure 32.2 (a,b) Drug-induced gingival overgrowth.

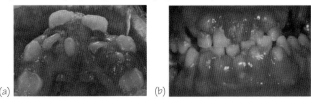

(a)

(b)

Figure 32.3 The normal gingival anatomy.

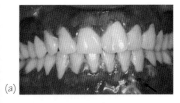

- Non-keratinised oral mucosa
- Mucogingival junction
- Attached gingiva
- Free gingiva
- Gingival groove

Sebaceous glands (Fordyce spots)

Figure 32.6 Lichen planus: (a) desquamative gingivitis – arrow depicts suture from biopsy; (b) plaque-like lichen planus; (c) reticular lichen planus; and (d) erosive lichen planus. Source: Courtesy of Professor I.L.C. Chapple.

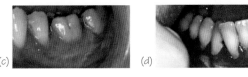

(a)

(b)

(c)

(d)

Figure 32.4 Sarcoidosis. Source: Courtesy of Professor I.L.C. Chapple.

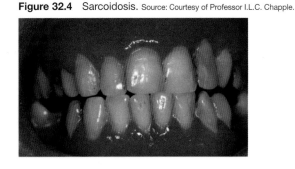

Figure 32.5 Varicella zoster. Source: Courtesy of Professor I.L.C. Chapple.

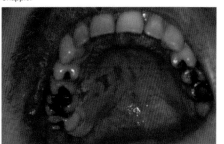

Figure 32.7 Leukoplakia: (a) localised veruccous leukoplakia; and (b) generalised homogenous leukoplakia. Source: Courtesy of Professor I.L.C. Chapple.

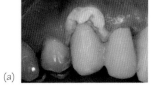

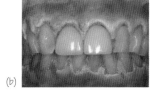

(a)

(b)

Figure 32.8 A surgical sieve utilising a mnemonic: 'HINTED'.
Source: Courtesy of Professor I.L.C. Chapple.

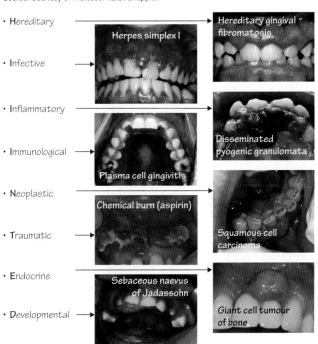

- Hereditary
- Infective
- Inflammatory
- Immunological
- Neoplastic
- Traumatic
- Endocrine
- Developmental

Herpes simplex I

Plasma cell gingivitis

Chemical burn (aspirin)

Sebaceous naevus of Jadassohn

Hereditary gingival fibromatosis

Disseminated pyogenic granulomata

Squamous cell carcinoma

Giant cell tumour of bone

Non-plaque-induced gingival conditions were classified for the first time in 1999 by an international workshop in peri-odontology and subsequently revised by the 2018 World Workshop Classification (Table 32.1), but the system is by no means comprehensive. Given the heterogeneity of the constituent cells of the gingivae (epithelial, endothelial, fibroblast, adipocytes, inflammatory-immune cells) and the various disorders associated with mixed tissues (ranging from genetic conditions to specific infections, inflammatory-immune and reactive lesions, trauma, pigmentation and neoplasms), it is estimated that well over 100 systemic or local non-plaque-induced conditions may involve the gingivae.

Diagnostic Process

Establishing a differential diagnosis for such a large number of conditions is challenging and a procedural algorithm to approach this is illustrated in Fig. 32.1. It is important to:

1 adopt a forensic approach to history taking and examination procedures
2 keep an open mind about potential causes
3 use every piece of available information (visual and tactile).

It is important to take a detailed history.

- *The complaint*: is often key to establishing a differential diagnosis. For example, gingival 'pain' or 'soreness' tends to indicate ulcerative or erosive conditions (viral or immune-mediated lesions are likely) such as lichen planus, pemphigoid or erythema multiforme.
- *History of the complaint*: this is extremely important in the diagnostic pathway. For example, the temporal relationship between the onset of symptoms and a patient commencing a course of medication could be the diagnostic key. Drug-induced pigmentation or ulceration, lichenoid drug reactions or drug-influenced gingival enlargement (Fig. 32.2) are all examples. Gingival overgrowths have variable appearances, ranging from fibrous (e.g. Dilantin® therapy for epilepsy) to vascular (e.g. calcium channel-blocking drugs that modify a plaque-induced inflammatory response).
- *Past or present medical history*: a positive medical history often leads directly or indirectly to a diagnosis. A history of atopy may indicate an allergic aetiology to the condition (e.g. plasma cell gingivitis). The presence of mucocutaneous diseases such as epidermolysis bullosa or lichen planus may explain oral blistering, erosions or scarring. Connective tissue diseases (e.g. systemic sclerosis) or inflammatory conditions (e.g. angio-oedema) may all present with gingival manifestations.
- *Drug history*: prescription drugs can produce side-effects following correct use (e.g. pigmentation with minocycline) or incorrect use (e.g. aspirin burns following topical application) and recreational drugs may cause ulcerative/necrotic lesions (e.g. cocaine).
- *Sexual history*: this may be necessary if sexually transmitted diseases (herpes simplex 2 or syphilis) or HIV are suspected. This should only be performed where there is a high index of suspicion and should be done sensitively and in the presence of a chaperone.
- *Family history*: may be important for conditions like hereditary gingival fibromatosis (autosomal dominant mutation of Son of Sevenless gene, 2p21-p22 or 5q13-q22).
- *Extraoral examination*: of clothed patients requires the oral physician to observe the face, neck, hands/arms and legs/shins for peripheral signs of lesions that may be relevant to the gingival pathology. Examples are enlarged lymph nodes in infectious conditions; purple/pruritic lesions on flexor surfaces of arms and shins in lichen planus; target lesions in erythema multiforme;

telangiectasia/spider naevi in liver disease or CREST syndrome (calcinosis, Raynaud's, oesophagitis, Sjögren syndrome, telangiectasia), now called progressive systemic sclerosis.

- *Intraoral examination*: should be systematic and thorough. The identification of non-gingival involvement may be essential in establishing a diagnosis. Definitive diagnosis may require biopsy or assimilation of several strands of information from clinical tests. Always ignore the obvious pathology initially and return to it at the end of the examination, as patients may have multiple pathology. Good knowledge of normal gingival anatomy is essential (Fig. 32.3), as lesions involving attached and free gingiva are unlikely to be plaque induced. For example, the erythema in Fig. 32.4 crosses the mucogingival junction and deep biopsy revealed granulomas of sarcoidosis. Equally, consider nerve distributions carefully – some antiretroviral drugs used in the management of HIV disease cause a painful trigeminal neuropathy. The ulceration in Fig. 32.5 is limited to the maxillary division of the trigeminal nerve and does not cross the midline (it was a varicella zoster infection – shingles).
- *Revisitation of a history*: issues highlighted by the examination process frequently necessitate a revisitation of the clinical or medical history, e.g. primary biliary cirrhosis is associated with Sjögren syndrome; chronic active hepatitis may associate with lichen planus.

Clinical investigations

A differential diagnosis should always list in order of most likely to least likely, the presumptive diagnoses. Clinical investigations such as biopsy or blood tests then help establish a definitive diagnosis.

When and where to biopsy

Biopsies are generally necessary:

- for the diagnosis of conditions or lesions that have variable clinical but classic histological features (e.g. lichen planus – Fig. 32.6).
- where the consequences of a positive histological diagnosis have implications for other body systems (e.g. sarcoidosis, vesiculo-bullous diseases).
- where a sinister lesion is suspected (Fig. 32.7). As gingival tissues always exhibit plaque-induced inflammation, which can mask classic histological features of other conditions, always try to biopsy non-gingival sites. This is essential in cases of 'desquamative gingivitis' where differential diagnoses may include lichen planus, pemphigoid, pemphigus or lupus (Fig. 32.6a).

The surgical sieve

A surgical sieve utilising a mnemonic, e.g. 'HINTED', may be helpful in stimulating thought processes towards formulating a differential diagnosis (Fig. 32.8).

Key points

- Adopt a forensic and systematic approach to questioning
- Keep an open mind throughout
- Use every piece of visual information available
- Consider links to existing medical conditions
- Consider the likelihood of multiple pathology
- Try to avoid gingival biopsies and utilise adjacent sites if possible
- If in doubt about a diagnosis, refer

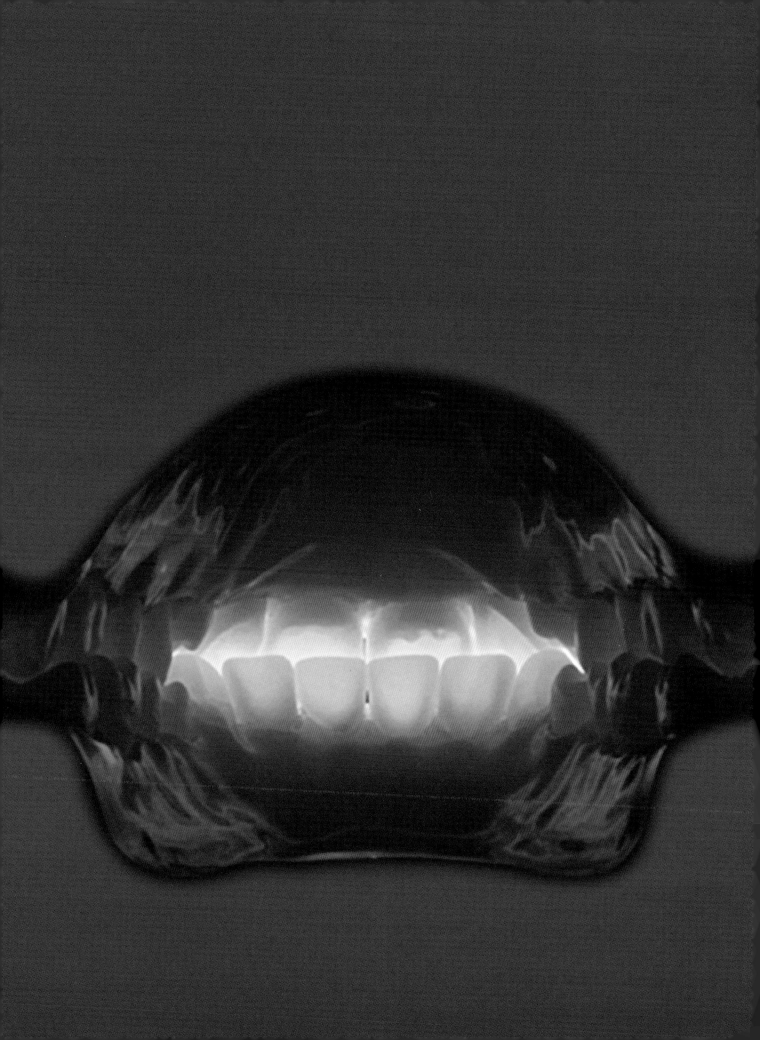

33 Gingival recession

Figure 33.1 Aetiology of gingival recession.

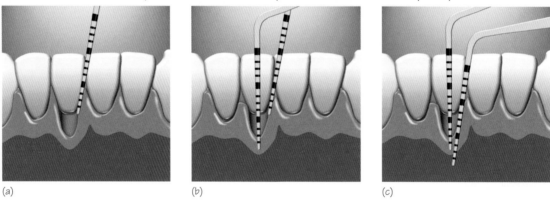

Trauma
- Toothbrushing
- Factitious injury
- e.g. finger nail picking at gingival margin
- Poorly designed/maintained P/P
- Direct trauma from malocclusion
- Class II division 2 with complete overbite
- Chemical trauma
  - Topical cocaine

Associated with pathological alveolar bone loss
- Periodontal disease
- Associated with tissue destruction
- Associated with treatment of periodontal disease
- Smoking

Plaque and local plaque retention factors
- High muscle attachment
- Frenal pull
- Subgingival margins
- Calculus

Orthodontic movements
- Lower incisor proclination
- Arch expansion

Thin periodontal phenotype
- Gingival tissue
- Keratinised tissue width
- Bone

Figure 33.2 Classification of recession lesions. (a) Recession type 1 (RT1): gingival recession with no loss of interproximal attachment. Interproximal CEJ (cement enamel junction) not clinically detectable at the mesial and distal aspects of the tooth. (b) Recession type 2 (RT2): gingival recession associated with loss of interproximal attachment. The amount of interproximal clinical attachment loss (measured from the interproximal CEJ to the depth of the interproximal sulcus/pocket) is ≤ buccal attachment loss (from the buccal CEJ to the apical end of the buccal sulcus/pocket). (c) Recession type 3 (RT3): gingival recession associated with loss of interproximal attachment. The amount of interproximal clinical attachment loss (from the interproximal CEJ to the apical end of the sulcus/pocket) is higher than the buccal attachment loss (from the buccal CEJ to the apical end of the buccal sulcus/pocket).

(a) (b) (c)

Figure 33.3 Pedicle grafts: laterally repositioned rotational flap. The flap is taken from an adjacent site to cover the localised area of recession.

Surgical root coverage techniques

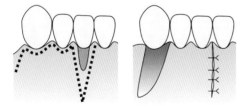

Figure 33.4 Pedicle grafts: double papilla rotational flap. Coverage is achieved from adjacent donor sites on either side of the area of recession.

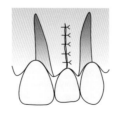

Figure 33.5 Free grafts: free epithelialised gingival graft. At the recipient site, the epithelium and outer part of the connective tissue are removed by split dissection around and below the recession defect. The graft is taken from the remote donor site and sutured securely at the recipient site.

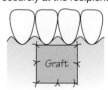

Graft

Periodontology at a Glance, Second Edition. Valerie Clerehugh, Aradhna Tugnait, Michael R. Milward, and Iain L. C. Chapple.
© 2024 John Wiley & Sons Ltd. Published 2024 by John Wiley & Sons Ltd.

Figure 33.6 Free grafts: free epithelialised gingival graft. (a) Site shown preoperatively. (b) The tissue graft sutured in place. (c) The site shown four months postoperatively. Source: Courtesy of Mr P.J. Nixon.

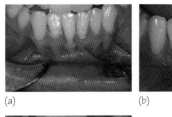
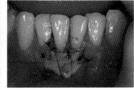

(a)

(b)

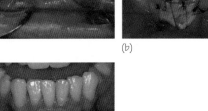

(c)

Figure 33.7 Free grafts: subepithelial connective tissue graft. A free connective tissue graft is taken from the palate. The tissue is sutured at the prepared recipient site. The graft is then covered by a flap (commonly a coronally advanced flap) so that the graft gains nutrition from the underlying periosteum and deep connective tissue and the overlying flap.

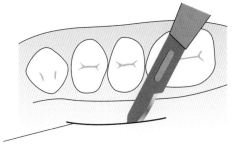

Single visible incision for envelope flap, to give access to underlying connective tissue

Figure 33.8 Free grafts: subepithelial connective tissue graft. (a) Procedure for coverage of recession at UL3, sulcular incision. (b) Creation of tunnel to receive graft. (c) Closure of palatal donor site following removal of subepithelial connective tissue graft. (d) Graft inserted and stabilised at recipient site with closure of flap with sling sutures. (e) UL3 10 months postoperatively. Source: Courtesy of Mr J. Chesterman.

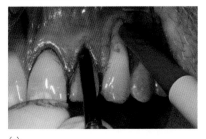
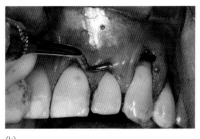
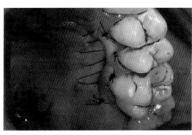

(a)

(b)

(c)

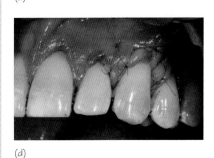
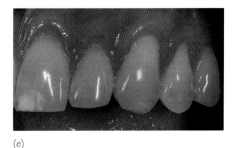

(d)

(e)

Gingival recession is defined as the apical shift of the gingival margin caused by different periodontal conditions/diseases. It is associated with clinical attachment loss and can occur on all tooth surfaces (buccal, lingual and interproximal) (Jepsen *et al.*, 2018). Aetiological factors associated with gingival recession are shown in Fig. 33.1. Periodontal phenotype is the term used to encompass both the gingival phenotype (gingival thickness, keratinised tissue width) and bone morphotype (thickness of the buccal bone plate) (Jepsen *et al.*, 2018). A thin phenotype increases risk of developing gingival recession (Chambrone & Tatakis, 2016). The gingival tissue can be assessed by observing a periodontal probe after this is inserted into the sulcus; if the probe is visible then the gingival tissue is ≤1 mm and thin.

Consequences of gingival recession

Unlike many other oral problems, patients are very often aware of gingival recession. Patients may potentially experience the following problems associated with recession.

- Pain from exposed dentine.
- Aesthetic concerns.
- Plaque retention and gingival inflammation.
- Root caries.
- Tooth surface loss (abrasion).

Management

A history and examination are carried out to identify aetiological factors and a diagnosis of gingival recession is made. Recession can be measured in millimetres with a periodontal probe; study models and photographs can be useful for records. Recession can be classified based on interdental clinical attachment loss (Cairo *et al.*, 2014) (Fig. 33.2). Management can be divided into the management of:

- aetiological factors associated with recession
- consequences of recession.

Management of aetiological factors associated with recession

- Oral hygiene advice: advise an atraumatic brushing technique using:
  - manual toothbrushing
  - electric toothbrushing.
- Smoking cessation advice.
- Advice relating to traumatic habits.
- Orthodontic treatment planning. If this is likely to create a dehiscence, review the volume of soft tissue at the site and consider grafting prior to unfavourable orthodontic movements.
- Removable partial denture design and restorations:
  - good support of dentures
  - placement of supragingival restorations where possible
  - regular review and maintenance.
- Treatment of periodontal disease.

Management of consequences of recession

- Dentine hypersensitivity: caused by exposed and open dentinal tubules.
  - Dietary advice.
  - Antisensitivity dentifrices; active agents interfere with nerve transmission in the dentinal tubules or form a coating over the outer surface of the teeth to occlude open dentinal tubules.
  - Topical products for professional application: (i) containing fluoride (e.g. Duraphat®, Colgate-Palmolive, Guildford, UK), (ii) other (e.g. containing chlorhexidine and thymol), and (iii) sealants.
  - Restorations.
- Root caries.
  - Prevention: diet, oral hygiene instruction and fluoride application.
  - Reshaping of shallow lesions.
  - Restorations.
- Restoration of aesthetics.
  - Gingival veneer: silicone mask to disguise interdental spaces (note this will act as a plaque retention factor).
  - Restorations: these can camouflage the exposed root surface in some cases; pink porcelain or composite can try to disguise exposed roots.
  - Root coverage by surgical techniques (see following section).

Recession can be monitored to ensure there is no further progression. In many cases where there are no consequences to the presence of the recession defect, sites are accepted and kept under review. In particular situations, root coverage to eliminate or reduce the recession defect may be appropriate.

Mucogingival surgery and the surgical management of gingival recession

Mucogingival surgery is a term used for surgical manipulation of the attached gingivae and vestibular tissues and so includes those techniques for management of gingival recession.

A high frenal attachment can sometimes impede oral hygiene measures. Where local hygiene measures have failed, a frenectomy may be advocated if it will give greater access to the site for cleaning.

Surgical root coverage

The main techniques are as follows.

- Pedicle grafts:
  - rotational flaps: these have largely been superseded by newer techniques
  - advanced flaps: coronally advanced flap. Often used with enamel matrix derivatives, connective tissue graft or acellular dermal matrix allograft material.
- Guided tissue regeneration. Used with or without enamel matrix derivatives.
- Free grafts:
  - epithelialised gingival grafts
  - subepithelial connective tissue graft.

Pedicle grafts
Rotational flaps

These have been used historically for covering small areas of gingival recession where a donor site is locally available but have been largely superseded by newer techniques (see next sections). For the laterally repositioned flap (Fig. 33.3), a split-thickness flap is created by sharp dissection at the donor site and advanced to the new location. Two flaps are raised in the double papilla flap technique (Fig. 33.4). Flaps gain nutrition from the base of the pedicle flap and from the prepared recipient site of periosteum surrounding the denuded area of root.

Advanced flaps

A mucosal flap can be raised beyond the mucogingival junction and moved coronally because of the elasticity of the tissue. Single or multiple defects can be covered. A systematic review and meta-analysis showed that for a single site of gingival recession, the coronally advanced flap with subepithelial connective tissue graft (see Free grafts below) gives the best and most stable root coverage (Dai *et al.*, 2019).

Guided tissue regeneration

The principles are discussed in Chapter 26 and the technique is used in conjunction with traditional flaps.

Free grafts

A free graft is taken from a remote site of keratinised tissue, usually the palate, to cover the area of recession (Figs 33.5, 33.6). A template can be used to take the correct amount of graft tissue.

The subepithelial connective tissue graft is harvested from the palate by a 'trap door' approach (Figs 33.7, 33.8) and generally leaves a less invasive wound and gives a better aesthetic result. The recipient site must be prepared to receive the graft and the graft carefully stabilised with sutures. A tunnel technique can be used where a sulcular incision is made beyond the mucogingival line and without raising the papillae. The graft is then placed within this tunnel to cover the sites of gingival recession. Enamel matrix derivative (EMD) can be used as an adjunct and may enhance the stability of the results of coronally advanced flap alone (Dai *et al.*, 2019). The predictability of root coverage is dependent on several factors including the anatomy of the recession defects (Fig. 33.2) with greater success of modern surgical techniques in the hands of skilled practitioners.

Allografts

These have the advantage that the patient does not require a surgical procdure to harvest the graft so surgery is only required at the site of recession. Acellular dermal connective tissue is derived from human donor skin tissue and can be used in place of the subepithelial connective graft.

34 Gingival enlargement

Figure 34.1 Gingival enlargement. (a) Gingival enlargement in a patient in the second trimester of pregnancy. The gingivae are very inflamed and bleed easily and are associated with the presence of generalised plaque deposits. (b) Drug-influenced gingival enlargement associated with the calcium channel blocking drug nifedipine. Note the enlarged interdental papillae and the deposits of gingival plaque.

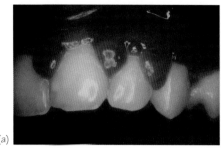
(a)

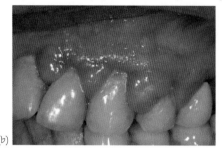
(b)

Figure 34.2 Causes of gingival enlargement.

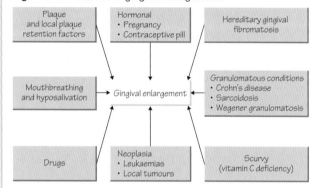

- Plaque and local plaque retention factors
- Hormonal
  - Pregnancy
  - Contraceptive pill
- Hereditary gingival fibromatosis
- Mouthbreathing and hyposalivation
- Gingival enlargement
- Granulomatous conditions
  - Crohn's disease
  - Sarcoidosis
  - Wegener granulomatosis
- Drugs
- Neoplasia
  - Leukaemias
  - Local tumours
- Scurvy (vitamin C deficiency)

Figure 34.3 Main drugs associated with drug-influenced gingival enlargement.

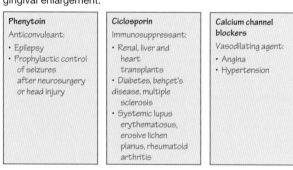

Phenytoin	Ciclosporin	Calcium channel blockers
Anticonvulsant: • Epilepsy • Prophylactic control of seizures after neurosurgery or head injury	Immunosuppressant: • Renal, liver and heart transplants • Diabetes, behçet's disease, multiple sclerosis • Systemic lupus erythematosus, erosive lichen planus, rheumatoid arthritis	Vasodilating agent: • Angina • Hypertension

Figure 34.4 Characteristics of drug-influenced gingival enlargement. The features listed may be seen in drug-influenced gingival enlargement but some are also found in gingival enlargement related to other aetiological factors.

- Interdental areas
- Anterior gingivae more than posterior
- Labial more than lingual
- Mandible more than maxilla
- Dense, firm, lobulated
- Pseudopocketing
- Lobulated masses separated by grooves
- Interproximal enlargement may cause tooth migration
- If plaque induced inflammation present:
  - Bleeding
  - Oedema
  - Redness
- Higher prevalence in young age groups
- Onset within 3 months of drug use
- Not associated with attachment loss (though can be found in a periodontium with or without bone loss)

Figure 34.5 Management of gingival enlargement.

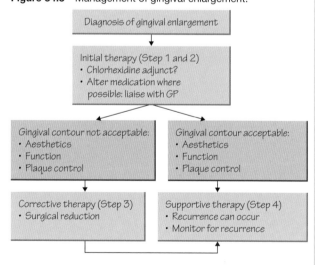

- Diagnosis of gingival enlargement
- Initial therapy (Step 1 and 2)
  - Chlorhexidine adjunct?
  - Alter medication where possible: liaise with GP
- Gingival contour not acceptable:
  - Aesthetics
  - Function
  - Plaque control
- Gingival contour acceptable:
  - Aesthetics
  - Function
  - Plaque control
- Corrective therapy (Step 3)
  - Surgical reduction
- Supportive therapy (Step 4)
  - Recurrence can occur
  - Monitor for recurrence

Periodontology at a Glance, Second Edition. Valerie Clerehugh, Aradhna Tugnait, Michael R. Milward, and Iain L. C. Chapple.
© 2024 John Wiley & Sons Ltd. Published 2024 by John Wiley & Sons Ltd.

Figure 34.6 Surgical management of drug-influenced gingival enlargement. (a) Preoperatively, the gingivae appear pink and fibrous with marked enlargement of the interdental papillae of the lower anterior teeth. (b) Gingivectomy incision to resect excess tissue (see Chapter 25 and Figure 25.1). (c) Tissue healing one month post surgery. Source: Courtesy of Mr J. Chesterman.

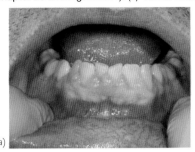 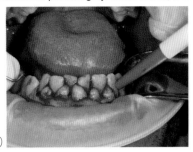 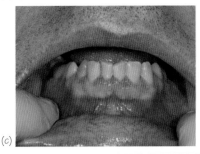

(a)   (b)   (c)

Gingival enlargement or gingival overgrowth is a term given to the development of increased gingival bulk that can arise from a number of causes. In many cases there is associated plaque-related inflammation. This may be involved in the development of the overgrowth, but the enlarged tissue contour is difficult to clean and so also acts as a local plaque retention factor.

The appearance of the enlargement varies. The tissues may be red, swollen and inflamed and tend to bleed easily, or may be pink and fibrous if associated with increased collagen formation (Fig. 34.1). If the gingival tissue is invaded by neoplastic cells or granulomas then it may appear more solid but may still present with a superimposed inflammatory component. The clinical appearance cannot be considered as diagnostic of any particular aetiology. Referral for further investigations should be considered if there are systemic signs of ill health or concerns about the possible diagnosis.

Problems experienced by patients with gingival enlargement include:

- the poor appearance of the gingivae
- functional discomfort if the gingiva extends onto the occlusal surfaces
- difficulty in plaque removal.

Causes of gingival enlargement

Readers are referred to textbooks in oral medicine for greater depth on this subject (Chapple & Hamburger, 2006). Drug-influenced gingival enlargement is covered in the following section, while the other main causes are listed below and shown in Fig. 34.2.

Sex steroid hormones

This is most commonly associated with pregnancy (see Fig. 31.9a).

- It is plaque related.
- It ranges in prevalence and severity.
- It commences in the second month and peaks in the eighth month.
- Increased progesterone alters the microcirculation.
- Subgingival microflora may be altered.
- A pregnancy epulis can develop in some cases (marked swelling of the interdental papilla; see Fig. 31.9b).

Leukaemias

In the leukaemias, white blood cells are abnormal.

- The white cells are unable to control infection at the gingival margins.
- The white cells infiltrate the gingival tissue, causing swelling.

Hereditary gingival fibromatosis

- This is associated with several hereditary disorders.
- The most common is an autosomal dominant syndrome. Other features are hypertrichosis, epilepsy, hearing loss and intellectual disability.
- Gingival overgrowth can precede eruption or occur in childhood.
- Marked overgrowth can bury the teeth.

Granulomatous conditions
Crohn's disease

- This affects the ileocaecal region.
- Abdominal pain, constipation or diarrhoea can occur.
- Oral lesions may precede abdominal symptoms:
  - gingival swelling and reddening
  - cobblestone thickening of the buccal mucosa
  - lip swelling
  - ulcers
  - glossitis.

Granulomatosis with polyangiitis (Wegener)

- This is characterised by granulomatous inflammation of the nasopharynx, pulmonary cavitation and glomerulonephritis.
- The gingivae are swollen with a granular surface clasically described as 'strawberry gingivae'. Giant cells are seen histologically.

Sarcoidosis

- Non-caseating granulomas are found in the lungs, lymph nodes and other sites such as the mouth.
- The gingivae, lips, palate and buccal mucosa can be involved.

Scurvy

The gingivae are grossly enlarged in advanced disease.

Drug-influenced gingival enlargement

This is associated mainly with the following agents.

- Anticonvulsants: phenytoin.
- Immunosppressants: ciclosporin.
- Calcium channel blockers:
  - nifedipine
  - diltiazem
  - amlodipine.

Figure 34.3 shows the main uses of these drugs. A wide range in the prevalence of the condition has been described for all of these drugs. Other drugs for which drug-influenced gingival enlargement has been described as a side-effect are sodium valproate and erythromycin.

Figure 34.4 lists the main characteristics of drug-influenced gingival enlargement.

Role of plaque in drug-influenced gingival enlargement

There is an association between oral hygiene and gingival inflammation and the severity of drug-induced gingival enlargement. However, it is not clear to what extent plaque contributes to the tissue changes or if it accumulates because of the excessive tissue contour.

Risk factors

- There is an association between age and the severity of enlargement for ciclosporin.
- Males seem to be more severely affected.
- There is an increased prevalence and severity of gingival enlargement with combinations of the associated drugs:
  - ciclosporin and amlodipine
  - ciclosporin and nifedipine.
- Other medication can affect severity.
  - There is reduced severity in transplant patients with prednisolone and azathioprine.
  - Increased enlargement is seen with phenytoin given with other anticonvulsants: phenobarbitone and carbamazepine.
- Genetic factors: HLA-B37 may protect from enlargement.

Drug variables

- A threshold of drug is probably required to initiate enlargement.
- Drug dosages are a poor predictor of gingival changes.
- The extent of enlargement and dose are not always closely related.
- Other measures such as the degree of drug protein binding or bioavailability may be appropriate.
- It is not clear if salivary concentrations of the drugs are correlated with the degree of gingival enlargement.

Management

Management of gingival enlargement is summarised in Fig. 34.5 and follows the principles of the stepwise approach covered in Chapter 19. Initial therapy (Step 1 and 2) is directed at the removal of plaque, calculus and local factors. Chlorhexidine mouthrinse can be a useful adjunct in the management of gingival enlargement. Appropriate and potentially urgent referral will be necessary if the oral symptoms are the first presenting sign of an undiagnosed systemic condition.

Where the enlargement is related to an underlying systemic condition, medical management will often lead to an improvement in the gingival overgrowth. Liaison with the general medical practitioner and any specialists is therefore appropriate to consider prescribing alternative drugs. Tacrolimus has been given to renal and cardiac transplant patients as an alternative to ciclosporin. It is not associated with gingival enlargement and rapid resolution or substantial reductions of the ciclosporin-induced enlargement have been reported following a change to tacrolimus. However, this drug does have several other non-oral side-effects.

Depending on the aetiology, surgical intervention to remove excess tissue or recontour the gingivae may be considered when non-surgical therapy does not bring about sufficient resolution of the gingival enlargement (Step 3, Fig. 34.6). Supportive therapy (Step 4) is important for long-term stability though recurrence of gingival enlargement is possible. However, where this is drug influenced recurrence is common if the drugs cannot be changed.

Key points

- There are several causes of gingival enlargement, although the clinical appearance is not generally diagnostic
- In most cases there is associated plaque-related inflammation
- Drug-influenced gingival enlargement is associated mainly with:
  - phenytoin
  - ciclosporin
  - calcium channel blockers
- Following the identification of aetiological factors, management is organised into:
  - initial therapy (Step 1 and 2) including control of plaque and review of medication with medical team
  - corrective therapy including surgical reduction as required (Step 3)
  - supportive therapy including monitoring for recurrence (Step 4)

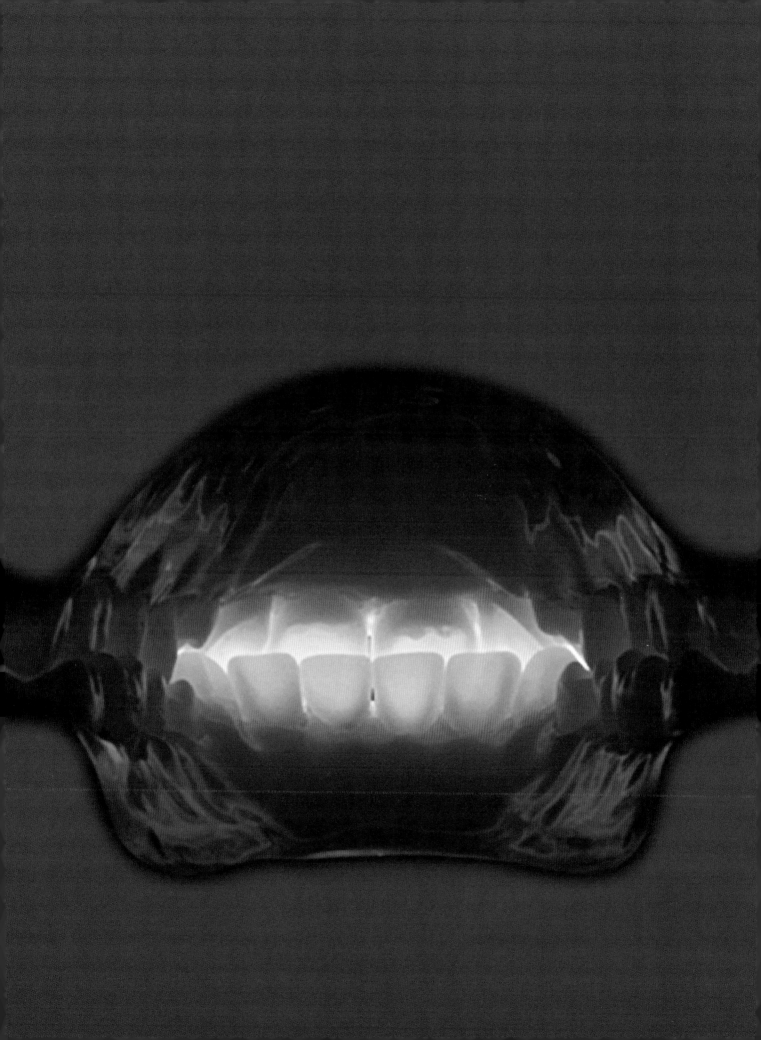

35 Periodontitis

Figure 35.1 (a) Section through tooth with incipient (initial Stage I) periodontitis. (b) Section through tooth with established periodontitis.

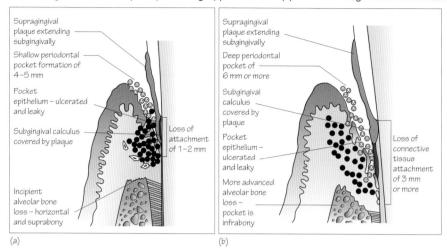

(a)
- Supragingival plaque extending subgingivally
- Shallow periodontal pocket formation of 4–5 mm
- Pocket epithelium – ulcerated and leaky
- Subgingival calculus covered by plaque
- Loss of attachment of 1–2 mm
- Incipient alveolar bone loss – horizontal and suprabony

(b)
- Supragingival plaque extending subgingivally
- Deep periodontal pocket of 6 mm or more
- Subgingival calculus covered by plaque
- Pocket epithelium – ulcerated and leaky
- More advanced alveolar bone loss – pocket is infrabony
- Loss of connective tissue attachment of 3 mm or more

Figure 35.2 Incipient (initial Stage I) periodontitis. (a) Subgingival calculus on mesio-buccal UR6 (arrow). (b) Subgingival calculus on mesio-buccal UL6 (arrow) and supragingival calculus on UL7. (c) Right horizontal bitewing showing slight horizontal bone loss and calculus mesio-buccal UR6 (arrow). (d) Left horizontal bitewing showing slight horizontal bone loss and calculus mesio-buccal UL6 (arrow).

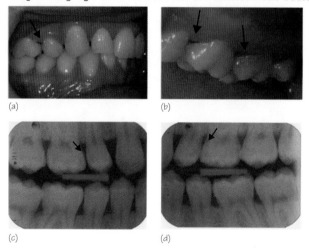

(a) (b)
(c) (d)

Figure 35.3 Smoking-related periodontitis. (a) Calculus labial LL1. (b) Subgingival calculus visible as dark shadow palatal upper incisors (arrows). (c) Right horizontal bitewing showing subgingival calculus. (d) Left horizontal bitewing, mesial overhang and vertical bone loss UL8; furcation involvement LL8. (e) Supragingival calculus lingual lower anteriors (arrow).

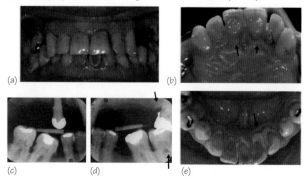

(a) (b)
(c) (d) (e)

Periodontology at a Glance, Second Edition. Valerie Clerehugh, Aradhna Tugnait, Michael R. Milward, and Iain L. C. Chapple.
© 2024 John Wiley & Sons Ltd. Published 2024 by John Wiley & Sons Ltd.

Figure 35.4 (a–c) Slight drifting of incisors, diastemas present between upper incisors. (d) Right vertical bitewing. (e) Left vertical bitewing showing vertical bone loss between UL6 and UL7 (arrow).

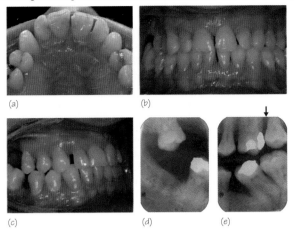

(a) (b) (c) (d) (e)

Figure 35.5 (a–c) Severe drifting of UL1 due to bone loss leading to lip trapping. (d) Scanora® panoramic radiograph showing bone loss and periodontal-endodontic lesions on UL6 and LR2 which were both extracted.

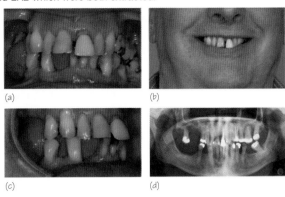

(a) (b) (c) (d)

Figure 35.6 Inflammation and blunting of papilla between UL2 and UL3.

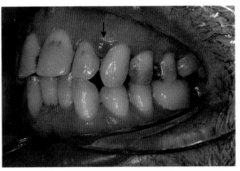

Figure 35.7 Suppuration. (a) Palatal suppuration. (b,c) Periapicals of crowned incisor teeth showing horizontal bone loss.

(a) (b) (c)

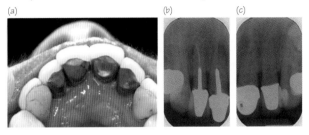

Figure 35.8 (a,b) Pretreatment inflammation and swelling. (c) Posttreatment image showing resolution.

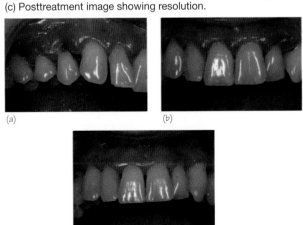

(a) (b) (c)

Figure 35.9 (a) Pretreatment, showing inflammation and swelling around upper anterior teeth. (b) Posttreatment resolution of inflammation with recession and exposure of crown margin of UL1 which is now supragingival. Due to poor aesthetics, crown can be replaced.

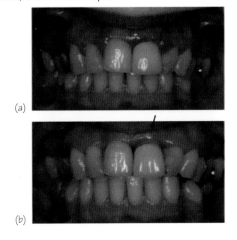

(a) (b)

A new classification for periodontitis was developed by the World Workshop on the Classification of Periodontal and Peri-Implant Diseases and Conditions and published in 2018, hence it is referred to as the '2018 classification'. Based on emerging scientific evidence and current knowledge of pathophysiology, three forms of periodontitis were identified: necrotising periodontitis (Chapter 39); periodontitis as a direct manifestation of systemic disease (Chapter 2); and the conditions previously called chronic or aggressive periodontitis in the 1999 International Workshop classification are now grouped under the single category of 'periodontitis'. As part of the revision of the 2018 classification, the Workshop agreed on a system of staging and grading of periodontitis which could be adapted as new evidence emerged.

Periodontitis is a complex multifactorial disease that has been defined as an inflammatory disease affecting the supporting tissues around teeth which can cause irreversible loss of periodontal ligament and alveolar bone, tooth mobility and, if left untreated, ultimately tooth loss (Fine *et al*., 2018). It is caused by an aberrant immune response to resident microbial communities on the teeth, which extend subgingivally. Normally the host lives symbiotically with the biofilm, but an individual can convert to an aberrant and dysbiotic microbiome and host response, resulting in periodontal destruction.

Features of periodontitis

Key features of periodontitis (Fig. 35.1) are as follows.
- Interproximal clinical attachment loss (CAL).
- Bone loss, visible on radiographs, which may be horizontal pattern (Figs 35.1a, 35.2, 35.7) or vertical (infrabony) (Figs 35.1b, 35.3, 35.4).
- True pocket formation of 4 mm or more.

Clinical presentation may also include the following.
- Poor plaque control; supragingival and subgingival calculus are frequently found (Figs 35.2, 35.3). There is a variable subgingival plaque microflora.
- Drifting of incisors (Figs 35.4, 35.5); bleeding on probing; inflammation (Figs 35.6, 35.8, 35.9); mobility; recession (Figs 35.3, 35.5); furcation defects (Fig. 35.3); suppuration (Fig. 35.7); halitosis.

Based on the new classification, periodontitis should be staged and graded.

Staging and grading (see Chapter 36)

- Staging reflects disease severity at presentation and complexity of overall patient management. It takes account of CAL, amount and % of bone loss, probing depth, presence and extent of angular defects, furcation involvement, tooth mobility and tooth loss due to periodontitis. It has four categories: I, initial; II, moderate; III, severe with potential for additional tooth loss; IV, advanced with extensive tooth loss and potential for loss of dentition.
- Periodontitis can also be further classified according to extent and distribution: localised, less than 30% sites affected; generalised, ≥30% affected; molar-incisor distribution.

- Grading reflects the patient's susceptibility to disease and takes account of periodontitis progression, patient health status and risk factors which may influence treatment response, specifically smoking and diabetes control. There are three rates of progression (A slow; B moderate; C rapid).

The British Society of Periodontology and Implant Dentistry has provided a workable framework for the implementation of the new staging and grading system into clinical practice (see Appendix 3 and Chapter 36) and published some clinical scenarios of its application (Dietrich *et al*., 2019).

Periodontitis can manifest in the incipient stages in teenagers (Figs 35.1a, 35.2; Chapter 41). Interproximal CAL of 1–2 mm may be found, commonly on maxillary first molars and mandibular incisors in the initial stages, but any teeth can become affected (Fig. 35.1a, 35.2). Early crestal alveolar bone loss, typically horizontal, may be present (Fig. 35.2 c,d). The prevalence, extent and severity of CAL increase slowly throughout the teens, in association with plaque and subgingival calculus (typically Stage I, Grade A). With increasing age, the cumulative effects of attachment loss, pocket formation and alveolar bone loss become more apparent (Fig. 35.1b) and can affect a sizeable proportion of the adult population (Chapter 3).

Grade modifiers, risk factors

Smoking and diabetes (if poorly controlled, HbA1c >7.5%) are cited as risk factors and grade modifiers (Grade B and C).

Typical features of patients who smoke (Fig. 35.3) include more severe CAL, pockets and radiographic bone loss than in same-age peers with similar plaque levels, therefore expect higher staging levels. Gingiva are pale and fibrous with less bleeding on probing due to fewer blood vessels and the vasoconstrictive effects of nicotine on the vasculature. Maxillary anterior and palatal surfaces are more adversely affected; anterior recession may be present.

Treatment response is poorer.

If BPE = 4 or * in an adolescent, look for modifying factors or suspect a rapidly progressing form of periodontitis (Grade C, Stage III or IV), consistent with the condition previously known as localised aggressive periodontitis (Chapter 41).

Management

Management follows the stepwise approach outlined below but covered in more detail in Chapter 19 which is based on the European step 3 (S3)-level treatment guideline (Sanz *et al*., 2020) and the BSP implementation of this (Kebschull & Chapple, 2020; West *et al*., 2021) (Fig. 19.5; see also Appendix 4).

Step 1 Building foundations for optimal treatment outcomes

Step 1 aims to control the plaque biofilm and may lead to behaviour change/motivation. It includes:
- tailored OHI
- professional mechanical plaque removal (PMPR) to remove supragingival and subgingival plaque and calculus on the tooth crown
- risk factor (RF) control.

Step 2 Subgingival biofilm and calculus control/removal

Step 2 is the cause-related phase of therapy and aims to control the subgingival plaque biofilm. It includes:

* subgingival PMPR
* possible adjunctive therapies for gingival inflammation.

Step 3 Management of non-responding sites (≥4 mm with BOP or ≥6 mm)

Step 3 is directed at treating non-responding sites to gain access to further subgingival instrumentation and may involve:

* repeated non-surgical subgingival PMPR for residual pockets of 4–5 mm with BOP
* surgical interventions for PDs ≥6 mm.

Step 4 Maintenance/supportive periodontal therapy (SPT)

Step 4 aims to maintain periodontal stability through SPT in all treated periodontitis patients, recognising they are 'periodontitis patients' for life. It combines:

* preventive/therapeutic interventions from Steps 1–3 if needed
* regular recall intervals tailored to patient's individual needs
* management of recurrent disease with an updated diagnosis and treatment plan
* compliance with OHI, healthy lifestyle, PMPR and ongoing RF control.

For stage IV periodontitis the focus shifts from the treatment of periodontitis to restoration of severe periodontitis cases.

Key points

* Periodontitis is a complex multifactorial inflammatory disease due to a dysbiotic microbiome and host response leading to irreversible periodontal destruction
* It can begin in adolescence and progress into adulthood
* Staging reflects severity and complexity of periodontitis and ranges from I to IV
* Grading reflects susceptibility and rate of progression of periodontitis and is in three levels (A, B, C)
* Treatment is based on the European S3-level treatment guideline and BSP's implementation of this

36 Staging and grading

Figure 36.1 BSP implementation of staging and grading in clinical practice. Source: Adapted from Dietrich *et al.* (2019), Table 2.

Staging of Periodontitis	Stage I Early/Mild	Stage II Moderate	Stage III Severe	Stage IV Very Severe
Interdental bone loss*	< 15 % or < 2 mm**	Coronal third of root	Mid third of root	Apical third of root***
* Maximum bone loss in % of root length ** Measurement in mm from CEJ if only bitewing radiograph available (bone loss) or no radiographs clinically justified (CAL) *** Stage IV can be assigned if tooth loss likely to have been due to bone loss in apical third of root				
Extent	Describe as: Localised (up to 30% of teeth) Generalised (more than 30% of teeth) Molar/incisor pattern			
Grading of Periodontitis	Grade A Slow		Grade B Moderate	Grade C Rapid
% Bone loss/Age	< 0.5		0.5–1.0	>1.0
Risk Factor Assessment	eg Smoking (≥ 10 cigarettes/day)		eg Diabetes mellitus (if sub-optimal control)	
Assessment of Current Periodontal Status	Currently Stable BOP < 10% PPD ≤ 4 mm No BOP at 4 mm sites		Currently In Remission BOP ≥ 10% PPD ≤ 4 mm No BOP at 4 mm sites	Currently Unstable PPD ≥ 5 mm or PPD ≥ 4 mm & BOP

Figure 36.2 Clinical decision-making algorithm. Source: Courtesy of corresponding author Professor I.L.C. Chapple.

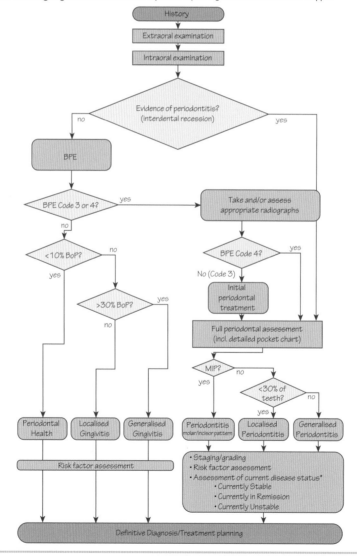

Periodontology at a Glance, Second Edition. Valerie Clerehugh, Aradhna Tugnait, Michael R. Milward, and Iain L. C. Chapple.
© 2024 John Wiley & Sons Ltd. Published 2024 by John Wiley & Sons Ltd.

As part of the 2018 classification emanating from the World Workshop on the Classification of Periodontal and Peri-Implant Diseases and Conditions held in 2017, the Workshop agreed on a system of staging and grading of periodontitis (Chapter 35) once a diagnosis of periodontitis had been confirmed (Chapter 19) which could be adapted as new evidence emerged (Tonetti *et al.*, 2018). For a consensus definition of what constitutes a periodontitis case, please see Chapters 3, 9 and Fig 9.6.

Staging and grading

Staging

Staging should be undertaken first and reflects the severity of periodontitis at initial presentation and is also linked to the complexity of case management.

- Stage I, early/mild
- Stage II, moderate
- Stage III, severe
- Stage IV, very severe

In order to facilitate implementation of the staging system into general dental practice, the British Society of Periodontology and Implant Dentistry (BSP) proposed a simplified staging grid based on radiographic bone loss alone (% bone loss in relation to root length, at worst site in the mouth), since CAL is not routinely measured in clinical practice and certain complexity measures such as tooth loss due to periodontitis and alveolar ridge defects may be poorly defined/difficult to discern in practice (Dietrich *et al.*, 2019) (Fig. 36.1).

The extent should also be added to the stage as a descriptor.

- Localised, up to 30% of teeth.
- Generalised, more than 30% of teeth.
- Molar/incisor pattern.

A key underlying principle of staging is that patients cannot regress to a lower stage of periodontitis due to treatment; this means that periodontal parameters that would be significantly affected by treatment such as PPD or BOP cannot be used to determine disease stage.

Pragmatically, for some patients, especially those with early-stage, incipient periodontitis, available radiographs may be limited to posterior bitewings, with no radiographs in anterior sextants; if periapicals or panoramic radiographs are not clinically justified, then the clinician can take a measurement in mm from the CEJ using bitewings or measure CAL; a measure of <2 mm radiographic bone loss or 1–2 mm CAL would be stage I. The clinician can assign stage IV if tooth loss is deemed likely to have been due to advanced periodontal bone loss affecting the apical third of the root (Fig. 36.1).

Grading

Grading takes account of the patient's susceptibility to disease, historical disease experience and the rate of progression of periodontitis. Grades can be modfied by the presence of risk factors. Periodontal disease experience at presentation has been recognised as the best predictor of future disease in the absence of treatment (Machtei *et al.*, 1999).

Various measures of disease susceptibilty were discussed at the 2017 World Workshop (Tonetti *et al.*, 2018). The BSP implementation group deemed that the ratio of % bone loss/age was the most pragmatic measure and suitable for use in clinical practice; however, of three thresholds considered, a different threshold of % bone loss/age to that proposed by Tonetti *et al.* (2018) was concluded to be more appropriate for clinical practice by Dietrich *et al.* (2019), and has been adopted by the BSP for implementation in the UK (Fig. 36.1).

- Grade A, slow <0.5
- Grade B, moderate 0.5-1.0
- Grade C, rapid > 1.0

The objective of grading is to use available information to determine the likelihood of the periodontitis case progressing at a greater rate than would be typical for the majority of the population or responding less predictably or favourably to standard therapy.

Grading is assigned based on the assessment of radiographic bone loss on the worst affected tooth in the dentition. Grade A is assigned if the maximum amount of radiographic bone loss as a % of root length is less than half the patient's age (e.g. less than 30% in a 60 year old, less than 40% in an 80 year old, less than 15% in a 30 year old, less than 10% in a 20 year old). Grade C is assigned if the maximum amount of radiographic bone loss as a % of root length exceeds the patient's age (e.g. more than 30% in a 29 year old; more than 50% in a 49 year old; more than 20% in a 19 year old). Grade B is assigned otherwise.

Risk factor assessment should be undertaken as it is essential for treatment planning and patient management. The presence of periodontal risk factors can be used to modify the grade to a higher score, e.g. smoking 10 or more cigarettes per day, or suboptimal diabetes control, based on the HbA1c and current recommended guideline by bodies such as the National Institute for Health and Care Exellence (NICE).

The staging and grading system does not account for the current health/disease status (stable/in remission/unstable) so the BSP implementation plan has included this by incorporating the presence of true pockets and bleeding on probing (reflecting inflammation) as they drive clinical treatment planning (Fig. 36.1).

Holistically, a clinical decision-making algorithm is available to guide clinicians on reaching a definitive diagnosis and treatment plan, incorporating the type and extent of disease, periodontitis staging and grading, current disease status and risk factor assessment, beginning with the history and examination, BPE screening and showing when it may be appropriate to take radiographs and conduct a full periodontal assessment (Fig. 36.2).

A pragmatic, workable framework for the implementation of the 2018 classification's staging and grading system into clinical practice has been published by the BSP (www.bsperio.org.uk/publications) (see Appendix 3) and various clinical scenarios of its application have been published (Dietrich *et al.*, 2019; Wadia *et al.*, 2019; Walter *et al.*, 2019a,b,c,d).

Key points

- Staging reflects severity and complexity of periodontitis and ranges from I to IV
- Grading reflects susceptibility and rate of progression of periodontitis and is in three levels (A, B, C)
- A clinical decision-making algorithm is available to guide clinicians on reaching a definitive diagnosis and treatment plan, incorporating the type and extent of disease, periodontitis staging and grading, current disease status and risk factor assessment

37 Periodontal management of patients who smoke

Figure 37.1 Health problems related to cigarette smoking.

Cancers due to smoking:	Other diseases:
• Lung	• Chronic obstructive pulmonary disease
• Oral	• Pneumonia
• Throat	• Heart disease, angina
• Oesophagus	• Cerebrovascular disease
• Bladder	• Osteoporosis
• Kidney	• Infertility, impotence
• Stomach	• Skin wrinkling
• Pancreas	• Macular degeneration (retina)
• Leukaemia	• Low birth weight baby
	• Periodontal diseases, NG
	• Passive smoking effects
(a)	(b) • Poorer mental health/well-being

Figure 37.2 Clinical appearance and characteristics in a cigarette smoker.

Clinical appearance in smoker	Clinical characteristics of smoker
• Fibrotic 'tight' gingiva, rolled margins	• Relatively earlier onset
• Less gingival redness and bleeding	• Rapid disease progression
• More severe, widespread disease than same age non-smoking control	• Greater severity and extent of disease (pockets, clinical attachment loss, bone loss)
• Anterior, maxilla, palate are worst areas affected	• More tooth loss
• Anterior recession, open embrasures	• Poorer response to non-surgical therapy
• Nicotine staining	• Recurrence within 1 year of surgery – ?avoid surgery
(a) • Calculus	(b) • Increased % are refractory to treatment

Figure 37.3 Male with smoking-related periodontitis. (a) Drifting and diastema between UR1 and UL1. (b) Panoramic radiograph showing generalised bone loss and an endodontic-periodontal lesion on LR5 which was subsequently extracted. (c) Palatal effects of smoking. (d) Palatal view of nicotine staining and inflamed, rolled gingival margins. (e) Fibrotic, pale gingiva. (f) Following extraction of LR5. (g) Recession and nicotine staining. (h) Nicotine-stained supragingival calculus.

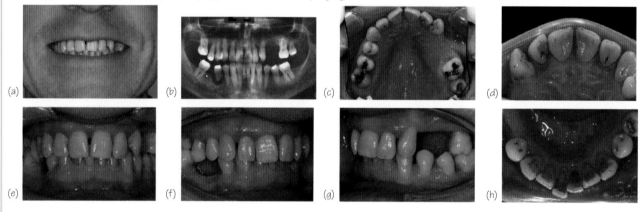

Figure 37.4 (a) Female with smoking-related periodontitis. (b) Upper and lower partial dentures *in situ*; staining and generalised recession. (c) Shortened dental arch following several extractions; denture-related stomatitis. (d) Marked recession/clinical attachment loss (e) Heavily nicotine-stained supragingival calculus on the lingual of the lower incisors.

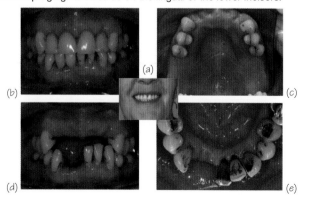

Figure 37.5 Quit smoking.

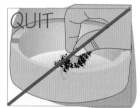

Periodontology at a Glance, Second Edition. Valerie Clerehugh, Aradhna Tugnait, Michael R. Milward, and Iain L. C. Chapple.
© 2024 John Wiley & Sons Ltd. Published 2024 by John Wiley & Sons Ltd.

Figure 37.6 (a) The three As. (b) Ask. (c) Advise. (d) Act. (e) Quitting methods.

The three As for the Dental Team
- Ask all patients about tobacco use as part of the medical history

After clinical examination, for at-risk patients:
- ADVISE on methods to quit
- ACT on their response

Based on guidance in: Smoking and Tobacco Use, Delivering Better Oral Health 4th Edition, Public Health England, Chapter 11, updated 9 November 2021. Available at: https://www.gov.uk/government/publications/delivering-better-oral-health-an-evidence-based-toolkit-for-prevention. Accessed on 17/11/22

(a)

ASK
- Ask all patients about their smoking status as part of medical history: 'Do you smoke?'
  - Record information in the clinical notes
  - Current, former, never smoker
- If current smoker, record:
  - How many cigarettes smoked daily / how much tobacco smoked
  - How many years smoked
  - Pattern of smoking e.g. on waking, socially

(b)

ADVISE ON METHODS OF QUITTING
- Do not ask patients if they want to quit as this leads to defensiveness
- Avoid detailed questions
- Give brief information on methods of quitting
  - Use clear, strong and personalised language
  - Highlight oral health effects of tobacco
  - Emphasise benefits of quitting

(c)

ACT ON RESPONSE
Interested?
- Acknowledge that e-cigarettes can help quit
- Recommend nicotine replacement therapies
- Refer or signpost to local resources
- Record response in clinical notes

ACT ON RESPONSE
Not interested?
- Give the patient control
- Let them know
  - it's their choice
  - help always available
  - to say if they change mind
  - if wish to quit in the future
    - you can refer them to stop smoking services
    - or, they can contact directly
- Record in clinical notes
- Ask at future visits

(d)

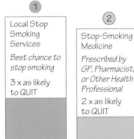
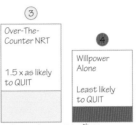

1. Local Stop Smoking Services — Best chance to stop smoking — 3 x as likely to QUIT

2. Stop-Smoking Medicine — Prescribed by GP, Pharmacist, or Other Health Professional — 2 x as likely to QUIT

3. Over-The-Counter NRT — 1.5 x as likely to QUIT

4. Willpower Alone — Least likely to QUIT

*Based on guidance in Fig 11.3 in Delivering Better Oral Health 4th Edition, Public Health England, updated 9 November 2021

(e)

Figure 37.7 Three steps to stop smoking.

1. PREPARING TO STOP
   - Set quit date
     - Vital to want to stop
   - List and re-read the benefits of stopping
2. STOPPING
   - Aim to get through the first day without smoking
   - Have strategies to relieve craving
     - e.g. Deep breaths until craving gone, chew sugar-free gum
3. STAYING STOPPED
   - Be aware that most people need several attempts to stop
     - Should not give up trying to quit
   - It can take up to 3 months to become a non-smoker
     - Usually takes less time
   - Physical craving often disappears in less than a week
     - Psychological dependence can last longer

Figure 37.8 Resources and support to stop smoking in the UK and the US.

RESOURCES AND SUPPORT
UK
- Free Smokefree National Helpline 0300 123 1044
- Websites:
  - Better Health Quit Smoking: https://www.nhs.uk/better-health/quit-smoking/
  - National Institute for Health and Care Excellence (NICE): https://www.nice.org.uk/guidance/ng209
  - NHS A-Z: https://www.nhs.uk/conditions/stop-smoking-treatments/
  - NHS Live Well: https://www.nhs.uk/live-well/quit-smoking/
  - Tommy's Pregnancy Hub: https://www.tommys.org/pregnancy-information/im-pregnant/smoking-and-pregnancy
US
- Free National Quitline 1-800-QUIT-NOW for national portal to state-based quitline services: https://www.cdc.gov/tobacco/features/quitlines/index.html
- Websites:
  - Smoking cessation evidence and resources (US Department of Health and Human Services, Agency for Healthcare Research and Quality): https://www.ahrq.gov/evidencenow/projects/heart-health/evidence/smoking.html
  - Smokefree: https://smokefree.gov

All websites accessed 17 Nov 2022

Table 37.1 Direct benefits of stopping smoking.

Time after cessation	Direct benefits
2 days	Sense of taste and smell improved
One month	Skin clearer, more hydrated
3 months	Improved breathing, no cough or wheeze Improved lung function (up to 10%) Risk of mouth and throat cancer reduced Most smoking related oral white patches gone
6 months	Gingival circulation improved
One year	Risk of heart attack reduced to half that of a smoker
10 years	Risk of lung cancer reduced by half
15 years	Risk of heart attack same as never-smoker Risk of tooth loss same as never-smoker

Table 37.2 Indirect benefits of stopping smoking.

Reasons to stop	Indirect benefits
Passive smoking	No longer causing harm to others through passive smoking, especially babies/children: – Sudden infant death syndrome – Asthma, ear and chest infections
Children	Less likely children will go on to smoke – Children of smokers are three times more likely to smoke
Unborn baby	Limiting harm to unborn baby – Most harmful effects in second and third trimester; risk of low birth weight baby – Quitting in first 3 months reduces risk to normal
Costs	Savings from not buying cigarettes

Tobacco smoking is a major cause of death and morbidity (Fig. 37.1) throughout the world. According to the World Health Organization (2022), tobacco kills up to half of its users and in 2020, 22.3% of the global population used tobacco; smoking-related diseases accounted for 8 million deaths annually. In the UK, although the prevalence of smoking has declined from 20.2% in 2011 to 13.8% of the population aged 18 years or more in 2020 (ONS, 2020), it remains the largest cause of preventable death and disease in the UK (Public Health England, 2021); the prevalence is highest in the 25–34-year-old age band (18.3%, around 1.5 million people) and continues to be higher in men (15.5%) than women (12.1%). The proportion of cigarette smokers who have quit continues to rise; of those who smoked regularly but do not currently smoke, 64.0% said they had quit in 2020. According to the Centers for Disease Control and Prevention (CDC, 2022) in the United States, cigarette smoking accounts for more than 480 000 deaths every year (~1 in 5) and, as in the UK, is the leading cause of preventable disease, disability and death in the US. Current smoking in adults aged ≥18 years declined from 20.9% in 2005 to 12.5% in 2020.

Nicotine

Tobacco smoke contains around 4000 chemicals, including nicotine (which is highly addictive), tar (which deposits in the lungs and contains carcinogens), carbon monoxide (which binds to haemoglobin in the blood, thus preventing carriage of sufficient oxygen) and oxidant gases (which make the blood more likely to clot and increase the risk of heart attack or stroke). Nicotine increases the heart rate and causes a rise in noradrenaline and dopamine in the brain, which in turn creates a positive mood swing. When the nicotine effects begin to wear off, this is accompanied by feelings of irritability, anxiety and craving for another cigarette. Nicotine causes dehydration of the skin and can increase certain forms of high blood pressure.

Smokeless tobacco

There are over 30 types of smokeless products, including dry chewing tobacco (part of 'betel quid' or 'paan') and sucked and inhaled tobacco (nasal snuff). Many forms are highly carcinogenic and almost all types cause oral cancer. They contain at least as much nicotine as smoked tobacco and so are highly addictive.

Clinical periodontal management

As well as the general health risks, tobacco smoking is associated with a greater risk of periodontitis (Chapters 10, 11), necrotising gingivitis (NG) (Chapter 39) and oral cancer. The effects are thought to be both local and systemic (Chapter 8). The level of risk relates to the number of pack-years (i.e. packs of cigarettes smoked daily multiplied by the number of years smoked). Periodontal diseases manifest at an earlier age in smokers, are more severe and exhibit several characteristic clinical features (Figs 37.2–37.4).

Management follows the basic stepwise principles of periodontal therapy (Chapter 19). However, periodontal diseases have been found to be more refractory to treatment in smokers than non-smokers.

Use of local antimicrobials (Chapter 23) may provide small adjunctive clinical benefits over and above subgingival PMPR for the management of periodontitis, but clinical improvement is less than in a non-smoker. Some clinicians prefer not to undertake periodontal surgery or implant provision in smokers due to compromised clinical outcome. It is imperative that:

- patients are advised about the risks of smoking and encouraged to quit (Fig. 37.5)
- the provision of smoking cessation advice is recorded in the treatment notes for medicolegal reasons.

Smoking cessation

The National Institute for Health and Care Excellence (NICE, 2022) in the UK and the Department of Health and Human Services, Agency for Healthcare Research and Quality in the US advocate the delivery of brief smoking cessation interventions for every patient who smokes (Agency for Healthcare Research and Quality, 2021). People are three times more likely to quit if they use a combination of stop smoking aids, including e-cigarettes and other forms of nicotine replacement therapy, together with specialist help and support (Public Health England, 2021). Healthcare personnel, including the dental practitioner, hygienist, therapist, dental nurse and oral health educator, have a key role in this. Very brief advice (VBA) from the dental team can double the patient's success in quitting, using the three As approach (Public Health England, 2021) (Fig. 37.6a–d): (i) **A**sk about smoking; (ii) **A**dvise on the best way of stopping smoking with a combination of specialist support and medication; and (iii) **A**ct according to the patient's motivation to quit. However, many patients will need this VBA on a number of occasions before they are ready to act.

Stopping smoking

There are various quitting methods (Fig. 37.6e) but gaining support from local stop smoking services yields the best chance of success (×3). There are three important steps for the patient (Fig. 37.7).

- Preparing to stop.
- Stopping.
- Staying stopped.

The patient should remember the benefits of quitting (Tables 37.1, 37.2) and use all available resources (Fig. 37.8).

Nicotine replacement therapy or e-cigarettes

Due to nicotine's highly addictive properties, nicotine replacement therapy (NRT) is the most common form of smoking cessation treatment. There are various formulations but a key aspect of NRT is to achieve a sufficient dose, often by regular topping up, for a recommended tailored period which varies from six to 12 weeks depending on the selected therapy and whether the individual smokes less or more than 20 cigarettes per day, as per the British National Formulary (BNF, 2022).

Products medicinally licensed for use as a stop smoking aid and for harm reduction include:

- transdermal patches that release nicotine
- chewing gum
- sublingual tablets, lozenges, mouth spray
- inhalators or nasal sprays.

Common side-effects include dizziness, headache, hyperhidrosis, nausea, palpitations, skin reactions and vomiting, which may be alleviated by using a different dose or formulation.

Some find alternative remedies useful, e.g. hypnosis and acupuncture.

E-cigarettes (vapes), whilst not risk free, are less harmful than smoking and growing evidence suggests they can help smokers quit (NICE, 2022); they may contain nicotine or be nicotine free.

Medication

Bupropion and varenicline are drugs, each with various contraindications and side effects, which have been available on prescription from a medical practitioner to help patients who want to quit in combination with motivational support (Public Health England, 2021).

- Bupropion may work on brain pathways involved with addiction and reduces the urge to smoke, and hence aids withdrawal. The BNF issued safety information in November 2020 on the risk of serotonin syndrome with the use of bupropion with other serotonergic drugs.

- Varenicline aids smoking cessation by binding to nicotine receptors in the brain that are implicated in nicotine addiction, thus easing cravings and reducing the pleasurable effects of nicotine. However, according to NICE (2022), varenicline (Champix®) was currently unavailable until further notice in the UK.

Key points
- Tobacco smoking is a major risk factor for general and oral health problems, including periodontitis, necrotising gingivitis and oral cancer
- Patients should be advised of the risks of smoking and this should be recorded in the notes for medicolegal purposes
- Smoking cessation advice should be offered
- Helpful approaches include:
  - the 3 As (**A**sk; **A**dvise; **A**ct)
  - nicotine replacement therapy or medication
  - e-cigarettes

38 Periodontal management of patients with diabetes

Figure 38.1 Examples of insulin pens and cartridges for insulin injections. Tresiba® (Novo-Nordisk) is a long-acting basal insulin; Novopen Echo Plus® (Novo-Nordisk) is a smart insulin pen that records dosing information, e.g. with quick-acting insulin like Fiasp®.

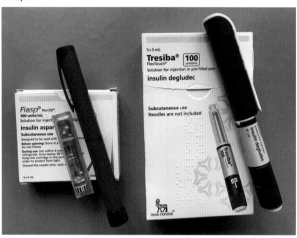

Figure 38.2 A healthy plate of food for people with diabetes: five daily portions of fruit and vegetables; bread, other cereals and potatoes should make up the bulk of the diet (usually low in fat, high in fibre); milk and dairy products in moderation; foods containing fat and sugar should be limited; meat, fish and alternatives in moderation for protein.

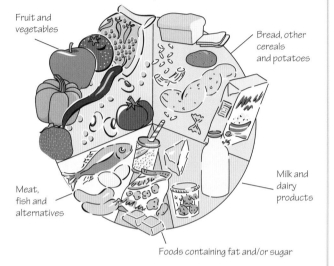

Figure 38.3 (a) Flash glucose monitoring system allows continuous glucose monitoring using a sensor which can be scanned using a smart phone. (b) Glucose monitor for home blood glucose testing.

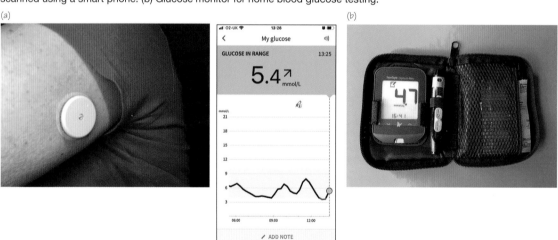

Figure 38.4 Possible complications of diabetes.

Macrovascular complications
- Cardiovascular disease (major cause of death) and peripheral vascular disease (amputations)
- Cerebrovascular disease and stroke

Microvascular complications
- Retinopathy (blindness)
- Nephropathy (renal failure)
- Neuropathy (painful nerve damage)

Figure 38.5   (a–g) A 35-year-old male with periodontitis related to smoking and poorly controlled type 1 diabetes (HbA1c >69 mmol/mol [8.5%]) with poor oral hygiene, calculus on labial LR1, LL1, diastema between UR1, UL1 and drifting. (c) Suppuration UR1. (d) Vertical bone loss UR1. (e) Horizontal and vertical bone loss. (f) Drifting UR1, UL1. (g) Nicotine staining.

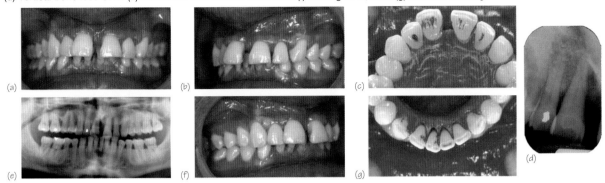

Figure 38.6   (a–d) A 35-year-old female with grade C, stage IV periodontitis who was a non-smoker and had poorly controlled type 1 diabetes (HbA1c >69 mmol/mol [8.5%]); LL1 had 100% bone loss and exfoliated spontaneously; plaque and calculus are visible on LR1 and LL2, but plaque levels are generally inconsistent with the severity of periodontal destruction.

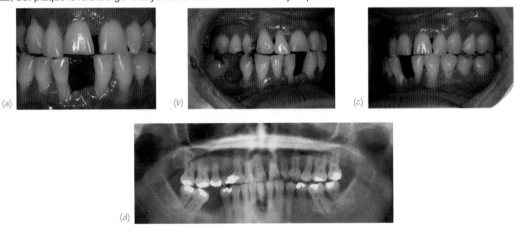

Figure 38.7   A 45-year-old male with very severe, stage IV periodontitis, poor oral hygiene and poorly controlled type 2 diabetes (home blood glucose persistently >10 mmol/l). (a) Inflamed, purplish-red gingivae and generalised subgingival calculus. (b,c) Periapicals show advanced bone loss. Source: Courtesy of P. Gregory.

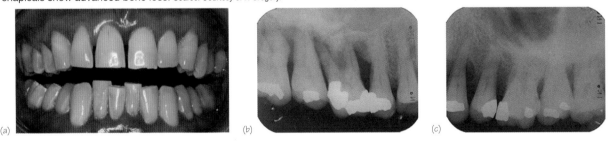

Figure 38.8   Glucose tablets.

Hypoglycaemia - blood glucose <4 mmol/l
- Patient may be pale, shaky, clammy, aggressive or confused
  - More likely to occur in Type 1 diabetes patient
- Give fast-acting oral glucose   eg glucose tablets/drink

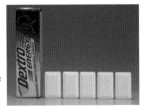

Figure 38.9   Glucagon injection.

Severe hypoglycaemia, loss of consciousness:
- Inject glucagon 1mg for adult (subcutaneous or intramuscular)
  - Give further oral carbohydrate on recovery
- If no recovery in 10 minutes and still unconscious, will need intravenous glucose
  - Call an ambulance

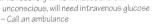

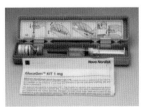

Diabetes mellitus is a common group of metabolic disorders characterised by chronic hyperglycaemia that results from insulin deficiency or impaired utilisation of insulin (insulin resistance). When poorly controlled, diabetes is a recognised risk factor for periodontal diseases and it has been hypothesised that a two-way relationship may exist (Chapters 10–12). Diabetes is one of the most common chronic diseases in the UK, with more than 4.9 million people affected and the prevalence is rising (Diabetes UK, 2021).

Diagnosis

There are four diagnostic tests for diabetes (WHO, 2019): (i) a random plasma glucose concentration of ≥11.1 mmol/l (200 mg/dl) with the clinical symptoms of diabetes (polyuria, polydipsia, blurred vision and unexplained weight loss); (ii) a fasting plasma glucose of ≥7.0 mmol/l (126 mg/dl) (normal level is <5.6 mmol/l or <100 mg/dl); (iii) a two-hour postload glucose of ≥11.1 mmol/l (200 mg/dl) after 75 g anhydrous glucose in a glucose tolerance test; or (iv) Hba1c ≥48 mmol/mol.

Classification

Classification of diabetes was revised in 2019 (WHO, 2019).
- Type 1 diabetes.
- Type 2 diabetes.
- Hybrid forms of diabetes.
- Other specific types, e.g. monogenetic defects of β-cell function including maturity-onset diabetes of the young; unclassified diabetes.
- Hyperglycaemia diagnosed during pregnancy, including gestational diabetes which may be transitional.

Type 1 diabetes

Type 1 diabetes affects approximately 8% of cases and is the most common form in children or adolescents, in whom it can present acutely. It can present at any age but incidence peaks in childhood and around puberty (NICE, 2023). It is characterised by destruction of the pancreatic β-cells which produce insulin which is mostly autoimmune mediated.

Treatment is by daily insulin injections using a combination of short/medium/long-acting formulations (Fig. 38.1) or pump therapy. Islet cell transplantation has been used successfully in some individuals worldwide but is not without risks and not routinely available (Anazawa et al., 2019). The first ever immunotherapy treatment to delay type 1 diabetes, teplizumab, was licensed in the US in November 2022, marking a big breakthrough, and it is undergoing regulatory approval for use in the UK. The key to success is a healthy diet, balancing dietary carbohydrate intake to injected insulin to achieve as normal a blood glucose as possible (Fig. 38.2). Blood glucose levels can be checked using home testing kits or by real-time or intermittently scanned (flash) continuous glucose monitoring systems (Fig. 38.3). The target plasma glucose level is 4–7 mmol/l (72–126 mg/dl) on waking and before meals and no more than 9 mmol/l (162 mg/dl) after meals.

Type 2 diabetes

This is associated with β-cell dysfunction and insulin resistance. It generally manifests in midlife in overweight, obese individuals with a sedentary lifestyle and constitutes 90–95% of cases. Up to 850 000 people are estimated to be living with undiagnosed type 2 diabetes in the UK (Diabetes UK, 2021). Genetic predisposition

is likely but not well understood. Certain ethnic groups (e.g. Asians) seem more susceptible. Onset can be insidious, by which time macrovascular and microvascular complications may already have occurred. Management is by diet (Fig. 38.2), exercise and, in some cases, oral hypoglycaemic drugs or even insulin injections to boost insulin levels.

In May 2022, the FDA approved a first-in-class new medication called Mounjaro® by Lilly (also known as tirzepatide) for type 2 diabetes management in conjunction with diet and exercise; it has been shown to improve glucose levels and also dramatically improve weight in clinical trials. A world-first study by Professor Roy Taylor in 2022 funded by Diabetes UK showed that after losing weight and harmful fat from the liver and pancreas following a structured low-calorie diet, 70% of participants went into remission.

Diabetes control/HbA1c

A glycated haemoglobin (HbA1c) blood test arranged by medical practitioners/diabetes specialists measures the proportion of glucose bound to the haemoglobin in the red blood cells and indicates diabetes control over the last 2–3 months. In the UK, the optimum target set by NICE is 48 mmol/mol (≤6.5% using old DCCT criteria), to minimize the risk of long-term complications, but the pragmatic treatment target monitored annually in the National Diabetes Core Audit/Paediatric Diabetes Audit is set at ≤58 mmol/mol (≤7.5% using old DCCT criteria); 2022 reports show that 34.8% of adults and 37.9% of children/adolescents achieved this target for type 1 diabetes in 2020/21 and 63.4% of adults for type 2 diabetes.

Complications of poor control

Macrovascular and microvascular complications are associated with poor diabetes control (Fig. 38.4). Periodontal disease has been suggested as a sixth complication.

Prevalence

- UK figures (Diabetes UK, 2021; Iacobucci, 2021) show that around 6% of the population have diabetes, of whom almost 4.1 million have been diagnosed with diabetes and an estimated 850 000 may have undiagnosed type 2 diabetes, representing a doubling in prevalence in the last 15 years.
- In the US in 2022, the CDC reported 37.3 million people (11.3% of the US population) had diabetes, of whom 28.7 million were diagnosed and 8.5 million estimated to have undiagnosed diabetes.
- Worldwide, in 2021, 539 million people were estimated to be living with diabetes, with approximately 240 million people undiagosed and 6.7 million deaths attributable to diabetes (International Diabetes Federation, 2021).

  Data indicate a continued global increase in diabetes prevalence, confirming diabetes as a significant global challenge to the health and well-being of individuals, families and societies.
- There are significant healthcare and cost implications.

Clinical periodontal management

Therapy

Well-controlled diabetes is not a significant risk factor for periodontal disease. If the diabetes is not well controlled, patients may present with a more severe, extensive form of periodontal disease than a non-diabetes-affected peer with similar plaque levels. Poorly controlled diabetes is well recognised as a systemic periodontal risk factor for periodontitis (Figs 38.5–38.7)

(Nascimento *et al.*, 2018) and forms an integral component of the staging and grading of periodontitis (Chapter 36). Hyperglycaemia is a stated risk factor for dental plaque-induced gingivitis in the 2018 classification of gingival diseases and conditions (Chapter 2).

Clinical periodontal care follows the stepwise principles of therapy (Chapter 19). At the start of therapy, the patient and their diabetes practitioner or specialist should be asked about the patient's diabetes control and, if available, the HbA1c sought. Some patients, medical practitioners and members of the diabetes care team may not be well informed about the bidirectional relationship between periodontal disease and diabetes mellitus (Stöhr *et al.*, 2021) and also (i) the adverse effects of poor diabetes control on periodontal health and (ii) the potential for non-surgical periodontal therapy to improve glycaemic control (NICE, 2022a, b; Di Domenico *et al.*, 2023) and reduce systemic inflammation in type 2 diabetes patients (Baeza *et al.*, 2020). Education and advice on this two-way relationship should be offered where appropriate. Screening of periodontitis patients for diabetes has been suggested (Baeza *et al.*, 2020).

An umbrella review of 16 systematic reviews showed that the effect of periodontal treatment plus adjunctive use of antibiotics/laser on glycaemic control was not statistically significant compared to non-surgical therapy alone (Di Domenico *et al.*, 2023) (Chapter 12).

Medical emergencies

The dental team should recognise the signs and symptoms of hypoglycaemia and be prepared to treat (Figs 38.8, 38.9). Hyperglycaemia may lead to ketoacidosis, but because of the time it takes to develop, it is less likely to present as an acute emergency; nevertheless, it is a serious condition needing medical intervention.

Key points
- Prevalence of diabetes is increasing worldwide
- Poorly controlled diabetes is a risk factor for periodontal diseases
- A two-way relationship exists between diabetes and periodontal diseases
- Periodontal infection/inflammation can adversely affect diabetes control
- Periodontal treatment may improve diabetes control
- The dental team should know how to manage hypoglycaemia in case it occurs during treatment

39 Necrotising periodontal diseases

Figure 39.1   Classification of necrotising periodontal diseases (NPDs). Source: Papapanou *et al*. (2018), adapted from Table 2.

Category	Patients	Predisposing conditions	Clinical condition
Necrotising periodontal diseases in chronically, severely compromised patients	In adults	HIV+/AIDS with CD4 counts <200 and detectable viral load	NG, NP, NS, Noma. Possible progression
		Other severe systemic conditions (Immunosuppression)	
	In children	Severe malnourishments	
		Extreme living conditions	
		Severe (viral) Infections	
Necrotising periodontal diseases in temporarily and/or moderately compromised patients	In gingivitis patients	Uncontrolled factors stress, nutrition, smoking, habits	Generalised NG. Possible progression to NP
		Previous NPD: residual craters	
		Local factors root proximity, tooth malposition	Localised NG. Possible progression to NP
			NG. Infrequent progression
	In periodontitis patients	Common predisposing factors for NPD	NP. Infrequent progression

Figure 39.3   Pseudomembranous slough palatal UR2 - UL2.

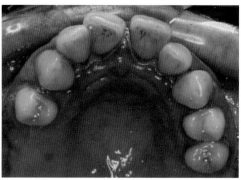

Figure 39.5   (a,b) NP in a male patient with HIV/AIDS leading to necrosis of the palatal tissue UL2 exposing bone.

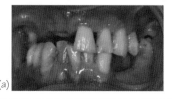
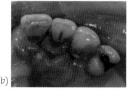

(a)   (b)

Figure 39.2   (a,b) NG showing marked necrosis and typical punched-out interdental papillae between the maxillary incisors and between LR2 and LR3.

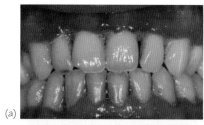

(a)

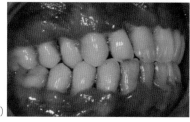

(b)

Figure 39.4   (a,b) Transition from NG to NP following the acute phase in 27-year-old male smoker: interdental necrosis, punched-out papillae and clinical attachment loss anteriorly; detachment of buccal gingiva LR2 - LL2; gross subgingival calculus deposits are now supragingival following apical migration of gingiva.

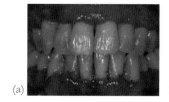
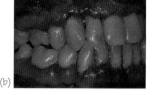

(a)   (b)

Figure 39.6   NP-like lesions on the lower incisors in a 15-year-old girl who used cocaine orally. Local application led to inflammation, recession and necrosis of the underlying bone. Source: Courtesy of Professor I.L.C. Chapple.

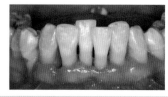

Following the 1999 International Workshop for the Classification of Periodontal Diseases and Conditions, it was recommended that necrotising ulcerative gingivitis and necrotising ulcerative periodontitis should be collectively called the necrotising periodontal diseases (NPDs). It was acknowledged that they may be different stages of the same infection. The term 'ulcerative' was subsequently eliminated as ulceration was deemed secondary to the necrosis (Herrera *et al.*, 2018). Necrotising stomatitis is thought to be an extension of the process below the mucogingival junction. NPDs remained a distinct periodontitis category with a new classification in the 2018 World Workshop classification (Figs 2.3a,b, 39.1); they have a characteristic clinical phenotype, which includes papilla necrosis, bleeding and pain, and are associated with host immune impairments (Herrera *et al.*, 2018; Papapanou *et al.*, 2018).

Necrotising gingivitis (NG)

Necrotising gingivitis has several distinctive features that distinguish it from plaque-induced gingivitis (Fig. 39.2). It is characterised by its rapid (acute) onset, and painful, ulcerated, necrotic gingivae which bleed with little provocation. The necrotic ulcers affect the interdental papillae and have a 'punched-out' appearance. They may

Periodontology at a Glance, Second Edition. Valerie Clerehugh, Aradhna Tugnait, Michael R. Milward, and Iain L. C. Chapple.
© 2024 John Wiley & Sons Ltd. Published 2024 by John Wiley & Sons Ltd.

be covered by a pseudomembranous grey slough, comprising fibrin, necrotic tissue, leukocytes, erythrocytes and bacteria (Fig. 39.3). Patients often present with a characteristic marked halitosis ('foetor ex ore'). Some may also have lymph nodes involvement.

Microbiology

Necrotising gingivitis has a specific fusiform/spirochaete bacterial aetiology. Four zones have been identified in the gingival lesion, the latter three of which are unique to NG:

- Bacterial zone.
- Neutrophil-rich zone.
- Necrotic zone.
- Spirochaetal infiltration zone.

Plasma cells have been observed in the deeper parts and IgG and C3 between epithelial cells.

The predominant cultivable flora comprises *Prevotella intermedia*, *Fusobacteria* spp., *Selenomonas* spp. and *Treponema* spp. Recent studies implicate a possible aetiological role for *Peptostreptococcus* spp. Knowledge is limited about the pathogenic mechanisms by which the bacterial flora produce the destructive lesions in NPD. Both spirochaetes and fusiforms can invade the tissues and liberate endotoxins, producing tissue destruction by: (i) direct toxic effects; and (ii) indirect effects from activating and modifying the host responses.

Predisposing factors

Certain factors predispose individuals to NG.

- Immune suppression including human immunodeficiency virus (HIV) infection.
- Smoking.
- Stress.
- Inadequate sleep.
- Poor diet or malnutrition.
- Heavy alcohol consumption.
- Pre-existing gingivitis, poor oral hygiene and previous history of NPD.

NPD was reported to be relatively common during World War II but nowadays it is unusual to find NPD in industrialised communities. Overall prevalence of NG has been reported to be 0.51–3.3% in general populations attending dental clinics; prevalence in students has been reported as 0.9–6.7%; but data are highly variable in African populations, for example (Herrera *et al.*, 2018). NG is more common in developing countries and has been reported in children, particularly if they are malnourished or following viral/protozoal infections. Prevalence for NG/NP is highly variable in HIV/AIDS patients. Whilst the acute nature of NG means there is no 'chronic' form, recurrence and progression can be a feature.

NG may present in HIV-positive individuals who are unaware of their status. If the history suggests this, the patient should be referred to their medical practitioner or specialist for further investigation and counselling.

Management

The painful nature of NG usually drives patients to seek treatment.

Local measures

- The removal of gross deposits of plaque and calculus, using local analgesia where necessary.
  - An ultrasonic scaler is useful, due to its flushing action.
  - Removal of the sloughed material will often reveal ulcerated, bleeding tissue.
- Gentle oral hygiene plus a chlorhexidine digluconate mouthwash (0.2% × 10 ml for one minute twice daily) to aid plaque control and help prevent secondary infection.

- Oxidising mouthwash (3% hydrogen peroxide with equal volume of warm water) to target the microbial flora.
- Review after 1–2 days.

Systemic measures

Due to the specific fusiform-spirochaete microflora and when there is lymph node involvement, systemic antimicrobials are effective (Chapter 23).

- Metronidazole 400 mg three times per day for three days in conjunction with debridement (pro-rata for children/adolescents).

After the acute phase

Appropriate nonsurgical periodontal therapy should be undertaken including, as appropriate, oral hygiene instruction; smoking cessation advice; thorough supra- and subgingival PMPR; professional medical advice on stress management; dietary advice; and counselling on recreational drug use. Some regeneration of the papillae can occur. Surgical soft tissue recontouring (gingivectomy) may correct the soft tissue craters and deformities. Flap surgery may be needed for deep defects.

If inadequately treated, the acute phase may subside, but recurrences can occur, leading to progressive tissue destruction and a shift from NG to NP (Fig. 39.4), particularly if the predisposing factors persist or in the presence of immunosuppression.

Necrotising periodontitis (NP)

Necrotising periodontitis is characterised by necrosis of the periodontal ligament and alveolar bone and may be a feature of HIV-infected patients (Fig. 39.5). NP-type lesions can be seen in patients using oral recreational drugs (Fig. 39.6).

Necrotising stomatitis (NS) and noma

Where the necrotising process extends more than 10 mm beyond the gingival margin or below the mucogingival junction, this is classified as NS. Specialist management is needed, involving broad surgical excision of the involved necrotic area and bone (usually maxilla) and extraction of affected teeth with packing of the defect and healing by secondary intention.

Noma (called cancrum oris in Africa) is a fulminating, disfiguring condition that may follow on from NP and NS in developing parts of the world.

Differential diagnosis

Differential diagnosis includes primary or recurrent herpetic gingivostomatitis which is a contagious condition of herpes simplex virus 1 aetiology, presenting with viral vesicles (yellow centre, red halo) on the gingiva or oral mucosa (see Fig. 41.7) and vesicular-bullous diseases

Key points

- Necrotising periodontal diseases (NPDs) comprise necrotising gingivitis (NG), necrotising periodontitis (NP) and necrotising stomatitis (NS)
- NPDs have a distinctive clinical phenotype, a specific fusiform/spirochaetal microflora and an association with host impairment
- NG is characterised by: ulcerated, necrotic gingivae; punched-out interdental papillae; bleeding; pain
- Only type of gingivitis for which antibiotics may be indicated
- Differential diagnosis includes primary herpetic gingivostomatitis
- NG predisposing factors include stress, smoking, poor diet, pre-existing gingivitis, poor oral hygiene and HIV infection
- NP is thought to be an extension of NG
- NS may be a late-stage development of NPD

40 Periodontal abscesses and endodontic-periodontal lesions

Figure 40.1 Classification of periodontal abscesses based on aetiological factors involved. Source: Adapted from Papapanou *et al*. (2018), Table 4.

Periodontal abscess in periodontitis patients (in a pre-existing periodontal pocket)	Acute exacerbations	Untreated periodontitis	
		Non-responsive to therapy periodontitis	
		Supportive periodontal therapy (SPT)	
	After treatment	Post-Professional Mechanical Plaque Removal (PMPR)	
		Post-surgery	
		Post-medications	Systemic antimicrobials Other drugs: nifedipine
Periodontal abscess in non-periodontitis patients (not mandatory to have a pre-existing periodontal pocket)	Impaction		Dental floss, orthodontic elastic, toothpick, rubber dam, popcorn hulls
	Harmful habits		Wire or nail biting and clenching
	Orthodontic factors		Orthodontic forces or cross-bite
	Gingival overgrowth		
	Alteration of root surface	Severe anatomic alterations	Invaginated tooth, dens evaginatus or odontodysplasia
		Minor anatomic alterations	Cemental tears, enamel pearls or developmental grooves
		Iatrogenic conditions	Perforations
		Severe root damage	Fissure or fracture, cracked tooth syndrome
		External root resorption	

Figure 40.2 Features of periodontal abscess (PA).

- Vital pulpal response
- Common features, depending on stage of periodontal abscess (PA):
- Ovoid swelling on lateral part of root
- Suppuration on probing
- Bleeding on probing
- Increased mobility
- Pain, easy to localise to tooth
- Tenderness
- Tooth may be 'elevated' from socket, feel 'high' on bite
- Patient may feel wants to bite down or grind tooth

Most PAs occur in periodontitis patients

In periodontitis patients, PA commonly occurs:
- In pre-existing deep periodontal pocket, with bone loss
- Associated with furcations, if affected tooth is a molar
- Associated with radiographic radiolucency in alveolar bone on lateral border of affected root

In non-periodontitis patients, PA may be associated with:
- Impacted foreign body
- Harmful habit
- Orthodontic factors
- Gingival enlargement
- Alterations of root surface

Figure 40.3 Early PA formation – pus not draining yet. (a) Features; (b) early PA on UR4.

(a) Features

- Redness and swelling of gingiva on affected tooth
- Swelling may be diffuse and not well localised yet
- Pus not draining through the pocket or through the swelling yet - no sinus tract
- Pain may be severe, constant, localised to tooth

(b)

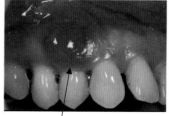

Early PA on UR4

Figure 40.4 PA with suppuration. (a) Features; (b) PA with suppuration and fluctuant swelling on LR5 in periodontitis patient; (c) associated bone loss LR5.

(a) Features

- Gingiva is red and swollen
- Swelling usually becomes more localised
  – Ovoid elevation of gingiva on lateral aspect of root
- Pus may be expressed from pocket on gentle pressure (suppuration) anywhere around the tooth
- Pus may point and drain through a fistula
  – Sinus tract may form
- Pain and discomfort ease when pus discharges

(b)

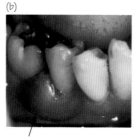

PA with suppuration and fluctuant swelling on LR5 in periodontitis patient

(c)

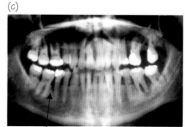

Associated bone loss LR5

Periodontology at a Glance, Second Edition. Valerie Clerehugh, Aradhna Tugnait, Michael R. Milward, and Iain L. C. Chapple.
© 2024 John Wiley & Sons Ltd. Published 2024 by John Wiley & Sons Ltd.

Figure 40.5 PA with systemic involvement. (a) Features; (b) extraoral swelling on angle of mandible.

(a) Features

- Occasionally see evidence of associated systemic involvement:
  - Extraoral swelling on affected side of mouth
  - Lymphadenopathy
  - Rarely cellulitis
  - Malaise
  - Raised temperature

(b)

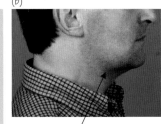

Extra-oral swelling on angle of mandible

Figure 40.6 Gingival abscess. (a) Features; (b) gingival abscess on UR6 mesio-palatal.

(a) Features

- Localised purulent infection that involves the marginal or interdental papilla
  - Localised, painful, rapidly expanding
  - Acute inflammatory response to foreign agents
  - Red, shiny, smooth
  - Fluctuant within 24–48 hours
  - Points and discharges spontaneously

(b)

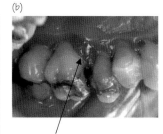

Gingival abscess on UR6 mesio-palatal

Figure 40.7 Classification of endodontic-periodontal lesions. Source: Adapted from Papapanou et al. (2018), Table 3.

Endo-periodontal lesions with root damage	Root fracture or cracking	
	Root canal / pulp chamber perforation	
	External root resorption	
Endo-periodontal lesions without root damage	Endo-periodontal lesions in periodontitis patients	Grade 1 - narrow deep periodontal pocket in 1 tooth surface
		Grade 2 - wide deep periodontal pocket in 1 tooth surface
		Grade 3 - deep periodontal pockets in >1 tooth surface
	Endo-periodontal lesions in non-periodontitis patients	Grade 1 - narrow deep periodontal pocket in 1 tooth surface
		Grade 2 - wide deep periodontal pocket in 1 tooth surface
		Grade 3 - deep periodontal pockets in >1 tooth surface

Figure 40.8 Endodontic-periodontal lesion (EPL) Grade 1, on LL3 in periodontitis patient. (a) Note swelling prior to treatment; (b) after endodontic treatment on LL3 with periapical radiolucency (shown) which resolved after several months; (c) healing of EPL after endodontic treatment and periodontal therapy on LL3.

(a)

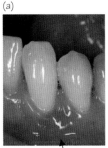

Note swelling prior to treatment

(b)

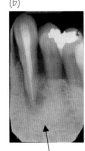

After endodontic treatment on LL3 with periapical radiolucency (shown) which resolved after several months

(c)

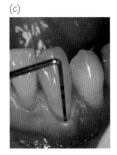

Healing of EPL after endodontic treatment and periodontal therapy on LL3

Figure 40.9 EPL Grade 3, on LR4 in periodontitis patient. (a) Swelling and suppuration; (b) radiolucency circumscribes root LR4.

(a)

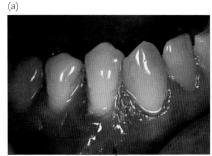

Swelling and suppuration

(b)

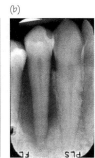

Radiolucency circumscribes root LR4

Periodontal abscess

A periodontal abscess (PA) is a localised purulent infection within the tissues adjacent to the periodontal pocket/sulcus that can lead to rapid and significant periodontal tissue destruction. It can present as an acute infection that interrupts the scheduled treatment plan and requires emergency management (Herrera *et al.*, 2018; Papapanou *et al.*, 2018).

Aetiology

There are several hypothesised causes.

- *Pocket occlusion*, due to: (i) incomplete removal of calculus; (ii) impaction of food or a foreign body; (iii) bacterial invasion after instrumentation.

Occlusion of the pocket orifice leads to reduced clearance of bacteria and an accumulation of host cells; infection spreads into the supporting tissues and is localised. Tissue damage occurs due to lysosomal enzymes released from neutrophils taking part in host defences.

- *Furcation involvement*: abscesses commonly occur in furcations or in relation to anatomical defects in the furcation area such as enamel pearls.
- *Systemic antibiotic therapy*: in patients with untreated periodontitis, superinfection with opportunistic organisms may occur following systemic antibiotics.
- *Manifestation of systemic disease*: multiple or recurrent abscesses can occur where a patient is immunocompromised and may alert the clinician to an underlying or undiagnosed medical condition (e.g. undiagnosed or poorly controlled diabetes; chronic lymphocytic leukaemia).

A PA can occur in periodontitis patients in a pre-existing periodontal pocket before or after treatment, or in non-periodontitis patients (see Fig. 40.1 for full classification).

Microbiology of PA

The microbial profile resembles that reported in periodontitis. The most prevalent species are *Porphyromonas gingivalis*, *Prevotella intermedia*, *Prevotella melaninogenica*, *Fusobacterium nucleatum*, *Tannerella forsythia*, *Treponema* spp., *Campylobacter* spp., *Capnocytophaga* spp., *Aggregatibacter actinomycetemcomitans* or Gram-negative enteric rods.

Features

Although there are some common features (Fig. 40.2), features of a periodontal abscess may vary according to the stage of development (early, pus not draining yet, see Fig. 40.3; with suppuration, see Fig. 40.4; with systemic involvement, see Fig. 40.5).

Differential diagnosis

It is important to consider the differential diagnosis, which may be non-periodontal, including the following possibilities.

- Gingival abscess (Fig. 40.6).
- Pericoronal abscess (pericoronitis) (non-periodontal).
  - Localised, purulent infection in the tissues surrounding a partially erupted tooth, commonly mandibular third molars; possible red, swollen gingival flap.

- Periapical periodontitis (non-periodontal).
  - Characterised by pulpal necrosis; tooth non-vital; periapical tissue involvement; periapical radiolucency; tooth tender to percussion, pain may be difficult to localise.
- Endodontic-periodontal lesion (EPL) (Figs 40.7, 40.8, 40.9).
- Other pathology (non-periodontal), e.g. cyst, tumour or osteomyelitis.

Confirmation of the diagnosis is reached after a thorough history and examination, consideration of the clinical and radiographic features and the results of any special tests.

Management

Acute phase

Treatment should be directed at relief of pain and controlling the acute infection to avoid destruction of vital periodontal tissues and averting systemic involvement.

- Relieve the occlusion: grind opposing tooth.
- Advise hot salt mouthwashes several times daily for 2–3 days to encourage drainage.
- Advise pain killers, e.g. ibuprofen (200 mg × 2 every 4–6 hours, maximum six per 24 hours) or paracetamol (500 mg × 2 every 4–6 hours, maximum eight per 24 hours).

Further measures depend on the stage of PA formation.

1 *Early stage, pus not draining (Fig. 40.3)*. If it is not possible to achieve drainage, severe pain is present and there is a risk of spread of infection, systemic antibiotics may be prescribed – see below.
2 *Pus draining/suppuration (Fig. 40.4)*. Achieve drainage through local gentle debridement through the pocket, being cautious to avoid further damage to vital periodontal ligament cells; or incision and drainage through the swelling. It is *not* generally appropriate to prescribe antibiotics if drainage has been achieved and there is no evidence of systemic involvement or spread of infection.
3 *Systemic involvement (Fig. 40.5)*. Incision and drainage may be appropriate. Where local measures are not sufficient and systemic involvement has been identified, systemic antimicrobials may be indicated (see British National Formulary): phenoxymethyl penicillin 500 mg four times daily, or alternatively amoxicillin 500 mg three times daily (or, if penicillin allergy, clarithromycin 500 mg twice daily) for up to five days, with a review at three days; plus metronidazole 400 mg three times per day if signs of spreading infection, e.g. lymph node involvement; doses should be pro rata according to age in younger age groups.

Review after a few days. Consider the prognosis and treatment options and whether non-surgical or surgical periodontal therapy is indicated.

Endodontic-periodontal lesions

There are many channels of communication between periodontal and pulpal tissues via lateral and accessory canals or the apical foramina. An endodontic-periodontal lesion (EPL) is defined as a pathological communication between the pulpal and periodontal tissues at a given tooth that may occur in an acute or chronic form (Papapanou *et al.*, 2018) and should be classified according to the signs and symptoms that directly impact prognosis and treatment (Fig. 40.7). According to the 2018 classification, the history of the lesion, whether primary endodontic, primary periodontal or combined, is deemed irrelevant, as irrespective of the primary source, both the root canal (first) and periodontal tissues (second) would require treatment (Herrera *et al.*, 2018).

Prognosis needs to be assessed (hopeless, poor, favourable) and the decision taken whether to maintain or extract the tooth. Success and the overall prognosis depend on (i) the ability to eliminate the bacteria in the root canal and gain a good coronal seal (Fig. 40.8) and (ii) the outcome of periodontal therapy, which relates to the severity, extent and complexity of the periodontal involvement of the tooth. Where there is severe periodontal involvement, bone loss and grade III mobility, prognosis may be deemed poor or even hopeless (see Fig. 40.9).

Key points

- Periodontal abscess (PA) is a localised purulent infection within the tissues adjacent to the periodontal pocket that can lead to rapid and significant periodontal tissue destruction
- PA can occur as an acute infection requiring emergency management
- A thorough history and examination are needed to reach the diagnosis after consideration of differential diagnosis
- PA management depends on the stage of development
- Endodontic-periodontal lesion (EPL) is a pathological communication between the pulpal and periodontal tissues at a given tooth that may occur in an acute or chronic form
- EPL should be classified according to the signs and symptoms that directly impact prognosis and treatment
- Endodontic treatment should be undertaken before periodontal treatment

41 Periodontal diseases in children and adolescents

Table 41.1 Gingival condition in 5–15 year olds in the 2013 Child Dental Health Survey (2003 data in parentheses).

Age (years)	% with visible gingival inflammation		% with gingival bleeding on any index teeth		% with visible plaque		% with visible calculus	
	2013	(2003)	2013	(2003)	2013	(2003)	2013	(2003)
5	22	(32)	–	–	46	(50)	9	(6)
8	46	(64)	–	–	71	(77)	28	(24)
12	60	(66)	–	–	64	(74)	39	(32)
15	52	(53)	40	(45)	50	(64)	46	(40)

Figure 41.1 Classification of periodontal diseases and conditions for children and adolescents.

Classification (Caton et al., 2018)

Periodontal Health, Gingival Diseases/Conditions
- Periodontal health and gingival health
- Gingivitis, dental plaque biofilm-induced
- Gingival diseases, non dental plaque biofilm-induced

Periodontitis
- Necrotising periodontal diseases
- Periodontitis
- Periodontitis as a manifestation of systemic disease

Other Conditions Affecting the Periodontium
- Systemic diseases/conditions affecting the periodontal supporting tissues
- Periodontal abscesses and endodontic-periodontal lesions
- Mucogingival deformities and conditions
- Traumatic occlusal forces
- Tooth and prosthesis related factors

Figure 41.2 Simplified BPE screening in children and adolescents.

- Simplified BPE (sBPE)
  - Index teeth (WHO partial recording for adolescents) UR6,UR1, UL6 LR6, LL1, LL6
- sBPE codes 0,1,2 ages 7-11 years (mixed dentition stage)
- Full range sBPE codes 0,1,2,3,4,* ages 12+ years (permanent teeth erupted)

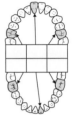

Ainamo, Nordblad, Kallio. Use of the CPITN in populations under 20 years of age. Int Dent J 1984:34:285-291

Figure 41.4 Plaque-induced gingivitis in a 15-year-old Asian girl.

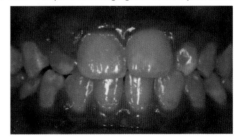

Figure 41.3 Plaque-induced gingivitis in a 16-year-old girl.

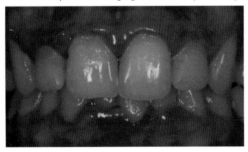

Figure 41.6 Plaque-induced gingivitis and local contributing factors. (a) Localised recession. (b) Frenal attachments near gingival margin. (c) Teenage girl with amelogenesis imperfecta and gross supragingival calculus. (d) Incompetent lips and mouth breather exacerbating gingivitis anteriorly in 12-year-old boy.

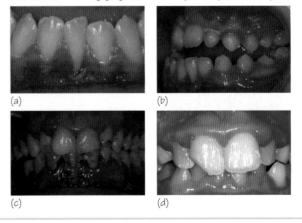

(a)   (b)

(c)   (d)

Figure 41.5 (a) Plaque-induced gingivitis and supragingival calculus on labial of lower incisors in a 10-year-old Asian girl. (b) Lingual lower anteriors with supragingival calculus.

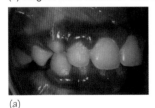
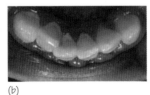

(a)   (b)

Periodontology at a Glance, Second Edition. Valerie Clerehugh, Aradhna Tugnait, Michael R. Milward, and Iain L. C. Chapple.
© 2024 John Wiley & Sons Ltd. Published 2024 by John Wiley & Sons Ltd.

Figure 41.7 Non-plaque-induced gingival condition: primary herpetic gingivostomatitis – herpes simplex virus 1 vesicles on the gingiva (a,b) and tongue (c). Source: Courtesy of Dr S. Kindelan.

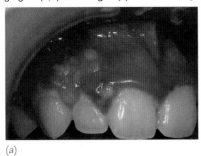

(a)

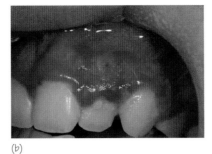

(b)

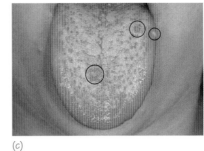

(c)

Figure 41.8 Non-plaque-induced gingival condition: neutropenia in a young child with severe gingival inflammation and mobile primary incisors. Source: Courtesy of Dr S. Kindelan.

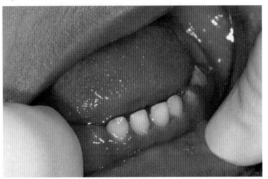

Figure 41.9 Non-plaque-induced gingival condition: histoplasmosis in a severely immunocompromised young child with bone marrow rejection. There is a fungal infection, deep mycoses, *Histoplasma capsulatum*. Source. Courtesy of Professor I L C Chapple.

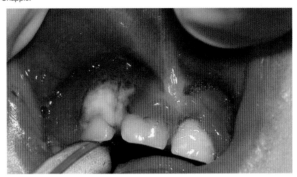

Figure 41.10 (a) The results of a five-year study of clinical attachment loss (CAL) in 14–19-year-old adolescents in Rochdale, UK. (b) Incipient (Grade I) periodontitis in a 19-year-old. Source: Clerehugh *et al*. (1990)/John Wiley & Sons.

(a)

5-year study of 167 14- to 19-year-olds, UK				
Mean age (years)		14.3	16.0	19.6
Prevalence (% subjects with CAL)	≥1 mm	3	37	77
	= 2 mm	0	3	14
Extent (% sites with CAL)	> 1 mm	0.3	7.2	31.3
	= 2 mm	0.0	0.3	3.1
Mean CAL (mm)		<0.01	0.08	0.35

(b)

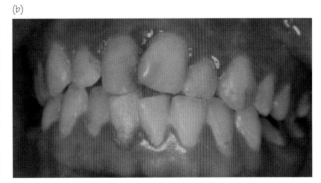

Figure 41.11 (a–c) Periodontitis, molar-incisor pattern, Stage III, Grade C, in a 12-year-old girl of African origin.

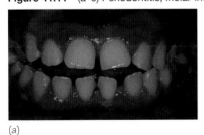

(a)

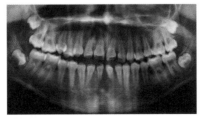

(b)

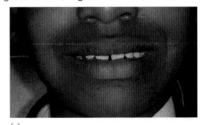

(c)

Figure 41.12 When to consider referral to a specialist in the younger age groups.

Stage II, III periodontitis not responding to treatment
Grade C or Stage IV periodontitis
Medical history that significantly affects periodontal treatment or requiring multi-disciplinary care
Periodontitis as a direct manifestation of systemic disease
Systemic/genetic diseases that can affect periodontal supporting tissues
Root morphology/furcation defects adversely affecting prognosis on key teeth
Non-plaque-induced conditions requiring complex or specialist care
Cases requiring diagnosis/management of rare/complex clinical pathology
Drug-induced gingival overgrowth needing surgery
Cases requiring evaluation for periodontal surgery

Figure 41.13 Papillon–Lefèvre syndrome in a nine-year-old boy with (a,b) acutely inflamed gingiva, and (c) severe periodontal destruction and bone loss of the permanent dentition, having lost all the primary dentition already. (d) Hyperkeratosis of the soles of the feet – the hands, knees and elbows are also affected.

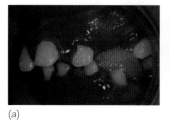
(a)

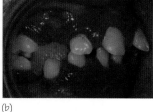
(b)

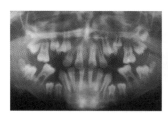
(c)

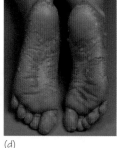
(d)

Many different periodontal problems manifest in children and adolescents (Clerehugh *et al.*, 2004) and all the categories of periodontal diseases and conditions that apply to adults from the 2018 classification emanating from the 2017 World Workshop on the Classification of Periodontal and Peri-implant Diseases and Conditions (Caton *et al.*, 2018) also apply to the younger age groups (Fig. 41.1). Periodontal screening is an important prerequisite in the dental examination of the child (Clerehugh, 2008; Clerehugh & Kindelan, 2021) (Fig. 41.2; Chapter 17).

Gingivitis

Data from the 2013 Child Dental Health Survey (Pitts *et al.*, 2015) support previous global findings that plaque biofilm-induced gingivitis is very common in the younger age groups (Figs 41.3, 41.4, 41.5). This survey was based on a representative sample of 13 628 school children aged 5, 8, 12 and 15 years attending state and independent schools in England, Wales and Northern Ireland, with 9,66 dental examinations completed (Table 41.1).

Local contributing factors

Various local contributing factors can influence the prevalence, severity and extent of plaque biofilm-induced gingivitis in the young (Fig. 41.6). Plaque biofilm-induced gingivitis can usually be treated readily in the primary dental care setting (Chapters 14, 31).

Non-plaque-induced gingival lesions

Non-plaque-induced gingival lesions (Figs 41.7–41.9) may be less common in the younger age groups and more difficult to diagnose and treat, in which case referral is indicated (Chapter 32).

Periodontitis

Incipient (Stage I) periodontitis

Although study methodology has varied, data from the UK, USA and other countries support the conclusion that periodontitis can begin to develop and progress in adolescents (Chapter 35). A five-year longitudinal study in the UK (Clerehugh *et al.*, 1990) showed that 3% of 167 14-year-old adolescents had incipient clinical attachment loss (CAL) of 1 mm or more on the mesiobuccal surface of at least one first molar, premolar or central incisor tooth, rising to a prevalence of 37% at age 16 years and 77% at age 19 years (Fig. 41.10) indicating Stage 1 periodontitis.

A simplified Basic Periodontal Examination (sBPE) code of 3 is consistent with shallow pockets of 4 or 5 mm and would be expected in an individual with incipient periodontitis, especially on the proximal surfaces of first molars and incisors. Confirmation of true pockets is by CAL measures and, where appropriate, alveolar bone loss, especially on serial bitewing radiographs. The presence of subgingival calculus has been found to be associated with subsequent development of CAL in adolescents (Clerehugh *et al.*, 1990). Periodontal pathogens typical of adults are also found in the subgingival plaque in adolescents (Clerehugh *et al.*, 1997): *Porphyromonas gingivalis*, *Prevotella intermedia* and *Aggregatibacter actinomycetemcomitans*. The presence of *Tannerella forsythia* (formerly *forsythensis*) has been associated with subsequent CAL in a three-year longitudinal study in adolescents (Hamlet *et al.*, 2004).

Grade C or Stage II, III or IV periodontitis

A BPE code of 4 in a young person under 18 years of age should be a red flag to proceed to staging and grading (Chapter 36). Although current evidence from the 2017 World Workshop (Caton *et al.*, 2018) does not support the distinction between the conditions previously classified as chronic and aggressive periodontitis in the 1999 classification (Lang *et al.*, 1999), it is important for the dental practitioner to be able to identify those under-18s at an incipient (early) stage of periodontitis who are amenable to treatment in general dental practice (typically Stage I, Grade A) and those minority of cases with a more severe, rapidly progressing, destructive form of periodontitis, typically Stage II, III or IV, Grade C (Fig. 41.11) who may need referral for specialist treatment (Wadia *et al.*, 2019; Walter *et al.*, 2019) (Fig. 41.12).

Periodontitis as a manifestation of systemic disease

A small number of young people may present with periodontitis as a manifestation of haematological disorders (acquired neutropenia, leukaemia) or genetic disorders including: (i) Down syndrome (characterised by: trisomy chromosome 21; destructive periodontitis; primary and permanent dentitions affected; tendency for shortened roots; early tooth loss possible; neutrophil defects; abnormal T-cell function; abnormal collagen synthesis); (ii) Papillon–Lefèvre syndrome (Fig. 41.13) (features include loss of function mutations in cathepsin C gene; palmar-plantar hyperkeratosis; periodontitis occurs prepubertally; autosomal recessive gene; treatment complex; poor success rates); (iii) Chediak–Higashi syndrome (rare autosomal recessive condition; neutrophil and monocyte function affected; severe inflammation and periodontal destruction); (iv) Ehlers–Danlos syndrome (types IV and VIII, features: autosomal dominant disorder; severe periodontitis; defective collagen synthesis; skin hyperextensibility, joint mobility; excessive bruising due to fragile blood vessels); (v) hypophosphatasia (childhood form, features include: defect in alkaline phosphatase; premature loss of primary teeth due to cementum hypoplasia/aplasia). Early referral is indicated.

Other classifications

Various other periodontal conditions may affect children and adolescents and key features of their diagnosis and management are covered in the following chapters of the book and also elsewhere (Clerehugh et al., 2004).

- Necrotising periodontal diseases: Chapter 39.
- Abscesses of the periodontium: Chapter 40.
- Periodontitis associated with endodontic lesions: Chapter 40.
- Development of acquired deformities and conditions: Chapters 15, 33, 34.

Treat or refer the child/adolescent?

This depends on the practitioner's experience, the patient and the complexity of the case (Fig. 41.12; Chapter 43).

Key points

- Many periodontal diseases can occur in children/adolescents within the 2018 classification emanating from the 2017 World Workshop on the Classification of Periodontal Diseases and Peri-implant Diseases and Conditions
- Periodontal screening using Simplified BPE (sBPE) on index teeth is important
- Plaque biofilm-induced gingivitis is common in under-18s and local contributing factors may apply
- Non-plaque-induced gingival conditions are less common
- Incipient (Stage I) periodontitis may develop in adolescence
- Vigilance for Stage II, III or IV, Grade C periodontitis is essential in young people
- The decision to treat or refer depends on dentist factors, patient-centred factors and the complexity of the case

42 Periodontal management of the older adult

Figure 42.1 Shared features of frailty and periodontal diseases.
Source: Adapted from Clark *et al.* (2021), Fig. 1.

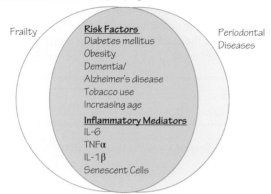

Frailty

Periodontal Diseases

Risk Factors
Diabetes mellitus
Obesity
Dementia/
Alzheimer's disease
Tobacco use
Increasing age
Inflammatory Mediators
IL-6
TNFα
IL-1β
Senescent Cells

Figure 42.2 (a–d) Female patient aged 73 years, with a restored mouth, a history of periodontitis, supragingival calculus on the lower anteriors, generalised recession, marginal gingival inflammation and erosion due to a lemon-sucking habit.

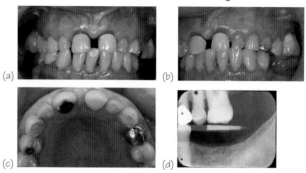

(a)   (b)
(c)   (d)

Figure 42.3 (a) A 'biologically young' patient aged 73 years. (b) Orthopantomogram radiograph prior to extraction of UR6 and UL7; root caries and apical pathology LL6 prior to root filling. (c–g) Restored dentition; tooth wear (attrition, abrasion), especially in the upper incisors; generalised periodontitis; recession and CAL; maintaining in Step 4 of periodontal therapy. Source: Courtesy of Dr M. Kellett.

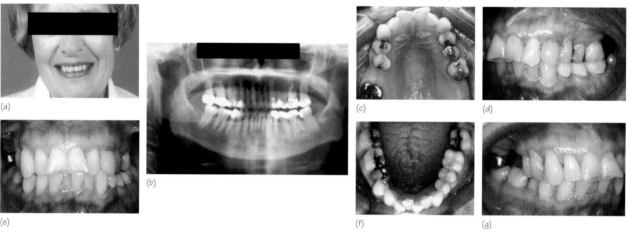

(a)
(b)
(c)   (d)
(e)
(f)   (g)

Figure 42.4 Root caries on the cervical mesial surface of UL7 with several mm of CAL in a 72-year-old male.

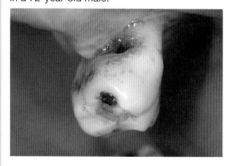

Figure 42.5 Attributes that in older adults may be (a) unaffected or enhanced, or (b) reduced.

(a)	(b)
Long term memory	Short term memory
Speaking ability, vocabulary	Visual, auditory, taste perception
Experience, positive attitude	Coordination
Reliability	Adaptability
Stability	Muscular strength
Simple learning skills	Complex learning skills
Ability to discriminate	Immune status, host resistance, medical well-being

Periodontology at a Glance, Second Edition. Valerie Clerehugh, Aradhna Tugnait, Michael R. Milward, and Iain L. C. Chapple.
© 2024 John Wiley & Sons Ltd. Published 2024 by John Wiley & Sons Ltd.

The definition of the 'older adult' varies in different countries and cultures. In developed, westernised communities it is commonly taken as the age of retirement from work. However, the biological age of the patient can vary from their actual chronological age. Patients well into their 70s and beyond may be spritely, active and young at heart in spite of advancing years.

Epidemiology of periodontal diseases

Some age changes occur in the epithelium, periodontal ligament and connective tissues, and the prevalence of periodontal diseases increases with age. Accordingly, it has been questioned whether:

- the worsening periodontal condition is an inevitable consequence of getting older (i.e. age related), or,
- the worsening periodontal condition is associated with other factors or characteristics in older adults (i.e. age associated).

A review of 14 cross-sectional and eight longitudinal studies of older adults from 1971 to 1995 supported the view that periodontal disease progression is age associated (Beck, 1996).

Risk factors for progression included smoking; oral hygiene habits (irregular flossing); length of time since last dental visit (more than three years); presence of periodontal pathogens (including *Porphyromonas gingivalis* and *Prevotella intermedia*); educational status; financial status; and health (depression). Type 2 diabetes is also an acknowledged risk factor.

A systematic review of 47 studies from 1965 to 2004 concluded that socioeconomic variables associated with periodontal diseases were of less importance than smoking, but in non-smokers, educational status could have an impact on periodontal diseases (Klinge & Norlund, 2005). Literacy issues have also been flagged (Jones & Wehler, 2005). A comparison of surveys in Germany and the United States demonstrates a relative improvement in the periodontal health of older adults in recent decades, but prevalence estimates for periodontitis remain high (Lopez et al., 2017) and access to dental care will be an ongoing concern.

Billings et al. (2017) deem exposures other than age are pivotal in determining periodontitis susceptibilty. Clark *et al.* (2021) concluded there is probably a bidirectional relationship between periodontal disease and frailty, defined as 'a clinically recognizable state of increased vulnerability, resulting from aging-associated decline in reserve and function across multiple physiologic systems such that the ability to cope with every-day or acute stressors is compromised'. Both frailty and periodontal diseases have strong associations with inflammatory dysregulation and other age-related pathophysiological changes (Fig. 42.1). A systematic review by Preshaw *et al.* (2017) concluded that immune senescence (the process of altered immune functioning) alters with increasing age, but that age-associated mechanistic changes are complex and incompletely understood; it is unclear how these relate to periodontal disease susceptibility (see also Chapter 11).

The UK Adult Dental Health Survey in 2009 (Fuller *et al.*, 2011; White *et al.*, 2011) showed an improving picture of tooth retention (1998 data in parentheses for comparison):

- 40% (versus 30%) of 65–74 year olds and 32% (versus 10%) of those aged 75 years or older had 21 or more of their own teeth
- 70% (versus 42%) of those aged 75 years or older still had some of their own teeth.

Because of increased tooth retention, maintaining periodontal health is an increasing issue. Shallow pocket, but not deep pocket, prevalence improved since 1998. For 65–74 year olds:

- 67% had clinical attachment loss (CAL) of 4 mm or more; 22% had CAL ≥6 mm
- 60% had shallow pockets of 4 mm or more; 14% had deep pockets ≥6mm.

For 75–84 year olds:

- 76% had CAL ≥4 mm; 25% had CAL ≥6 mm; pocket data were similar to 65–74 year olds.

Periodontal problems in older adults

Adults who have retained their teeth into old age must have maintained a reasonably favourable balance between host defences, bacterial challenge and an ecologically conducive oral environment. Therefore, they can be assumed to have a degree of resistance to periodontal diseases, unless some new periodontal risk factor or upset in the balance occurs.

Periodontal problems likely to be seen in the older adult (Figs 42.2–42.4) include: gingivitis; periodontitis; CAL and gingival recession; tooth wear – abrasion, attrition, erosion; dentine hypersensitivity; root caries.

Due to the cumulative effects of periodontal diseases, both CAL and recession are common and therefore the root surfaces are more susceptible to root caries, especially if the elderly adult lives alone and has frequent sucrose-containing snacks. Some lesions are very visible, whilst others are located subgingivally on approximal surfaces and are difficult to diagnose.

Older adults may experience oral dryness due to the polypharmacy of drugs that many take. Physical disability (e.g. arthritis) often compromises tooth cleaning ability, whilst depression can make patients less inclined to engage in oral hygiene routines; infirmity can jeopardise attendance; and mental disability (e.g. Alzheimer's disease) can create confusion over advice given. Medical disorders including cardiovascular disease, stroke, type 2 diabetes, respiratory ailments and digestive problems become increasingly common with advancing years. A thorough history (particularly the medical and social history) and examination are important.

Periodontal management

Periodontal management follows the usual stepwise principles of therapy, using the skills of the whole dental team according to need. Certain attributes may be enhanced or diminished with age (Fig. 42.5).

There are no conclusive data that age *per se* affects plaque build-up, gingival inflammation, reduction in inflammation following treatment or response to surgical therapy. However, several immune functions may be altered in association with ageing (Preshaw et al., 2017) and periodontal deterioration may relate to cellular senescence, an emerging field, or deterioration of type 1 collagen with age (Lopez *et al.*, 2017).

The treatment philosophy influences the treatment provided. Papapanou *et al.* (1990) and Wennstrom *et al.* (1990) proposed two approaches to treatment outcomes. To reach age 75 with one-third of the root length, few patients would need treatment. To remove all signs of periodontal disease, 70% would need treatment for bleeding on probing, 28% for shallow pockets and less than 5% for deep pockets with bleeding on probing. Ultimately, the outcome of periodontal therapy needs to be realistic and agreed with the patient, and the patient should have similar expectations and choices as younger patients unless there are medical, physical or other risk factors or barriers.

Key points

- Biological age can differ from chronological age
- Periodontal diseases are age associated, not age related
- Risk factors include tobacco smoking, poorly controlled type 2 diabetes and education
- Clinical attachment loss and recession are common
- Medical history and polypharmacy will influence management
- Treatment goals need to be realistic and agreed with the patient

43 The delivery of periodontal care

Figure 43.1 Key roles of some of the periodontal team.

Dentist
- Co-ordinates patient care
- Responsible for overall care and working of the team
- Discusses diagnosis and prognosis and options with patient
- Draws up treatment plan
- Identifies which team members will play a role
- Writes prescriptions to team members
- Indicates recall schedule
- Assesses response to treatment, further treatment needs including referral to specialist

Dental hygienist/hygiene therapist
- Provides non-surgical periodontal therapy
- Records indices to plan treatment and monitoring patient response

Specialist periodontist
- Diagnoses and treatment plan for referred cases
- Undertakes management of complex cases
- May provide advice to referring dentist
- May undertake complex treatment, e.g. periodontal surgery

Figure 43.2 Making the decision to treat or refer.

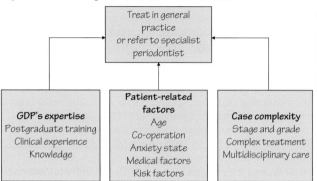

Figure 43.3 (a) Level 1 complexity. (b) Level 2 complexity. (c) Level 3 complexity. (d) Management for all levels of complexity. (e) Modifying factors relevant to periodontal treatment.

Periodontal Treatment Assessment	Comprehensive interpretation of medical, social, behavioural factors relevant to periodontal health
Level 1 Complexity	Diagnosis and management of patients with uncomplicated periodontal diseases including but not limited to:
• All patients • Treatment ideally performed in general practice	• Evaluation of periodontal risk, diagnosis of periodontal condition and design of initial care plan within the • context of overall oral health needs. • Measurement and accurate recording of periodontal indices. • Communication of nature of condition, clinical findings, • risks and outcomes • Designing care plan and providing treatment • Assessment of patient understanding, willingness and capacity to adhere to advice and care plan • Evaluation of outcome of periodontal care and provision of supportive periodontal care program • On-going motivation and risk factor management including plaque biofilm control • Avoidance of antibiotic use except in specific conditions necrotizing periodontal diseases or acute abscess with systemic complications) unless recommended by specialist as part of comprehensive care plan • Preventive and supportive care for patients with implants • Palliative periodontal care and periodontal maintenance

(a)

Periodontal Treatment Assessment	Comprehensive interpretation of medical, social, behavioural factors relevant to periodontal health
Level 2 Complexity	Management of Patients:
• Treatment may be provided by oral healthcare professionals in general dental practice or referred. • There may be instances where periodontal/ peri-implant treatment may need to be delivered by a specialist as part of a more complex integrated treatment strategy.	• Who following primary care periodontal therapy have stage II, III or IV periodontitis (>30% bone loss) periodontitis and residual true pocketing of 6 mm and above? • With Grade C periodontitis as determined by a specialist at referral. • With furcation defects and other complex root morphologies when strategically important and, realistic and delegated by a specialist. • With gingival enlargement non-surgically, in collaboration with medical colleagues. • Who require pocket reduction surgery when delegated by a specialist? • With certain non-plaque-induced periodontal diseases e.g. virally induced diseases, auto-immune diseases, abnormal pigmentation, vesiculo-bullous disease, periodontal manifestations of gastrointestinal and other systemic diseases and syndromes, under specialist guidance. • With peri-implant mucositis.

(b)

Periodontology at a Glance, Second Edition. Valerie Clerehugh, Aradhna Tugnait, Michael R. Milward, and Iain L. C. Chapple.
© 2024 John Wiley & Sons Ltd. Published 2024 by John Wiley & Sons Ltd.

Figure 43.3 (Continued)

Periodontal Treatment Assessment	Comprehensive interpretation of medical, social, behavioural factors relevant to periodontal health
Level 3 Complexity • Patients are usually referred once the lifestyle or behavioural risk factors have been addressed and appropriate nonsurgical treatment undertaken in general practice.	Triage and Management of patients: • With Grade C or Stage IV periodontitis (bone loss > 2/3 root length) and true pocketing of 6 mm or more. • Requiring periodontal surgery. • Furcation defects and other complex root morphologies not suitable for delegation. • With non-plaque induced periodontal diseases not suitable for delegation to a practitioner with enhanced skills. • Patients who require multi-disciplinary specialist care (Level 3). • Where patients of level 2 complexity do not respond to treatment. • Non-plaque induced periodontal diseases including periodontal manifestations of systemic diseases, to establish a differential diagnosis, joint care pathways with relevant medical colleagues and where necessary, manage conditions collaboratively with practitioners with enhanced skills if appropriate & provide advice and treatment planning to colleagues. • With peri-implantitis

(c)

All cases of periodontitis of any level of complexity should have initial care (including treatment) and if unsuccessful, referral may then be indicated.

Patients with modifying factors may require movement to the next level of care, including those where behaviour change is challenging. Evidence for the latter will be required to accompany referral letters.

Patients with Grade C Periodontitis should be referred after initial preventive advice on risk factor management and oral hygiene instruction.

(d)

Modifying Factors Relevant to Periodontal Treatment

• Co-ordinated medical or dental multi-disciplinary care
• Regular tobacco smoking and tobacco substitute products that deliver nicotine, e.g. vaping
• Dental special care for the acceptance or provision of treatment
• Concurrent mucogingival disease, e.g. erosive lichen planus
• Medical history that significantly affects clinical management:

   • Patients with a history of head/neck radiotherapy or intravenous bisphosphonate therapy
   • Patients who are significantly immunocompromised or immunosuppressed
   • Patients with a significant bleeding dyscrasia/disorder
   • Patients with a potential drug interaction

(e)

Figure 43.4 Complexity levels by stage and grade of periodontitis from Commissioning Standard for Restorative Dentistry.
Source: Adapted from Dietrich et al. (2019).

Grade		Stage			
		I	II	III	IV
	A	Level 1	Level 1	Level 2	Level 3
	B	Level 1	Level 2	Level 3	Level 3
	C	Level 2	Level 3	Level 3	Level 3

Figure 43.5 Key information to include in a referral to a specialist.

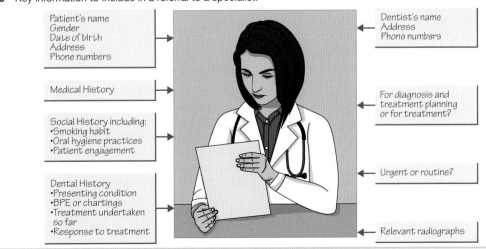

Patient's name, Gender, Date of birth, Address, Phone numbers

Medical History

Social History including: •Smoking habit •Oral hygiene practices •Patient engagement

Dental History •Presenting condition •BPE or chartings •Treatment undertaken so far •Response to treatment

Dentist's name, Address, Phone numbers

For diagnosis and treatment planning or for treatment?

Urgent or routine?

Relevant radiographs

Periodontal diseases are generally chronic conditions and patients are best managed by a team approach. For many patients, the management of their periodontal condition can be solely carried out in a primary care setting where the dentist will take on the role of team leader, planning and co-ordinating the patient's treatment. The team may also include a dental hygienist or dental therapist who may be responsible for delivery of much of the initial phase of treatment and supportive care. Oral health educators may deliver the oral health message which should be supported by other members of the team to ensure a consistent message. The dental receptionist, dental nurses, dental technician and practice manager may all contribute to the patient's care, the exact nature of the contribution depending on the local organization and national regulations.

Consultation with the medical practitioner may be required for some patients. Referral to a specialist periodontist may be appropriate for some patients, and treatment may be delivered within the specialist referral centre or jointly with the general practice. Key roles of some of the dental team are summarised in Fig. 43.1.

The decision to treat or refer a patient will be dependent on three broad issues (Fig. 43.2). Any decision is made on a case-specific basis, using current local, national and international Guideline to inform that decision. Figure 43.3 presents levels of complexity of care linked to specialist referral taken from Guideline of the British Society of Periodontology and Implant Dentistry for patient referral for periodontal treatment and maintenance (2020). Figure 43.4 shows complexity levels by stage and grade of periodontitis using the British Society of Periodontology and Implant Dentistry implementation of the 2018 Classification of Periodontal Disease and Conditions (Dietrich et al., 2019).

The referral process

The referral letter

Most patients are referred to a specialist by a written referral letter. The quality of referral letters is variable but use of a pro forma or template can prevent key pieces of information being omitted. Figure 43.5 shows a checklist for information to include in a referral letter. The dentist should ensure that the patient understands why they are to be referred and consents to the referral.

Radiographs

Every attempt should be made to limit the radiation dose to the patient (Chapter 18) so where possible, the dentist should send relevant radiographs as part of a referral. Digital imaging enables the images to be sent without the radiographs leaving the practice but care must be taken to ensure compliance with data protection regulations when dealing with patient information. Sight of previous radiographs may reduce the need for further exposures and help to assess the progress of the disease if sequential radiographs are available.

Starting periodontal therapy

For almost all cases of periodontitis, initial therapy should be provided and evaluated by the dentist and their team in primary care before considering a referral. If the patient has Grade C periodontitis, the dentist should commence initial preventive advice to manage risk factors and potentially start treatment but send an early referral without necessarily evaluating response. The dentist should indicate the provisional diagnosis in the referral letter and flag the urgency of the case. Some of the non-plaque-induced lesions (Chapter 32) require an immediate referral for diagnosis and management in a specialist centre.

The specialist's reply

Following the patient's visit to the specialist, the dentist should receive a reply to the original referral letter. This will generally include:

* a summary of the clinical findings
* a diagnosis and treatment plan
* clear indication of which parts of the treatment plan are to be carried out in the specialist centre and which in primary practice.

It is important that the patient, referring dentist and specialist are clear as to where the different parts of treatment will be delivered. Generally, routine dental care including treatment integral to the periodontal treatment plan, such as extractions or modification of plaque retentive restorations, and the long-term management of the patient will fall to the referring practitioner. As periodontal therapy can extend over some time, it is important that the patient understands that regular dental examinations should continue alongside any specialist periodontal provision.

Discharge from the specialist to referring dentist

On completion of the corrective phase of treatment, the patient is evaluated and supportive therapy is planned. Where the corrective phase of treatment has been provided in the specialist setting, the periodontist may wish to review the treatment response but then the patient will usually be discharged back to the referring practitioner. A letter of discharge should advise the dentist on the plan for supportive care, including sites requiring particular attention.

After an intensive period of treatment when the patient may have been very compliant, it is easy for the patient to lapse into old habits and feel that the periodontal problem has been solved. It is also often hard for the patient to maintain the high standards of hygiene required when the frequency of appointments decreases and the patient moves into the supportive phase of care. It is therefore important in this phase to be vigilant for any disease recurrence and review the patient's compliance with oral home care.

Medico-legal implications

Undiagnosed and untreated periodontal disease is one of the fastest growing areas of dental complaints and subsequent litigation. Commonly patients complain that they were not made aware of having periodontal disease or that the severity and consequences were not adequately explained. The UK Dental Defence Union reports that between 2008 and 2012 it paid out over £2.8m in compensation and a similar amount in legal fees for claims relating to periodontal disease (Dental Defence

Union, 2014). It is therefore important that the periodontal situation is explained clearly to patients and that communication within the dental team supports this. Accurate records should include appropriate periodontal screening and chartings as well as the advice given, such as smoking cessation and preventive advice, as well as the outcome of discussions with the patient. Patient compliance with advice should also be noted.

Key points

- Each member of the dental team has a valuable role to play
- The decision to refer a patient may depend on the dentist's expertise, patient-related factors and the complexity of the case
- Referral letters should contain key facts about the patient and condition
- Previous relevant radiographs should be made available to the specialist where possible
- Good diagnosis, communication and record keeping are imperative

Appendix 1: Unabridged Figure 2.2 (b): 2018 Classification of gingival diseases: non-dental plaque-induced

Gingival diseases:non-dental-plaque -induced:

A Genetic/developmental disorders
- i Hereditary gingival fibromatosis

B Specific infections
- i Bacterial origin
  - a *Neisseria gonorrhoea*
  - b *Treponema pallidum*
  - c *Mycobacterium tuberculosis*
  - d Streptococcal gingivitis
- ii Viral origin
  - a Coxsackie virus (hand-foot-and-mouth disease)
  - b Herpes simplex I & II (primary or recurrent)
  - c Varicella zoster (chicken pox & shingles – V nerve)
  - d Molluscum contagiosum
  - e Human papilloma virus (squamous cell papilloma; condyloma acuminatum; verruca vulgaris; focal epithelial hyperplasia)
- iii Fungal origin
  - a Candidosis
  - b Other mycoses, e.g., histoplasmosis, aspergillosis

C Inflammatory and immune conditions
- i Hypersensitivity reactions
  - a Contact allergy
  - b Plasma cell gingivitis
  - c Erythema multiforme
- ii Autoimmune diseases of skin and mucous membranes
  - a Pemphigus vulgaris
  - b Pemphigoid
  - c Lichen planus
  - d Lupus erythematosus
    Systemic lupus erythematosus
    Discoid lupus erythematosus
- iii Granulomatous inflammatory lesions (orofacial granulomatoses)
  - a Crohn's disease
  - b Sarcoidosis

D Reactive processes
- i Epulides
  - a Fibrous epulis
  - b Calcifying fibroblastic granuloma
  - c Vascular epulis (pyogenic granuloma)
  - d Peripheral giant cell granuloma

E Neoplasms
- i Premalignancy
  - a Leukoplakia
  - b Erythroplakia
- ii Malignancy
  - a Squamous cell carcinoma
  - b Leukaemic cell infiltration
  - c Lymphoma
    Hodgkin's
    Non-Hodgkin's
  - d Chondrosarcoma

F Endocrine, nutritional & metabolic diseases
- i Vitamin deficiencies
  - a Vitamin C deficiency (scurvy)

G Traumatic lesions
- i Physical/mechanical trauma
  - a Frictional keratosis
  - b Mechanically induced gingival ulceration
  - c Factitious injury (self-harm)
- ii Chemical (toxic) burn
- iii Thermal insults
  - a Burns to gingiva

H Gingival pigmentation
- i Melanoplakia
- ii Smoker's melanosis
- iii Drug-induced pigmentation (antimalarials, minocycline)
- iv Amalgam tattoo

Source: Adapted from Chapple *et al.* (2018), Table 2.

Periodontology at a Glance, Second Edition. Valerie Clerehugh, Aradhna Tugnait, Michael R. Milward, and Iain L. C. Chapple.
© 2024 John Wiley & Sons Ltd. Published 2024 by John Wiley & Sons Ltd.

Appendix 2: Unabridged Figure 2.4: 2018 Classification of systemic diseases and conditions that affect the periodontal supporting tissues

Classification	Disorders	ICD-10 code
1.	Systemic disorders that have a major impact on the loss of periodontal tissues by influencing periodontal inflammation	
1.1.	Genetic disorders	
1.1.1.	Diseases associated with immunologic disorders	
	Down syndrome	Q90.9
	Leukocyte adhesion deficiency syndromes	D72.0
	Papillon-Lefèvre syndrome	Q82.8
	Haim-Munk syndrome	Q82.8
	Chediak-Higashi syndrome	E70.3
	Severe neutropenia	
	Congenital neutropenia (Kostmann syndrome)	D70.0
	Cyclic neutropenia	D70.4
	Primary immunodeficiency diseases	
	Chronic granulomatous disease	D71.0
	Hyperimmunoglobulin E syndromes	D82.9
	Cohen syndrome	Q87.8
1.1.2.	Diseases affecting the oral mucosa and gingival tissue	
	Epidermolysis bullosa	
	Dystrophic epidermolysis bullosa	Q81.2
	Kindler syndrome	Q81.8
	Plasminogen deficiency	D68.2
1.1.3.	Diseases affecting the connective tissues	
	Ehlers-Danlos syndromes (types IV, VIII)	Q79.6
	Angioedema (C1-inhibitor deficiency)	D84.1
	Systemic lupus erythematosus	M32.9
1.1.4.	Metabolic and endocrine disorders	
	Glycogen storage disease	E74.0
	Gaucher disease	E75.2
	Hypophosphatasia	E83.30
	Hypophosphatemic rickets	E83.31
	Hajdu-Cheney syndrome	Q78.8
1.2.	Acquired immunodeficiency diseases	
	Acquired neutropenia	D70.9
	HIV infection	B24

Classification	Disorders	ICD-10 code
1.3.	Inflammatory diseases	
	Epidermolysis bullosa acquisita	L12.3
	Inflammatory bowel disease	K50, K51.9, K52.9
2.	Other systemic disorders that influence the pathogenesis of periodontal diseases	
	Diabetes mellitus	E10 (type 1), E11 (type 2)
	Obesity	E66.9
	Osteoporosis	M81.9
	Arthritis (rheumatoid arthritis, osteoarthritis)	M05, M06, M15-M19
	Emotional stress and depression	F32.9
	Smoking (nicotine dependence)	F17
	Medications	
3.	Systemic disorders that can result in loss of periodontal tissues independent of periodontitis	
3.1.	Neoplasms	
	Primary neoplastic diseases of the periodontal tissues	
	Oral squamous cell carcinoma	C03.0 – 1
	Odontogenic tumors	D48.0
	Other primary neoplasms of the periodontal tissues	C41.0
	Secondary metastatic neoplasms of the periodontal tissues	C06.8
3.2.	Other disorders that may affect the periodontal tissues	
	Granulomatosis with polyangiitis	M31.3
	Langerhans cell histiocytosis	C96.6
	Giant cell granulomas	K10.1
	Hyperparathyroidism	E21.0
	Systemic sclerosis (scleroderma)	M34.9
	Vanishing bone disease (Gorham-Stout syndrome)	M89.5

Source: Jepsen *et al.* (2018), Table 1, adapted from Albandar *et al.* (2018).

Periodontology at a Glance, Second Edition. Valerie Clerehugh, Aradhna Tugnait, Michael R. Milward, and Iain L. C. Chapple.
© 2024 John Wiley & Sons Ltd. Published 2024 by John Wiley & Sons Ltd.

Appendix 3: Implementing the 2018 Classification of periodontal diseases to reach a diagnosis in Clinical Practice

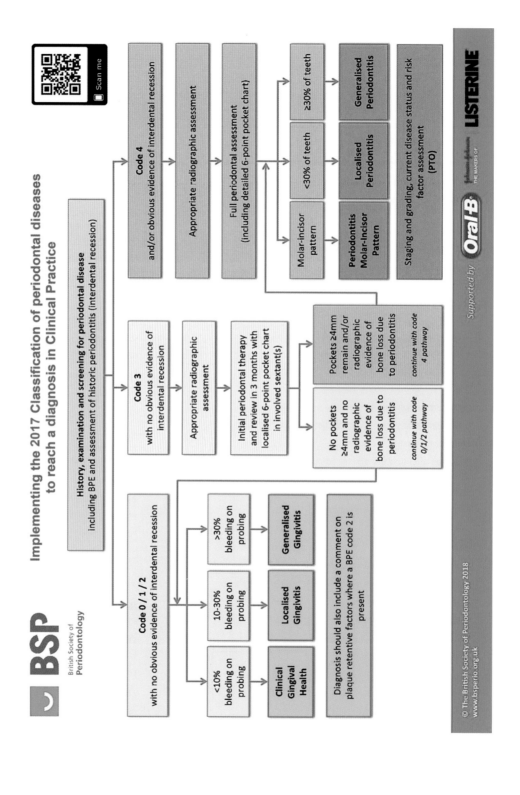

Implementing the 2017 Classification of periodontal diseases to reach a diagnosis in Clinical Practice

© The British Society of Periodontology 2018
www.bsperio.org.uk

Supported by Oral-B Johnson & Johnson THE MAKERS OF LISTERINE

Periodontology at a Glance, Second Edition. Valerie Clerehugh, Aradhna Tugnait, Michael R. Milward, and Iain L. C. Chapple.
© 2024 John Wiley & Sons Ltd. Published 2024 by John Wiley & Sons Ltd.

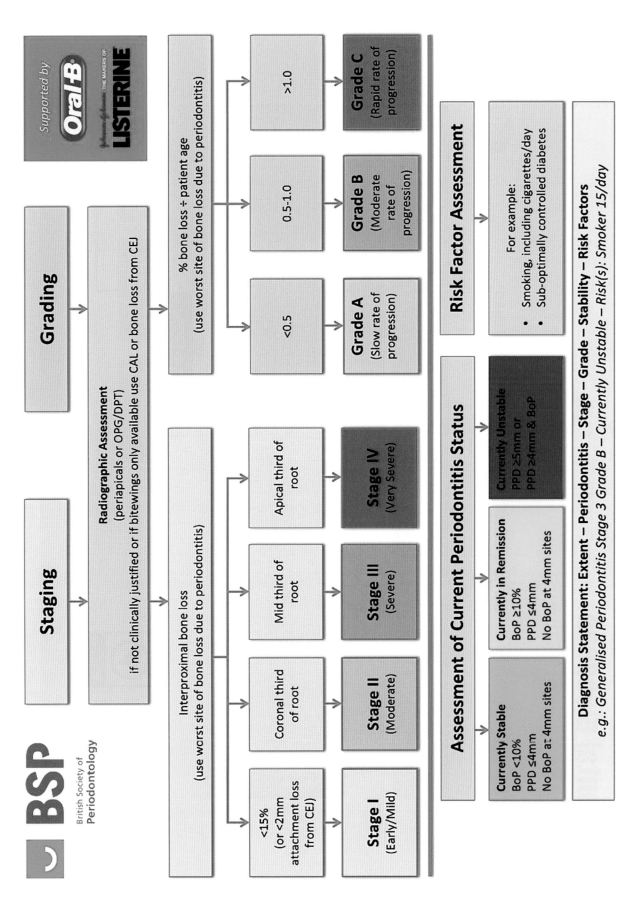

BSP
British Society of
Periodontology

Supported by
Oral-B® THE MAKERS OF **LISTERINE**

Staging

Radiographic Assessment
(periapicals or OPG/DPT)
if not clinically justified or if bitewings only available use CAL or bone loss from CEJ

Interproximal bone loss
(use worst site of bone loss due to periodontitis)

| <15% (or <2mm attachment loss from CEJ) | Coronal third of root | Mid third of root | Apical third of root |

| Stage I (Early/Mild) | Stage II (Moderate) | Stage III (Severe) | Stage IV (Very Severe) |

Grading

% bone loss ÷ patient age
(use worst site of bone loss due to periodontitis)

| <0.5 | 0.5-1.0 | >1.0 |

| Grade A (Slow rate of progression) | Grade B (Moderate rate of progression) | Grade C (Rapid rate of progression) |

Risk Factor Assessment

For example:
• Smoking, including cigarettes/day
• Sub-optimally controlled diabetes

Assessment of Current Periodontitis Status

Currently Stable
BoP <10%
PPD ≤4mm
No BoP at 4mm sites

Currently in Remission
BoP ≥10%
PPD ≤4mm
No BoP at 4mm sites

Currently Unstable
PPD ≥5mm or
PPD ≥4mm & BoP

Diagnosis Statement: Extent – Periodontitis – Stage – Grade – Stability – Risk Factors
e.g.: *Generalised Periodontitis Stage 3 Grade B – Currently Unstable – Risk(s): Smoker 15/day*

Appendix 4: BSP UK Clinical Practice guideline for the treatment of periodontal diseases

Supported by

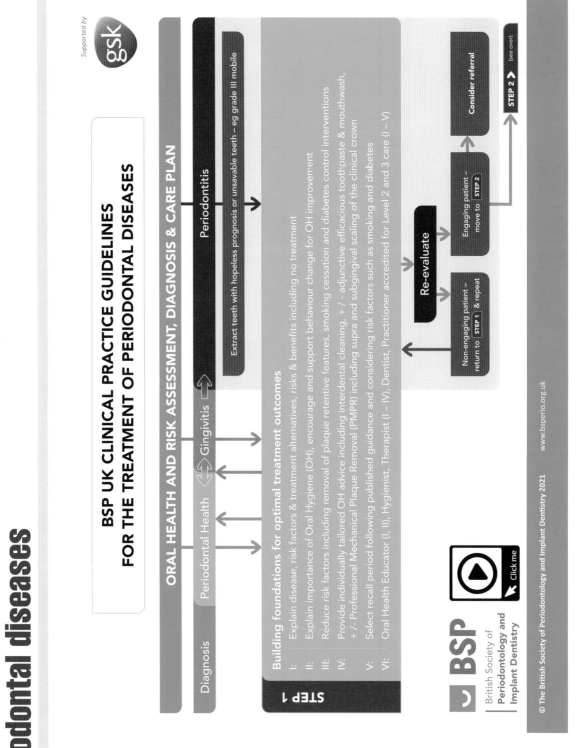

BSP UK CLINICAL PRACTICE GUIDELINES
FOR THE TREATMENT OF PERIODONTAL DISEASES

ORAL HEALTH AND RISK ASSESSMENT, DIAGNOSIS, DIAGNOSIS & CARE PLAN

Diagnosis — Periodontal Health ⇄ Gingivitis ⇄ Periodontitis

Extract teeth with hopeless prognosis or unsavable teeth – eg grade III mobile

Building foundations for optimal treatment outcomes

I: Explain disease, risk factors & treatment alternatives, risks & benefits including no treatment

II: Explain importance of Oral Hygiene (OH), encourage and support behaviour change for OH improvement

III: Reduce risk factors including removal of plaque retentive features, smoking cessation and diabetes control interventions

IV: Provide individually tailored OH advice including interdental cleaning, + / - adjunctive efficacious toothpaste & mouthwash, + /- Professional Mechanical Plaque Removal (PMPR) including supra and subgingival scaling of the clinical crown

V: Select recall period following published guidance and considering risk factors such as smoking and diabetes

VI: Oral Health Educator (I – II), Hygienist, Therapist (I – IV), Dentist, Practitioner accredited for Level 2 and 3 care (I – V)

STEP 1

Re-evaluate

Non-engaging patient – return to STEP 1 & repeat

Engaging patient – move to STEP 2

Consider referral

STEP 2 ▶ (see over)

BSP
British Society of
Periodontology and
Implant Dentistry

Click me

© The British Society of Periodontology and Implant Dentistry 2021   www.bsperio.org.uk

Periodontology at a Glance, Second Edition. Valerie Clerehugh, Aradhna Tugnait, Michael R. Milward, and Iain L. C. Chapple.
© 2024 John Wiley & Sons Ltd. Published 2024 by John Wiley & Sons Ltd.

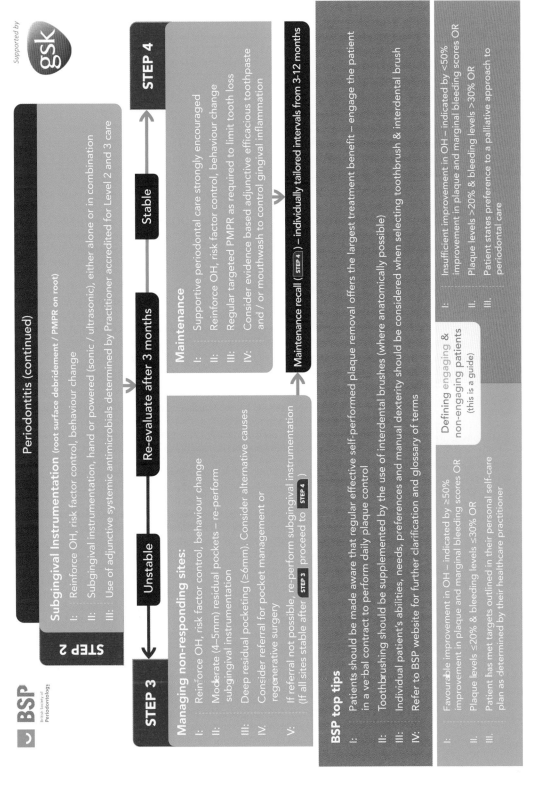

Periodontitis (continued)

STEP 2

Subgingival Instrumentation (root surface debridement / PMPR on root)

I: Reinforce OH, risk factor control, behaviour change

II: Subgingival instrumentation, hand or powered (sonic / ultrasonic), either alone or in combination

III: Use of adjunctive systemic antimicrobials determined by Practitioner accredited for Level 2 and 3 care

Re-evaluate after 3 months

Unstable → **STEP 3**

Stable → **STEP 4**

STEP 3

Managing non-responding sites:

I: Reinforce OH, risk factor control, behaviour change

II: Moderate (4–5mm) residual pockets – re-perform subgingival instrumentation

III: Deep residual pocketing (≥6mm). Consider alternative causes

IV: Consider referral for pocket management or regenerative surgery

V: If referral not possible, re-perform subgingival instrumentation after **STEP 3** proceed to **STEP 4** (If all sites stable after

STEP 4

Maintenance

I: Supportive periodontal care strongly encouraged

II: Reinforce OH, risk factor control, behaviour change

III: Regular targeted PMPR as required to limit tooth loss

IV: Consider evidence based adjunctive efficacious toothpaste and / or mouthwash to control gingival inflammation

Maintenance recall (STEP 4) – individually tailored intervals from 3-12 months

BSP top tips

I: Patients should be made aware that regular effective self-performed plaque removal offers the largest treatment benefit – engage the patient in a ve-bal contract to perform daily plaque control

II: Toothbrushing should be supplemented by the use of interdental brushes (where anatomically possible)

III: Individual patient's abilities, needs, preferences and manual dexterity should be considered when selecting toothbrush & interdental brush

IV: Refer to BSP website for further clarification and glossary of terms

Defining engaging & non-engaging patients (this is a guide)

I: Favourable improvement in OH – indicated by ≥50% improvement in plaque and marginal bleeding scores OR

II. Plaque levels ≤20% & bleeding levels ≤30% OR

III. Patient has met targets outlined in their personal self-care plan as determined by their healthcare practitioner

I: Insufficient improvement in OH – indicated by <50% improvement in plaque and marginal bleeding scores OR

II. Plaque levels >20% & bleeding levels >30% OR

III. Patient states preference to a palliative approach to periodontal care

Available at: www.bsperio.org.uk/professionals BSP UK Version of the S3-level Clinical Treatment Guideline for periodontitis Accessed 18/08/22

Appendix 5: References and further reading

Preface

Chen MX, Zhong YJ, Dong QQ, Wong HM, Wen YF. Global, regional, and national burden of severe periodontitis, 1990–2019: An analysis of the Global Burden of Disease Study 2019. *Journal of Clinical Periodontology* 2021; **48**(9): 1165–1188. https://doi.org/10.1111/jcpe.13506

World Health Organization. Oral Health fact sheet updated 18 Nov 2022. www.who.int/news-room/fact-sheets/detail/oral-health

Chapter 2

Albandar JM, Susin C, Hughes FJ. Manifestations of systemic diseases and conditions that affect the periodontal attachment apparatus: case definitions and diagnostic considerations. *Journal of Clinical Periodontology* 2018; **45**(Suppl. 20): S171–S189.

Armitage GC. Development of a classification system for periodontal diseases and conditions. *Annals of Periodontology* 1999; **4**: 1–6.

Berglundh T, Armitage G, Araujo M *et al*. Peri-implant diseases and conditions: consensus report of workgroup 4 of the 2017 World Workshop on the Classification of Periodontal and Peri-Implant Diseases and Conditions. *Journal of Clinical Periodontology* 2018; **45**(Suppl. 20): S286–S291.

Caton J, Armitage G, Berglundh T *et al*. A new classification scheme for periodontal and peri-implant diseases and conditions – introduction and key changes from the 1999 classification. *Journal of Clinical Periodontology* 2018; **45**(Suppl. 20): S1–S8.

Chapple ILC, Mealey BL, Van Dyke T *et al*. Periodontal health and gingival diseases and conditions on an intact and a reduced periodontium: consensus report of workgroup 1 of the 2017 World Workshop on the Classification of Periodontal and Peri-Implant Diseases and Conditions. *Journal of Clinical Periodontology* 2018; **45**(Suppl. 20): S68–S77.

Cortellini P, Bissada NF. Mucogingival conditions in the natural dentition: narrative review, case definitions, and diagnostic considerations. *Journal of Clinical Periodontology* 2018; **45**(Suppl. 20): S199–S206.

Ercoli C, Caton JG. Dental prostheses and tooth-related factors. *Journal of Clinical Periodontology* 2018; **45**(Suppl. 20): S207–S218.

Fan J, Caton JG. Occlusal trauma and excessive occlusal forces: narrative review, case definitions, and diagnostic considerations. *Journal of Clinical Periodontology* 2018; **45**(Suppl. 20): S207–S218.

Herrera D, Retamal-Valdes B, Alonso B, Feres M. Acute periodontal lesions (periodontal abscesses and necrotizing periodontal diseases) and endo-periodontal lesions. *Journal of Clinical Periodontology* 2018; **45**(Suppl. 20): S78–S94.

Jepsen S, Caton JG, Albandar J *et al*. Periodontal manifestations of systemic diseases and developmental and acquired conditions: consensus report of workgroup 3 of the 2017 World Workshop on the Classification of Periodontal and Peri-Implant Diseases and Conditions. *Journal of Clinical Periodontology* 2018; **45**(Suppl. 20): S219–S229.

Papapanou PN, Sanz M, Buduneli N *et al*. Periodontitis: consensus report of workgroup 2 of the 2017 World Workshop on the Classification of Periodontal and Peri-Implant Diseases and Conditions. *Journal of Clinical Periodontology* 2018; **45**(Suppl. 20): S162–S170.

Tonetti MS, Greenwell H, Kornman KS. Staging and grading of periodontitis: framework and proposal of a new classification and case definition. *Journal of Clinical Periodontology* 2018; **45**(Suppl. 20): S149–S161.

Trombelli L, Farina R, Silva CO, Tatakis DN. Plaque-induced gingivitis: case definition and diagnostic considerations. *Journal of Clinical Periodontology* 2018; **45**(Suppl. 20): S44–S66.

Chapter 3

Barnes GP, Parker WA, Lyon TC, Fulz RP. Indices used to evaluate signs, symptoms and etiologic factors associated with diseases of the periodontium. *Journal of Periodontology* 1986; **56**: 643–51.

Borrell LN, Papapanou PN. Analytical epidemiology of periodontitis. *Journal of Clinical Periodontology* 2005; **32**(Suppl. 6): 132–58.

Chen MX, Zhong YJ, Dong QQ, Wong HM, Wen YF. Global, regional, and national burden of severe periodontitis, 1990–2019: An analysis of the Global Burden of Disease Study 2019. *Journal of Clinical Periodontology* 2021; **48**(9): 1165–1188. https://doi.org/10.1111/jcpe.13506

Eke PI, Page RC, Wei L, Thornton-Evans G, Genco RJ. Update of the case definitions for population-based surveillance of periodontitis. *Journal of Periodontology* 2012; **83**(12): 1449–54.

Eke PI, Thornton-Evans GO, Wei L *et al*. Periodontitis in US adults: National Health and Nutrition Examination Survey 2009–2014. *Journal of the American Dental Association* 2018; **149**(7): 576–88.e6.

Frencken, JE, Sharma, P, Stenhouse, L, Green, D, Laverty, D, Dietrich, T. Global epidemiology of dental caries and severe periodontitis – a comprehensive review. *Journal of Clinical Periodontology* 2017; **44**(Suppl. 18): S94–S105.

Last JM. *A Dictionary of Epidemiology*, 4th edn. International Epidemiological Association, Oxford University Press, New York, 1995.

Leroy R, Eaton KA, Savage A. Methodological issues in epidemiological studies of periodontitis – how can it be improved? *BMC Oral Health* 2010; **10**: 8.

Löe H, Silness J. The gingival index, the plaque index and the retention index systems. *Journal of Periodontology* 1967; **38**: 610–17.

Nazir M, Al-Ansari A, Al-Khalifa K, Alhareky M, Gaffar B, Almas K. Global prevalence of periodontal disease and lack of its surveillance. *Scientific World Journal* 2020; Article ID 2146160.

Papapanou PN, Sanz M, Buduneli N *et al*. Periodontitis: consensus report of Workgroup 2 of the 2017 World Workshop on the Classification of Periodontal and Peri-Implant Diseases and Conditions. *Journal of Clinical Periodontology* 2018; **45** (Suppl. 20): S162–S170.

Relvas M, López-Jarana P, Monteiro L, Pacheco JJ, Braga AC, Salazar F. Study of prevalence, severity and risk factors of periodontal disease in a Portuguese population. *Journal of Clinical Medicine* 2022; **11**: 3728.

Tonetti MS, Greenwell H, Kornman KS. Staging and grading of periodontitis: framework and proposal of a new classification and case definition. *Journal of Clinical Periodontology* 2018; **45**(Suppl. 20): S149–S161.

Tu Y-K, Jackson M, Kellett M, Clerehugh V. Direct and indirect effects of interdental hygiene in a clinical trial. *Journal of Dental Research* 2008; **87**: 1037–42.

White D, Pitts N, Steele J, Sadler K, Chadwick B. *2: Disease and Related Disorders – A Report from the Adult Dental Health Survey 2009*. Health and Social Care Information Centre, London, 2011.

White DA, Tsakos G, Pitts NB *et al.* Adult Dental Health Survey 2009: common oral health conditions and their impact on the population. *British Dental Journal* 2012; **213**(11): 567–72.

World Health Organization. Oral Health fact sheet updated 18 Nov 2022. www.who.int/news-room/fact-sheets/detail/oral-health

Chapter 4

Hajishengallis G, Darveau RP, Curtis MA. The keystone-pathogen hypothesis. *Nature Reviews Microbiology* 2012; **10**(10): 717–25.

Lamont RJ, Hajishengallis G. Polymicrobial synergy and dysbiosis in inflammatory disease. *Trends in Molecular Medicine* 2015; **21**(3): 172–83.

Lamont RJ, Koo H, Hajishengallis G. The oral microbiota: dynamic communities and host interactions. *Nature Reviews Microbiology* 2018; **16**(12): 745–59.

Löe H, Theilade E, Jensen SB. Experimental gingivitis in man. *Journal of Periodontology* 1965; **36**: 177–87.

Loesche WJ. Chemotherapy of dental plaque infections. *Oral Science Reviews* 1976; **9**: 63–107.

Loesche WJ. Clinical and microbiological aspects of chemotherapeutic agents used according to the specific plaque hypothesis. *Journal of Dental Research* 1979; **58**: 2404–12.

Marsh PD. Sugar, fluoride, pH and microbial homeostasis in dental plaque. *Proceedings of the Finnish Dental Society* 1991; **87**: 515–25.

Marsh PD. Microbial ecology of dental plaque and its significance in health and disease. *Advances in Dental Research* 1994; **8**: 263–71.

Marsh PD. Dental plaque: biological significance of a biofilm and community life-style. *Journal of Clinical Periodontology* 2005; **32**(Suppl. 6): 7–15.

Marsh P. The role of biofilms in health and disease. In: *Practical Periodontics*, 2nd edn (Eaton K, Ower P, eds), pp. 41–55. Elsevier, Oxford, 2022.

Meuric V, Le Gall-David S, Boyer E, Acuña-Amador L, Martin B, Fong SB, BarloyHubler F, Bonnaure-Mallet M. 2017. Signature of microbial dysbiosis in periodontitis. *Appl Environ Microbiol* 83:e00462-17. https://doi .org/10.1128/AEM.00462-17.

Naginyte M, Do T, Meade J, Devine DA, Marsh PD. Enrichment of periodontal pathogens from the biofilms of healthy adults. *Scientfic Reports* 2019; **9**: 5491.

Theilade E. The non-specific theory in microbial etiology of inflammatory periodontal diseases. *Journal of Clinical Periodontology* 1986; **13**: 905–11.

Van Dyke TE, Bartold PM and Reynolds EC (2020) The nexus between periodontal inflammation and dysbiosis. *Front. Immunol.* 11:511. doi:10.3389/fimmu.2020.00511.

Wood SR, Kirkham J, Shore RC, Brookes SJ, Robinson C. Changes in the structure and density of oral plaque biofilms with increasing plaque age. *FEMS Microbiology Ecology* 2002; **39**: 239–44.

Chapter 5

Curtis MA, Slaney JM, Aduse-Opoku J. Critical pathways in microbial virulence. *Journal of Clinical Periodontology* 2005; **32**: 8–38.

Curtis MA, Diaz PI, Van Dyke TE. The role of the microbiota in periodontal disease. *Periodontology 2000* 2020; **83**: 14–25.

Dahlen G, Basic A, Bylund J. Importance of virulence factors for the persistence of oral bacteria in the inflamed gingival crevice and in the pathogenesis of periodontal disease. *Journal of Clinical Medicine* 2019; **8**(9): 1339.

Falkow S. Molecular Koch's postulates applied to microbial pathogenicity. *Reviews of Infectious Diseases* 1988; **10**(Suppl. 2): S274–S276.

Kilian M, Chapple ILC, Hannig M *et al.* The oral microbiome – an update for oral healthcare professionals. *British Dental Journal* 2016; **221**: 657–66.

Krishnan K, Chen T, Paster BJ. A practical guide to the oral microbiome and its relation to health and disease. *Oral Diseases* 2017; **23**(3): 276–86.

Marsh P. The role of biofilms in health and disease. In: *Practical Periodontics*, 2nd edn (Eaton K, Ower P, eds), pp. 41–55. Elsevier, Oxford, 2022.

Marsh PD, Lewis MAO, Rogers H, Williams DW, Wilson M. *Marsh and Martin's Oral Microbiology*, 6th edn. Elsevier, Edinburgh, 2016.

Pérez-Chaparro PJ, Gonçalves C, Figueiredo LC *et al.* Newly identified pathogens associated with periodontitis: a systematic review. *Journal of Dental Research* 2014; **93**(9): 846–58.

Schincaglia GP, Hong BY, Rosania A *et al.* Clinical, immune, and microbiome traits of gingivitis and peri-implant mucositis. *Journal of Dental Research* 2017; **96**(1): 47–55.

Socransky SS, Haffajee AD. Periodontal microbial ecology. *Periodontology 2000* 2005; **38**: 135–87.

Socransky SS, Haffajee AD, Cugini MA, Smith C, Kent Jr RL. Microbial complexes in subgingival plaque. *Journal of Clinical Periodontology* 1998; **25**: 134–44.

Teles RP, Haffajee AD, Socransky SS. Microbiological goals of periodontal therapy. *Periodontology 2000* 2006; **39**: 180–218.

Vartoukian SR, Adamowska A, Lawlor M *et al. In vitro* cultivation of 'unculturable' oral bacteria, facilitated by community culture and media supplementation with siderophores. *PLoS One* 2016; **11**(1): e0146926.

Zarco MF, Vess TJ, Ginsburg GS. The oral microbiome in health and disease and the potential impact on personalized dental medicine. *Oral Diseases* 2012; **18**: 109–20.

Chapter 6

Jin Y, Yip H-K. Supragingival calculus: formation and control. *Critical Reviews in Oral Biology and Medicine* 2002; **13**: 426–41.

Roberts-Harry EA, Clerehugh V. Subgingival calculus: where are we now? A comparative review. *Journal of Dentistry* 2000; **28**: 93–102.

Roberts-Harry EA, Clerehugh V, Shore RC, Kirkham J, Robinson C. Morphology and elemental composition of subgingival calculus in two ethnic groups. *Journal of Periodontology* 2000; **71**: 1401–11.

Chapter 7

Lamont RJ, Hajishengallis G. Polymicrobial synergy and dysbiosis in inflammatory disease. *Trends in Molecular Medicine* 2015; **21**: 172–83.

Ling MR, Chapple ILC, Matthews JB. Peripheral blood neutrophil cytokine hyperreactivity in chronic periodontitis. *Innate Immunity* 2015; **21**: 714–25.

Matthews JB, Wright HJ, Roberts A, Cooper PR, Chapple ILC. Hyperactivity and reactivity of peripheral blood neutrophils in chronic periodontitis. *Clinical and Experimental Immunology* 2007; **147**: 255–64.

Milward MR, Chapple ILC, Wright HJ, Millard JL, Matthews JB, Cooper P. Differential activation of NF-kB and gene expression in oral epithelial cells by periodontal pathogens. *Clinical and Experimental Immunology* 2007; **148**; 307–24.

Mitroulis I, Ruppova K, Wang B *et al.* Modulation of myelopoiesis progenitors is an integral component of trained immunity. *Cell* 2018; **172**: 147–61.e12

Roberts HM, Ling MR, Insall R *et al.* Impaired neutrophil directional chemotactic accuracy in chronic periodontitis patients. *Journal of Clinical Periodontology* 2015; **42**: 1–11.

van Staveren S, Ten Haaf T, Klöpping M *et al.* Multi-dimensional flow cytometry analysis reveals increasing changes in the systemic neutrophil compartment during seven consecutive days of endurance exercise. *PLoS One* 2018; **13**(10): e0206175.

White P, Sakellari D, Roberts H *et al.* Peripheral blood neutrophil extracellular trap production and degradation in chronic periodontitis. *Journal of Clinical Periodontology* 2016; **43**: 1041–9.

Chapter 8

Chapple ILC, Bouchard P, Cagetti MG *et al.* Interaction of lifestyle, behaviour or systemic diseases with dental caries and periodontal diseases: consensus report of group 2 of the joint EFP/ORCA workshop on the boundaries between caries and periodontal diseases. *Journal of Clinical Periodontology* 2017; **44**(Suppl. 18): 39–51.

Chapple ILC, Mealey BL, Van Dyke TE *et al.* Periodontal health and gingival diseases and conditions on an intact and a reduced periodontium: consensus report of workgroup 1 of the 2017 World Workshop on the Classification of Periodontal and Peri-Implant Diseases and Conditions. *Journal of Clinical Periodontology* 2018; **45**(Suppl. 20): S68–S77.

Economist Intelligence Unit. Time to take gum disease seriously. The societal and economic impact of periodontitis. EIU, 2021. https://impact.economist.com/perspectives/sites/default/files/eiu-efp-oralb-gum-disease.pdf

Kilian M, Chapple ILC, Hanig M *et al.* The oral microbiome, an update for oral healthcare professionals. *British Dental Journal* 2016; **221**: 657–66.

Konkel J, Chapple ILC. B-cells/T-cells. In: *Cell-to-Cell Communication: Cell Atlas – Visual Biology in Oral Medicine* (Gruber R, Stadlinger B, Terheyden H, eds), pp. 13–23. Quintessence, New Malden, 2022.

Ling MR, Chapple ILC, Matthews JB. Neutrophil superoxide release and plasma C-reactive protein levels pre- and post-periodontal therapy. *Journal of Clinical Periodontology* 2016; **43**: 652–8.

Matthews JB, Wright HJ, Roberts A, Cooper PR, Chapple ILC. Hyperactivity and reactivity of peripheral blood neutrophils in chronic periodontitis. *Clinical and Experimental Immunology* 2007; **147**: 255–64.

Page RC, Schroeder HE. Pathogenesis of inflammatory periodontal disease. A summary of current work. *Laboratory Investigation* 1976; **33**: 235–49.

Rothman KJ. Measuring interactions. In: *Epidemiology: An Introduction* (Rothman KJ, ed.), pp. 168–80. Oxford University Press, New York, 2002.

Schätzle M, Löe H, Bürgin W, Ånerud Å, Boysen H, Lang NP. Clinical course of chronic periodontitis I. The role of gingivitis. *Journal of Clinical Periodontology* 2003; **30**: 887–901.

Schätzle M, Löe H, Lang NP, Bürgin W, Ånerud Å, Boysen H. The clinical course of chronic periodontitis IV. Gingival inflammation as a risk factor in tooth mortality. *Journal of Clinical Periodontology* 2004; **31**: 1122–7.

Serhan CN, Chiang N, Van Dyke TE. Resolving inflammation: dual anti-inflammatory and pro-resolution lipid mediators. *Nature Reviews Immunology* 2008; **8**: 349–61.

Seymour GJ, Powell RN, Davies WIR. Conversion of a stable T-cell lesion to a progressive B-cell lesion in the pathogenesis of chronic periodontal disease: a hypothesis. *Journal of Clinical Periodontology* 1979; **6**: 267–77.

Chapter 9

Chapple IL, Van der Weijden F, Doerfer C *et al.* Primary prevention of periodontitis: managing gingivitis. *Journal of Clinical Periodontology* 2015; **42**(Suppl. 16): 71–6.

Chen MX, Zhong YJ, Dong QQ,Wong HM, Wen YF. Global, regional, and national burden of severe periodontitis, 1990–2019: An analysis of the Global Burden of Disease Study 2019. *Journal of Clinical Periodontology* 2021; **48**(9): 1165–1188. https://doi.org/10.1111/jcpe.13506

Gilthorpe MS, Zamzuri AT, Griffiths GS, Maddick IH, Eaton KA, Johnson NW. Unification of the "burst" and "linear" theories of periodontal disease progression: a multilevel manifestation of the same phenomenon. *Journal of Dental Research* 2003; **82**: 200–5.

Grant MM, Taylor JJ, Jaedicke K *et al.* Discovery, validation, and diagnostic ability of multiple protein-based biomarkers in saliva and gingival crevicular fluid to distinguish between health and periodontal diseases. *Journal of Clinical Periodontology* 2022; **49**: 622–32.

Hasturk H, Schulte F, Martins M *et al.* Safety and preliminary efficacy of a novel host-modulatory therapy for reducing gingival inflammation. *Frontiers in Immunology* 2021; **12**: 704163.

Jeffcoat MK, Reddy MS. Progression of probing attachment loss in adult periodontitis. *Journal of Periodontology* 1991; **62**: 185–9.

Kassebaum NJ, Bernabé E, Dahiya M, Bhandari B, Murray CJL, Marcenes W. Global burden of severe periodontitis in 1990–2010: a systematic review and meta-regression. *Journal of Dental Research* 2014; **93**: 1045–53.

Lang NP, Nyman S, Adler R, Joss A. Absence of bleeding on probing – a predictor of periodontal health. *Journal of Clinical Periodontology* 1990; **17**: 714–21.

Löe H, Anerud A, Boysen H, Morrison E. Natural history of periodontal disease in man. *Journal of Clinical Periodontology* 1986; **13**: 431–40.

Meyle J, Chapple I. Molecular aspects of the pathogenesis of periodontitis. *Periodontology 2000* 2015; **69**: 7–17.

Page RC, Kornman KS. The pathogenesis of human periodontitis: an introduction. *Periodontology 2000* 1997; 14: 9–11.

Papapanou P, Sanz M, Buduneli N *et al.* Periodontitis: Consensus report of workgroup 2 of the 2017 World Workshop on the Classification of Periodontal and Peri-Implant Diseases and Conditions. *Journal of Clinical Periodontology* 2018; **45**(Suppl. 20): S162–S170.

Serhan CN, Chiang N, Van Dyke TE. Resolving inflammation: dual anti-inflammatory and pro-resolution lipid mediators. *Nature Reviews Immunology* 2008; **8**: 349–61.

Socransky SS, Haffajee AD, Goodson JM, Lindhe J. New concepts of destructive periodontal disease. *Journal of Clinical Periodontology* 1984; **11**: 21–32.

Van Dyke TE. Proresolving lipid mediators: potential for prevention and treatment of periodontitis. *Journal of Clinical Periodontology* 2011; **38**(Suppl. 11): 119–25.

Van Dyke TE, Bartold PM, Reynolds EC. The nexus between periodontal inflammation and dysbiosis. *Frontiers in Immunology* 2020; **11**: 511.

Wennström JL, Tomasi C, Bertelle A, Dellasega E. Full-mouth ultrasonic debridement verses quadrant scaling and root planning as an initial approach in the treatment of chronic periodontitis. *Journal of Clinical Periodontology* 2005; **32**: 851–9.

Westfelt E, Rylander H, Dahlen G, Lindhe J. The effect of supragingival plaque control on the progression of advanced periodontal disease. *Journal of Clinical Periodontology* 1998; **25**: 536–41.

Chapter 10

Beck JD. Risk revisited. *Community Dentistry and Oral Epidemiology* 1998; **26**: 220–5.

Last JM. *A Dictionary of Epidemiology*, 4th edn. International Epidemiological Association, Oxford University Press, New York, 2001.

Chapter 11

Chapple ILC. Potential mechanisms underpinning the nutritional modulation of periodontal inflammation. *Journal of the American Dental Association* 2009; **1402**: 178–84.

Dommisch H, Kuzmanova D, Jonsson D, Grant M, Chapple ILC. Effect of micronutrient malnutrition on periodontal disease and periodontal therapy. *Periodontology 2000* 2018; **78**(1): 129–53.

Hazeldine J, Lord JM, Hampson P. Immunesenescence and inflammaging: a contributory factor in the poor outcome of the geriatric trauma patient. *Ageing Research Reviews* 2015; **24** (Pt B): 349–57.

Chapter 12

Armingohar Z, Jørgensen JJ, Kristoffersen AK, Abesha-Belay E, Olsen I. Bacteria and bacterial DNA in atherosclerotic plaque and aneurysmal wall biopsies from patients with and without periodontitis. *Journal of Oral Microbiology* 2014; **6**. doi: 10.3402/jom.v6.23408.

Chapple ILC, Mealey BL, Van Dyke TE *et al.* Periodontal health and gingival diseases and conditions on an intact and a reduced periodontium: consensus report of workgroup 1 of the 2017 World Workshop on the Classification of Periodontal and

Peri-Implant Diseases and Conditions. *Journal of Clinical Periodontology* 2018; **45**(Suppl. 20): S68–S77.

D'Aiuto F, Gkranias N, Bhowruth D *et al.* Systemic effects of periodontitis treatment in patients with type 2 diabetes: a 12 month, single-centre, investigator-masked, randomised trial. *Lancet Diabetes and Endocrinology* 2018; **6**: 954–65.

Herrera D, Sanz M, Shapira L *et al.* Association between periodontal diseases and cardiovascular diseases, diabetes and respiratory diseases: consensus report of the Joint Workshop by the European Federation of Periodontology (EFP) and the European arm of the World Organization of Family Doctors (WONCA Europe). *Journal of Clinical Periodontology* 2023; **50**(6): 819–41.

Molina A, Huck O, Herrera D, Montero E. The association between respiratory diseases and periodontitis: a systematic review and meta-analysis. *Journal of Clinical Periodontology* 2023; **50**(6): 842–87.

Taylor GW, Burt BA, Becker MP et al. Severe periodontitis and risk for poor glycemic control in patients with non-insulin-dependent diabetes mellitus. *Journal of Periodontology* 1996; **67**: 1085–93.

Yonel Z, Kocher T, Chapple ILC *et al.* Development and external validation of a multivariable prediction model to identify nondiabetic hyperglycemia and undiagnosed type 2 diabetes: Diabetes Risk Assessment in Dentistry Score (DDS). *Journal of Dental Research* 2023; **102**(2): 170–7.

Chapter 13

Amaliya A, Risdiana A, Van der Velden U. Effect of guava and vitamin C supplementation on experimental gingivitis: a randomizd clinical trial. *Journal of Clinical Periodontology* 2018; **45**: 959–67.

Chapple ILC, Milward MR, Dietrich T. The prevalence of inflammatory periodontitis is negatively associated with serum antioxidant concentrations. *Journal of Nutrition* 2007; **137**: 657–64.

Chapple ILC, Milward MR, Ling-Mountford N *et al.* Adjunctive daily supplementation with encapsulated fruit, vegetable and berry juice powder concentrates and clinical periodontal outcomes: a double blind RCT. *Journal of Clinical Periodontology* 2012; **39**: 62–72.

Graziani F, Discepoli N, Gennai S *et al.* The effect of twice daily kiwi fruit consumption on periodontal and systemic conditions before and after treatment: a randomized clincial trial. *Journal of Periodontology* 2018; **89**: 285–93.

Institute of Medicine. *Dietary Reference Intakes for Calcium and Vitamin D*. National Academies Press, Washington, DC, 2011.

National Institutes of Health, Office of Dietary Supplements. *Calcium Fact Sheet for Health Professionals* (2022). https://ods.od.nih.gov/factsheets/Calcium-HealthProfessional/

Nishida M, Grossi SG, Dunford RG, Ho AW, Trevisan M, Genco RJ. Calcium and the risk for periodontal disease. *Journal of Periodontology* 2000a; **71**: 1057–66.

Nishida M, Grossi SG, Dunford RG, Ho AW, Trevisan M, Genco RJ. Vitamin D and the risk for periodontal disease. *Journal of Periodontology* 2000b; **71**: 1215–23.

Weaver CM, Proulx WR, Heaney RP. Choices for achieving adequate dietary calcium with a vegetarian diet. *American Journal of Clinical Nutrition* 1999; **70**: S543–8.

Chapter 14

Andreasen JO. External root resorption: its implication in dental traumatology, paedodontics, periodontics, orthodontics and endodontics. *International Endodontic Journal* 1985; **18**: 109–18.

Caton JG, Armitage G, Berglundh T *et al.* A new classification scheme for periodontal and peri-implant diseases and conditions – introduction and key changes from the 1999 classification. *Journal of Clinical Periodontology* 2018; **45**(Suppl. 20): S1–S8.

Eismann D, Prusas R. Periodontal findings before and after orthodontic therapy in cases of incisor cross-bite. *European Journal of Orthodontics* 1990; **12**: 281–3.

Ercoli C, Caton JG. Dental prostheses and tooth-related factors. *Journal of Clinical Periodontology* 2018; **45**(Suppl. 20): S207–S218.

Jensen BL, Solow B. Alveolar bone loss and crowding in adult periodontal patients. *Community Dentistry and Oral Epidemiology* 1989; **17**: 47–51.

Jepsen, S, Caton, JG, Albandar J et al. Periodontal manifestations of systemic diseases and developmental and acquired conditions: consensus report of workgroup 3 of the 2017 World Workshop on the Classification of Periodontal and Peri-Implant Diseases and Conditions. *Journal of Clinical Periodontology* 2018; **45**(Suppl. 20): S219–S229.

Jernberg GR, Bakdash MB, Keenan KM. Relationship between proximal tooth open contacts and periodontal disease. *Journal of Periodontology* 1983; **54**: 529–33.

Morris HF. Veterans Administration Cooperative Studies Project No 147. Part VIII: plaque accumulation on metal ceramic restorations cast from noble and nickel-based alloys. A five year report. *Journal of Prosthetic Dentistry* 1989; **61**: 543–9.

Parsell DE, Steckfus CF, Stewart BM, Buchanan WT. The effect of amalgam overhangs on alveolar bone height as a function of patient age and overhanging width. *Operative Dentistry* 1997; **23**: 94–9.

Van der Velden U, Abbas F, Armand S *et al.* Java project on periodontal diseases. The natural development of periodontitis: risk factors, risk predictors and risk determinants. *Journal of Clinical Periodontology* 2006; **33**: 540–8.

Chapter 15

Dommisch H, Walter C, Difloe-Geisert JC, Gintaute A, Jepsen S, Zitzmann NU. Efficacy of tooth splinting and occlusal adjustment in patients with periodontitis exhibiting masticatory dysfunction: a systematic review. *Journal of Clinical Periodontology* 2021; **49**(Suppl. 24): 149–66.

Fox AM, Artese HP, Horliana AC, Pannuti CM, Romito GA. Occlusal adjustment associated with periodontal therapy – a systematic review. *Journal of Dentistry* 2012; **40**: 1025–35.

Jepsen S, Caton JG, Albandar J *et al.* Periodontal manifestations of systemic diseases and developmental and acquired conditions: consensus report of workgroup 3 of the 2017 World Workshop on the Classification of Periodontal and Peri-Implant Diseases and Conditions. *Journal of Clinical Periodontology* 2018; **45**(Suppl. 20): S219– S229.

Lindhe J, Ericsson I. The effect of elimination of jiggling forces on periodontally exposed teeth in the dog. *Journal of Periodontology* 1982; **53**: 562–7.

Lindhe J, Nyman S. A longitudinal study of combined periodontal and prosthetic treatment of patients with advanced periodontal disease. *Journal of Periodontology* 1979; **50**: 163–9.

Lindhe J, Nyman S, Ericsson I. Trauma from occlusion: periodontal tissues. In: *Clinical Periodontology and Implant Dentistry*, 5th edn (Lindhe J, Lang NP, Karring T, eds), pp. 349–62. Wiley-Blackwell, Oxford, 2008.

Polson AM, Zander HA. Effect of periodontal trauma upon infrabony pockets. *Journal of Periodontology* 1983; **54**: 586–91.

Weston P, Yaziz YA, Moles DR, Needleman I. Occlusal interventions for periodontitis in adults. *Cochrane Database of Systematic Reviews* 2008; **3**: CD004968.

Chapter 16

British Society of Periodontology (BSP). *Healthy Gums Do Matter*, 2nd edn, 2019. www.bsperio.org.uk/assets/downloads/NHS_HGdM_Quick_Ref_(Mar19).pdf

Chapple ILC, Mealey BL, Van Dyke T et al. Periodontal health and gingival diseases and conditions on an intact and a reduced periodontium: consensus report of workgroup 1 of the 2017 World Workshop on the Classification of Periodontal and Peri-Implant Diseases and Conditions. *Journal of Clinical Periodontology* 2018; **45**(Suppl. 20): S68–S77.

Dietrich T, Ower P, Tank M *et al.* Periodontal diagnosis in the context of the 2017 classification system of periodontal diseases and conditions – implementation in clinical practice. *British Dental Journal* 2019; **226**: 16–22.

Chapter 17

BSP guidance on interpretation of Basic Periodontal Examination (BPE) codes, published January 2019 available at: (https://www.bsperio.org.uk/assets/downloads/BSP_BPE_Guidelines_2019.pdf). Accessed 07 November 2023.

Clerehugh V. Periodontal diseases in children and adolescents. *British Dental Journal* 2008; **204**; 469–71.

Clerehugh V, Kindelan S. *Guidelines for Periodontal Screening and Management of Children and Adolescents Under 18 Years of Age.* 2021. www.bsperio.org.uk/publications and www.bspd.co.uk/Professionals/Resources/Clinical-Guidelines-and-Evidence-Reviews

Dietrich T, Ower P, Tank M et al. Periodontal diagnosis in the context of the 2017 classification system of periodontal diseases and conditions – implementation in clinical practice. *British Dental Journal* 2019; **226**: 16–22.

Faculty of General Dental Practitioners (UK). *Selection Criteria for Dental Radiography*, 3rd edn (Horner K, Eaton K, eds). FGDP, London, 2018. https://cgdent.uk/selection-criteria-for-dental-radiography/

Chapter 18

SEDENTEXCT. *Radiation Protection 172. Cone Beam CT for Dental and Maxillofacial Radiology: Evidence-Based Guidelines.* European Commission, Luxembourg, 2012. https://energy.ec.europa.eu/system/files/2014-11/172_1.pdf

Chapter 19

Caton JG, Armitage G, Berglundh T et al. A new classification scheme for periodontal and peri-implant diseases and conditions – introduction and key changes from the 1999 classification. *Journal of Clinical Periodontology* 2018; **45**(Suppl. 20): S1–S8.

Dietrich T, Ower P, Tank M et al. Periodontal diagnosis in the context of the 2017 classification system of periodontal diseases and conditions – implementation in clinical practice. *British Dental Journal* 2019; **226**: 16–22.

Figuero E, Roldán S, Serrano J, Escribano M, Martín C, Preshaw PM. Efficacy of adjunctive therapies in patients with gingival inflammation: a systematic review and meta-analysis. *Journal of Clinical Periodontology* 2020; **47**: 125–43.

Kebschull M, Chapple I. Evidence-based, personalised and minimally invasive treatment for periodontitis patients – the new EFP S3-level clinical treatment guidelines. *British Dental Journal* 2020; **229**(7): 443–9.

Sanz M, Herrera D, Kebschull M et al., for the EFP Workshop Participants and Methodological Consultants. Treatment of stage I–III periodontitis – the EFP S3 level clinical practice guideline. *Journal of Clinical Periodontology* 2020; **47**: 4–60.

West N, Chapple I, Claydon N et al., for the British Society of Periodontology and Implant Dentistry Guideline Group Participants. BSP implementation of European S3-level evidence-based treatment guidelines for stage I–III periodontitis in UK clinical practice. *Journal of Dentistry* 2021; **106**: 1–72.

Chapter 20

British Society of Periodontology (BSP). *UK Clinical Practice Guidelines for the Treatment of Periodontal Diseases: Flowchart.* 2021. www.bsperio.org.uk/assets/downloads/BSP_Treatment_Flow_Chart_16_For_Screen.pdf

Carra MC, Detzen L, Kitzmann J, Woelber JP, Ramseier CA, Bouchard P. Promoting behavioural changes to improve oral hygiene in patients with periodontal diseases: a systematic review. *Journal of Clinical Periodontology* 2020; **47**: 72–89.

Chapple ILC, Van der Weijden F, Doerfer C et al. Primary prevention of periodontitis: managing gingivitis. *Journal of Clinical Periodontology* 2015; **42**(Suppl. 16): S71–S76.

Gunsolley JG. A meta-analysis of six-month studies of antiplaque and antigingivitis agents. *Journal of the American Dental Association* 2006; **137**: 1649–57.

Kiyak HA, Persson RE, Persson GR. Influences on the perceptions of and responses to periodontal disease among older adults. *Periodontology 2000* 1998; **16**: 34–43.

Newton TJ, Asimakopoulou K. Managing oral hygiene as a risk factor for periodontal disease: a systematic review of psychological approaches to behaviour change for improved plaque control in periodontal management. *Journal of Clinical Periodontology* 2015; **42**(Suppl. 16): S36– S46.

Robinson P, Deacon SA, Deery C et al. Manual versus powered toothbrushing for oral health. *Cochrane Database of Systematic Reviews* 2005; **2**: CD002281.

Shou L. Behavioural aspects of dental plaque control: an oral health promotion perspective. In: *Proceedings of the European Workshop on Mechanical Plaque Control* (Lang NP, Attstrom R, Loe H, eds), pp. 297–99. Quintessence, Berlin, 1998.

Slot DE, Valkenburg C, Van der Weijden GA. Mechanical plaque removal of periodontal maintenance patients: a systematic review and network meta-analysis. *Journal of Clinical Periodontology* 2020; **47**: 107–24.

Tu Y-K, Jackson M, Kellett M, Clerehugh V. Direct and indirect effects of interdental hygiene in a clinical trial. *Journal of Dental Research* 2008; **87**: 1037–42.

Van der Weijden FA, Slot DE. Efficacy of homecare regimens for mechanical plaque removal in managing gingivitis a meta review. *Journal of Clinical Periodontology* 2015; **42**(Suppl. 16): S77–S91.

West N, Chapple I, Claydon N et al. BSP implementation of European S-3 level evidence-based treatment guidelines for stage I-III periodontitis in UK clinical practice. *Journal of Dentistry* 2021; **106**: 103562.

Yaacob M, Worthington HV, Deacon SA et al. Powered versus manual toothbrushing for oral health. *Cochrane Database of Systemic Reviews* 2014; **6**: CD002281.

Chapter 21

Badersten A, Nilveus R, Egelberg J. Effect of nonsurgical periodontal therapy. *Journal of Clinical Periodontology* 1984; **11**: 63–76.

British Society of Periodontology (BSP). *Glossary – BSP Implementation of the S3 Treatment Guidelines for Periodontitis.* 2021. www.bsperio.org.uk/assets/downloads/Glossary_-_BSP_Implementation_of_the_S3_Treatment_Guidelines_for_Periodontitis.pdf

Drisko CL. Scaling and root planing without over instrumentation: hand versus power-driven scalers. *Current Opinion in Periodontology* 1993; 78–88.

Drisko CL, Cochran DL, Blieden T et al. Position paper: sonic and ultrasonic scalers in periodontics. Research, Science and Therapy Committee of the American Academy of Periodontology. *Journal of Periodontology* 2000; **71**: 1792–801.

Eberhard J, Jepsen S, Jervøe-Storm PM, Needleman I, Worthington HV. Full-mouth treatment modalities (within 24 hours) for chronic periodontitis in adults. *Cochrane Database of Systematic Reviews* 2015; **4**: CD004622.

Graziani F, Cei S, Orlandi M et al. Acute-phase response following full-mouth versus quadrant non-surgical periodontal treatment: a randomized clinical trial. *Journal of Clinical Periodontology* 2015; **42**(9): 843–52.

Greenstein G. Nonsurgical periodontal therapy in 2000: a literature review. *Journal of the American Dental Association* 2000; **131**(11): 1580–92.

Guentsch A, Preshaw PM. The use of a linear oscillating device in periodontal treatment: a review. *Journal of Clinical Periodontology* 2008; **35**: 514–24.

Loos BG, Needleman I. Endpoints of active periodontal therapy. *Journal of Clinical Periodontology* 2020; **47**: 61–71.

Lovdal A, Arno A, Schei O, Waerhaug J. Combined effect of subgingival scaling and controlled oral hygiene on the incidence of gingivitis. *Acta Odontologica Scandinavica* 1961; **19**: 537–55.

Mongardini C, van Steenberghe D, Dekeyser C, Quirynen M. One stage full- versus partial-mouth disinfection in the treatment of chronic adult or generalized early-onset periodontitis. I. Long-term clinical observations. *Journal of Periodontology* 1999; **70**(6): 632–45.

Quirynen M, De Soete M, Boschmans G *et al.* Benefit of "one-stage full-mouth disinfection" is explained by disinfection and root planing within 24 hours: a randomized controlled trial. *Journal of Clinical Periodontology* 2006; **33**(9): 639–47.

Suvan J, Leira Y, Moreno F, Graziani F, Derks J, Tomasi C. Subgingival instrumentation for treatment of periodontitis. A systematic review. *Journal of Clinical Periodontology* 2020; **47**: 155–75.

Tunkel J, Heinecke A, Flemmig TF. A systematic review of efficacy of machine-driven and manual subgingival debridement in the treatment of chronic periodontitis. *Journal of Clinical Periodontology* 2002; **29**(Suppl. 3): 72–91.

Van Weijden F, Slot D. Oral hygiene in the prevention of periodontal diseases: the evidence. *Periodontology 2000* 2011; **55**: 104–23.

West N, Chapple I, Claydon N *et al.* BSP implementation of European S-3 level evidence-based treatment guidelines for stage I-III periodontitis in UK clinical practice. *Journal of Dentistry* 2021; **106**: 103562.

Chapter 22

Dietrich T, Ower P, Tank M *et al.* Periodontal diagnosis in the context of the 2017 classification system of periodontal diseases and conditions – implementation in clinical practice. *British Dental Journal* 2019; **226**: 16–22.

Loos BG, Needleman I. Endpoints of active periodontal therapy. *Journal of Clinical Periodontology* 2020; **47**: 61–71.

Magnusson I, Lindhe J, Yoneyama T, Liljenberg B. Recolonization of a subgingival microbiota following scaling in deep pockets. *Journal of Clinical Periodontology* 1984; **11**: 193–207.

Sanz M, Herrera D, Kebschull M *et al.*, for the EFP Workshop Participants and Methodological Consultants. Treatment of stage I–III periodontitis – the EFP S3 level clinical practice guideline. *Journal of Clinical Periodontology* 2020; **47**: 4– 60.

Segelnick SL, Weinberg MA. Re-evaluation of initial therapy: when is the appropriate time? *Journal of Periodontology* 2006; **77**: 1598–601.

West N, Chapple I, Claydon N *et al.* BSP implementation of European S-3 level evidence-based treatment guidelines for stage I-III periodontitis in UK clinical practice. *Journal of Dentistry* 2021; **106**: 103562.

Chapter 23

Caton J, Armitage G, Berglundh T *et al.* A new classification scheme for periodontal and peri-implant diseases and conditions – introduction and key changes from the 1999 classification. *Journal of Clinical Periodontology* 2018; **45**(Suppl. 20): S1–S8.

Donos N, Calciolari E, Brusselaers N, Goldoni M, Bostanci N, Belibasakis GN. The adjunctive use of host modulators in non-surgical periodontal therapy. A systematic review of randomized, placebo-controlled clinical studies. *Journal of Clinical Periodontology* 2019; **47**: 199–238.

Haas AN, de Castro GD, Moreno T *et al.* Azithromycin as an adjunctive treatment of aggressive periodontitis: 12-months randomized clinical trial. *Journal of Clinical Periodontology* 2008; **35**: 696–704.

Lopez NJ, Socransky SS, Da Silva I, Japlit MR, Haffajee AD. Effects of metronidazole plus amoxicillin as the only therapy on the microbiological and clinical parameters of untreated chronic periodontitis. *Journal of Clinical Periodontology* 2006; **33**: 648–60.

Matesanz-Perez P, Garcia-Gargallo M, Figuero E, Bascones-Martinez A, Sanz M, Herrera D. A systematic review on the effects of local antimicrobials as adjuncts to subgingival debridement, compared with subgingival debridement alone, in the treatment of chronic periodontitis. *Journal of Clinical Periodontology* 2013; **40**: 227–41.

Mombelli A, Schmid B, Rutar A, Lang NP. Persistence patterns of *Porphyromonas gingivalis, Prevotella intermedia/nigrescens*, and *Actinobacillus actinomycetemcomitans* after mechanical therapy of periodontal disease. *Journal of Periodontology* 2000; **71**: 14–21.

Rabelo CC, Feres M, Gonçalves C *et al.* Systematic antibiotics in the treatment of aggressive periodontitis. A systematic review and a Bayesian Network meta-analysis. *Journal of Clinical Periodontology* 2015; **42**: 647–57.

Salvi GE, Stähli A, Schmidt JC, Ramseier CA, Sculean A, Walter C. Adjunctive laser or antimicrobial photodynamic therapy to non-surgical mechanical instrumentation in patients with untreated periodontitis: a systematic review and meta-analysis. *Journal of Clinical Periodontology* 2020; **47**: 176–98.

Scottish Dental Clinical Effectiveness Programme. *Drug Prescribing for Dentistry*. 2021. www.sdcep.org.uk/media/ckgfnx3w/sdcep-drug-prescribing-ed-3-update-june-2021.pdf

Sgolastra F, Petrucci A, Gatto R, Monaco A. Effectiveness of systemic amoxicillin/metronidazole as an adjunctive therapy to full-mouth scaling and root planing in the treatment of aggressive periodontitis: a systematic review and meta-analysis. *Journal of Periodontology* 2012; **83**: 731–43.

West N, Chapple I, Claydon N *et al.* BSP implementation of European S-3 level evidence-based treatment guidelines for stage I-III periodontitis in UK clinical practice. *Journal of Dentistry* 2021; **106**: 103562.

Chapter 24

Varju I, Sotonyi P, Machovich R *et al.* Hindered dissolution of fibrin formed under mechanical stress. *Journal of Thrombosis and Haemostasis* 2011; **9**: 979–86.

West N, Chapple I, Claydon N *et al.* BSP implementation of European S-3 level evidence-based treatment guidelines for stage I-III periodontitis in UK clinical practice. *Journal of Dentistry* 2021; **106**: 103562.

Chapter 25

Cortellini P, Prato GP, Tonetti MS. The modified papilla preservation technique. A new surgical approach for interproximal regenerative procedures. *Journal of Periodontology* 1995; **66**: 261–6.

Chapter 26

Cortellini P, Buti J, Pini Prato G, Tonetti MS. Periodontal regeneration compared with access flap surgery in human intra-bony defects 20-year follow-up of a randomized clinical trial: tooth retention, periodontitis recurrence and costs. *Journal of Clinical Periodontology* 2017; **44**(1): 58–66.

Darby IB, Morris KH. A systematic review of the use of growth factors in human periodontal regeneration. *Journal of Periodontology* 2013; **84**(4): 465–76.

West N, Chapple I, Claydon N *et al.* BSP implementation of European S-3 level evidence-based treatment guidelines for stage I-III periodontitis in UK clinical practice. *Journal of Dentistry* 2021; **106**: 103562.

Chapter 27

Cortellini P, Buti J, Pini Prato G, Tonetti MS. Periodontal regeneration compared with access flap surgery in human intra-bony defects 20-year follow-up of a randomized clinical trial: tooth retention, periodontitis recurrence and costs. *Journal of Clinical Periodontology* 2017; **44**(1): 58–66.

West N, Chapple I, Claydon N *et al.* BSP implementation of European S-3 level evidence-based treatment guidelines for stage I-III periodontitis in UK clinical practice. *Journal of Dentistry* 2021; **106**: 103562.

Chapter 28

Chrcanovic BR, Albrektsson T, Wennerberg A. Smoking and dental implants: a systematic review and meta-analysis. *Journal of Dentistry* 2015; **43**(5): 487–98.

Kungsadalpipob K, Supanimitkul K, Manopattanasoontorn S *et al.* The lack of keratinized mucosa is associated with poor peri-implant tissue health: a cross-sectional study. *International Journal of Implant Dentistry* 2020; **6**: 28.

Chapter 29

Berglundh T, Armitage G, Araujo M *et al.* Peri-implant diseases and conditions: consensus report of workgroup 4 of the 2017 World Workshop on the Classification of Periodontal and Peri-Implant Diseases and Conditions. *Journal of Periodontology* 2018; **89**(Suppl. 1): S313– S318.

Costa FO, Takenaka-Martinez S, Cota LO, Ferreira SD, Silva GL, Costa JE. Peri-implant disease in subjects with and without preventive maintenance: a 5-year follow-up. *Journal of Clinical Periodontology* 2012; **39**(2): 173–81.

De Siena F, Francetti L, Corbella S, Taschieri S, Del Fabbro M. Topical application of 1% chlorhexidine gel versus 0.2% mouthwash in the treatment of peri-implant mucositis. An observational study. *International Journal of Dental Hygiene* 2013; **11**(1): 41–7.

Esposito M, Grusovin MG, Worthington HV. Treatment of peri-implantitis: what interventions are effective? A Cochrane systematic review. *European Journal of Oral Implantology* 2012; **5**(Suppl): S21–S41.

Heitz-Mayfield LJ, Mombelli A. The therapy of peri-implantitis: a systematic review. *International Journal of Oral & Maxillofacial Implants* 2014; **29**(Suppl): 325–45.

Heitz-Mayfield LJ, Salvi GE, Botticell, D, Mombelli A, Faddy M, Lang NP, for the Implant Complication Research Group. Anti-infective treatment of peri-implant mucositis: a randomised controlled clinical trial. *Clinical Oral Implants Research* 2011; **22**: 237–41.

Javed F, Al-Ghamdi AST, Ahmed A, Mikami T, Ahmed HB, Tenenbaum HC. Clinical efficacy of antibiotics in the treatment of peri-implantitis. *International Dental Journal* 2013; **63**: 169–76.

Lindhe J, Meyle J, Group D of European Workshop on Periodontology. Peri-implant diseases: consensus report of the Sixth European Workshop on Periodontology. *Journal of Clinical Periodontology* 2008; **35**(Suppl. 8): 282–5.

Renvert S, Roos-Jansåker AM, Claffey N. Non-surgical treatment of peri-implant mucositis and peri-implantitis: a literature review. *Journal of Clinical Periodontology* 2008; **35**: 305–15.

Roos-Jansåker AM, Lindahl C, Renvert H, Renvert S. Nine- to fourteen-year follow-up of implant treatment. Part II: presence of peri-implant lesions. *Journal of Clinical Periodontology* 2006; **33**(4): 290–5.

Salvi GE, Ramseier CA. Efficacy of patient-administered mechanical and/or chemical plaque control protocols in the management of peri-implant mucositis. A systematic review. *Journal of Clinical Periodontology* 2015; **42**(Suppl. 16): S187–S201.

Schwarz F, Becker K, Sager M. Efficacy of professionally administered plaque removal with or without adjunctive measures for the treatment of peri-implant mucositis. A systematic review and meta-analysis. *Journal of Clinical Periodontology* 2014; **42**(Suppl. 16): S202–S213.

Chapter 30

Public Health England. *Delivering Better Oral Health: An Evidence-based Toolkit for Prevention*, 4th edn. 2021. www.gov.uk/government/publications/delivering-better-oral-health-an-evidence-based-toolkit-for-prevention

Chapter 31

Chapple ILC, Mealey BL, Van Dyke T *et al.* Periodontal health and gingival diseases and conditions on an intact and a reduced periodontium: consensus report of workgroup 1 of the 2017 World Workshop on the Classification of Periodontal and Peri-Implant Diseases and Conditions. *Journal of Clinical Periodontology* 2018; **45**(Suppl. 20): S68–S77.

Dietrich T, Ower P, Tank M *et al.* Periodontal diagnosis in the context of the 2017 classification system of periodontal diseases and conditions – implementation in clinical practice. *British Dental Journal* 2019; **226**: 16–22.

Chapter 32

Chapple ILC, Hamburger JH. *Periodontal Medicine*. Quintessence, London, 2006.

Chapple ILC, Mealey BL, Van Dyke T *et al.* Periodontal health and gingival diseases and conditions on an intact and a reduced periodontium: consensus report of workgroup 1 of the 2017 World Workshop on the Classification of Periodontal and Peri-Implant Diseases and Conditions. *Journal of Clinical Periodontology* 2018; **45**(Suppl. 20): S68–S77.

Chapter 33

Aroca S, Molnar B, Windisch P *et al.* Treatment of multiple adjacent Miller class I and II gingival recessions with a Modified Coronally Advanced Tunnel (MCAT) technique and a collagen matrix or palatal connective tissue graft: a randomized, controlled clinical trial. *Journal of Clinical Periodontology* 2013; **40**: 713–20.

Cairo F, Nieri M, Pagliaro U. Efficacy of periodontal plastic surgery procedures in the treatment of localized gingival recessions. A systematic review. *Journal of Clinical Periodontology* 2014; **41**(Suppl. 15): S44–S62.

Chambrone L, Tatakis DN. Long-term outcomes of untreated buccal gingival recessions: a systematic review and meta-analysis. *Journal of Periodontology* 2016; **87**: 796–808.

Cortellini P, Tonetti M, Baldi C *et al.* Does placement of a connective tissue graft improve the outcomes of coronally advanced flap for coverage of single gingival recessions in upper anterior teeth? A multi-centre, randomized, double-blind, clinical trial. *Journal of Clinical Periodontology* 2009; **36**: 68–79.

Dai A, Huang JP, Ding PH, Chen LL. Long-term stability of root coverage procedures for single gingival recessions: a systematic review and meta-analysis. *Journal of Clinical Periodontology* 2019; **46**: 572–85.

Jepsen S, Caton JG, Albandar JM *et al.* Periodontal manifestations of systemic diseases and developmental and acquired conditions: consensus report of workgroup 3 of the 2017 World Workshop on the Classification of Periodontal and Peri-Implant Diseases and Conditions. *Journal of Clinical Periodontology* 2018; **45**: S219–S229.

Chapter 34

Chapple ILC, Hamburger JH. *Periodontal Medicine*. Quintessence, London, 2006.

Chapter 35

Dietrich T, Ower P, Tank M *et al.* Periodontal diagnosis in the context of the 2017 classification system of periodontal diseases and conditions – implementation in clinical practice. *British Dental Journal* 2019; **226**: 16–22.

Fine DH, Patil AG, Loos BG. Classification and diagnosis of aggressive periodontitis. *Journal of Clinical Periodontology* 2018; **45**(Suppl. 20): S95–S111.

Kebschull M, Chapple I. Evidence-based, personalised and minimally invasive treatment for periodontitis patients – the new EFP S3-level clinical treatment guidelines. *British Dental Journal* 2020; **229**(7):443–9.

Sanz M, Herrera D, Kebschull M *et al.*, for the EFP Workshop Participants and Methodological Consultants. Treatment of stage I–III periodontitis – the EFP S3 level clinical practice guideline. *Journal of Clinical Periodontology* 2020; **47**: 4–60.

West N, Chapple I, Claydon N *et al.* BSP implementation of European S-3 level evidence-based treatment guidelines for stage I-III periodontitis in UK clinical practice. *Journal of Dentistry* 2021; **106**: 103562.

Chapter 36

Dietrich T, Ower P, Tank M et al. Periodontal diagnosis in the context of the 2017 classification system of periodontal diseases and conditions – implementation in clinical practice. *British Dental Journal* 2019; **226**: 16–22.

Machtei EE, Hausmann E, Dunford R et al. Longitudinal study of predictive factors for periodontal disease and tooth loss. *Journal of Clinical Periodontology* 1999; **26**(6): 374–80.

Tonetti MS, Greenwell H, Kornman KS. Staging and grading of periodontitis: framework and proposal of a new classification and case definition. *Journal of Clinical Periodontology* 2018; **45**(Suppl. 20): S149–S161.

Wadia R, Walter C, Chapple ILC et al. Periodontal diagnosis in the context of the 2017 classification system of periodontal diseases and conditions: presentation of a patient with periodontitis localized to the molar teeth. *British Dental Journal* 2019; **226**: 180–2.

Walter C, Chapple ILC, Ower P et al. Periodontal diagnosis in the context of the 2017 classification system of periodontal diseases and conditions: presentation of a pair of young siblings with periodontitis. *British Dental Journal* 2019a; **226**: 23–6.

Walter C, Ower P, Tank M et al. Periodontal diagnosis in the context of the 2017 classification system of periodontal diseases and conditions: presentation of a middle-aged patient with localized periodontitis. *British Dental Journal* 2019b; **226**: 98–100.

Walter C, Chapple ILC, Ower P et al. Periodontal diagnosis in the context of the 2017 classification system of periodontal diseases and conditions: presentation of a patient with a history of periodontal treatment. *British Dental Journal* 2019c; **226**: 265–7.

Walter C, Chapple ILC, Ower P et al. Periodontal diagnosis in the context of the 2017 classification system of periodontal diseases and conditions: presentation of a patient with severe periodontitis following successful periodontal therapy and supportive periodontal treatment. *British Dental Journal* 2019d; **226**: 411–13.

Chapter 37

Agency for Healthcare Research and Quality (US Department of Health and Human Services). Smoking Cessation Evidence and Resources. www.ahrq.gov/evidencenow/projects/heart-health/evidence/smoking.html

British National Formulary (BNF). Nicotine. https://bnf.nice.org.uk/drugs/nicotine/

Centers for Disease Control and Prevention. Current cigarette smoking among adults in the United States. www.cdc.gov/tobacco/data_statistics/fact_sheets/adult_data/cig_smoking/index.htm

National Institute for Health and Care Excellence (NICE). Tobacco: preventing uptake, promoting quitting and treating dependence. NG209. www.nice.org.uk/guidance/ng209

Office for National Statistics (ONS). Smoking prevalence in the UK and the impact of data collection changes: 2020. www.ons.gov.uk/peoplepopulationandcommunity/healthandsocialcare/drugusealcoholandsmoking/bulletins/smokingprevalenceintheukandtheimpactofdatacollectionchanges/2020

Public Health England. *Delivering Better Oral Health*, 4th edn. www.gov.uk/government/publications/delivering-better-oral-health-an-evidence-based-toolkit-for-prevention

World Health Organization. Tobacco. Key Facts. www.who.int/news-room/fact-sheets/detail/tobacco

Chapter 38

Anazawa T, Okajima H, Masui T, Uemoto S. Current state and future evolution of pancreatic islet transplantation. *Annals of Gastroenterological Surgery* 2019; **3**: 34–42.

Baeza M, Morales A, Cisterna C et al. Effect of periodontal treatment in patients with periodontitis and diabetes: systematic review and meta-analysis. *Journal of Applied Oral Science* 2020; **28**: e20190248.

Diabetes UK. Diabetes diagnoses double in the last 15 years. 2021. www.diabetes.org.uk/about_us/news/diabetes-diagnoses-doubled-prevalence-2021

Di Domenico GL, Minoli M, Discepoli N, Ambrosi A, de Sanctis M. Effectiveness of periodontal treatment to improve glycemic control: an umbrella review. *Acta Diabetologica* 2023; **60**(1): 101–13.

Iacobucci G. One in 10 UK adults could have diabetes by 2030, warns charity. *British Medical Journal* 2021; **375**: n2453.

International Diabetes Federation. *Diabetes Around the World in 2021*, 10th edn. 2021. https://idf.org/aboutdiabetes/what-is-diabetes/facts-figures.html

Nascimento GG, Leite FRM, Vestergaard P, Scheutz F, López R. Does diabetes increase the risk of periodontitis? A systematic review and meta-regression analysis of longitudinal prospective studies. *Acta Diabetologica* 2018; **55**(7): 653–67.

National Diabetes Audit. Report 1: Care Processes and Treatment Targets 2020–21, Full Report. https://digital.nhs.uk/data-and-information/publications/statistical/national-diabetes-audit/core-report-1-2020-21

National Institute of Health and Care Excellence (NICE). 2022a. Periodontal treatment to improve diabetic control in children and young people with type 1 or type 2 diabetes. https://www.nice.org.uk/guidance/ng18/evidence/c-periodontal-treatment-to-improve-diabetic-control-in-children-and-young-people-with-type-1-or-type-2-diabetes-pdf-11129469949. Accessed 3 April 2024.

National Institute of Health and Care Excellence (NICE). 2022b. Periodontal treatment to improve diabetic control in adults with type 1 or type 2 diabetes. https://www.nice.org.uk/guidance/ng17/evidence/d-periodontal-treatment-to-improve-diabetic-control-in-adults-with-type-1-or-type-2-diabetes-pdf-11129467357. Accessed 3 April 2024.

National Institute of Health and Care Excellence (NICE). 2023. Diabetes Type 1 – how common is it? 2023. https://cks.nice.org.uk/topics/diabetes-type-1/background-information/incidence-prevalence/

National Paediatric Diabetes Audit (NPDA). Annual Report 2020–21: Care Processes and Outcomes. www.rcpch.ac.uk/sites/default/files/2022-04/National%20NPDA%20report%202020-21%20Summary%20Report.pdf

Stöhr J, Barbaresko J, Neuenschwander M et al. Bidirectional association between periodontal disease and diabetes mellitus: a systematic review and meta-analysis of cohort studies. *Scientific Reports* 2021; **11**: 13686.

World Health Organization. Classification of diabetes mellitus. 2019. www.who.int/publications/i/item/classification-of-diabetes-mellitus

Chapter 39

Herrera D, Retamal-Valdes B, Alonso B, Feres M. Acute periodontal lesions (periodontal abscesses and necrotizing periodontal diseases) and endo-periodontal lesions. *Journal of Clinical Periodontology* 2018; **45**(Suppl. 20): S78–S94.

Papapanou PN, Sanz M, Buduneli N et al. Periodontitis: consensus report of workgroup 2 of the 2017 World Workshop on the Classification of Periodontal and Peri-Implant Diseases and Conditions. *Journal of Clinical Periodontology* 2018; **45**(Suppl. 20): S162–S170.

Chapter 40

Herrera D, Retamal-Valdes B, Alonso B, Feres M. Acute periodontal lesions (periodontal abscesses and necrotizing periodontal diseases) and endo-periodontal lesions. *Journal of Clinical Periodontology* 2018; **45**(Suppl. 20): S78–S94.

Papapanou PN, Sanz M, Buduneli N et al. Periodontitis: consensus report of workgroup 2 of the 2017 World Workshop on the Classification of Periodontal and Peri-Implant Diseases and Conditions. *Journal of Clinical Periodontology* 2018; **45**(Suppl. 20): S162–S170.

Chapter 41

Caton JG, Armitage G, Berglundh T *et al.* A new classification scheme for periodontal and peri-implant diseases and conditions – introduction and key changes from the 1999 classification. *Journal of Clinical Periodontology* 2018; **45**(Suppl. 20): S1–S8.

Clerehugh V. Periodontal diseases in children and adolescents. *British Dental Journal* 2008; **204**: 469–71.

Clerehugh V, Kindelan S. Guidelines for periodontal screening and management of children and adolescents under 18 years of age. 2021. www.bspd.co.uk/Professionals/Resources/Clinical-Guidelines-and-Evidence-Reviews

Clerehugh V, Lennon MA, Worthington HV. Five-year results of a longitudinal study of early periodontis in 14 to 19-year-old adolescents. *Journal of Clinical Periodontology* 1990; **17**: 702–8.

Clerehugh V, Seymour GJ, Bird PS, Cullinan M, Drucker DB, Worthington HV. The detection of *Actinobacillus actinomycetemcomitans*, *Porphyromonas gingivalis* and *Prevotella intermedia* using an ELISA in an adolescent population with early periodontitis. *Journal of Clinical Periodontology* 1997; **24**: 57–64.

Clerehugh V, Tugnait A, Chapple ILC. *Periodontal Management of Children, Adolescents and Young Adults*. Quintessence, London, 2004.

Hamlet S, Ellwood R, Cullinan M *et al.* Persistent colonisation with *Tannerella forsythensis* and loss of attachment in adolescents. *Journal of Dental Research* 2004; **83**: 232–5.

Lang N, Bartold PM, Cullinan M *et al.* Consensus report: aggressive periodontitis. *Annals of Periodontology* 1999; **4**: 53.

Pitts N, Chadwick B, Anderson T. Child Dental Health Survey 2013. Report 2: Dental Disease and Damage in Children, England, Wales and Northern Ireland. 2015. https://digital.nhs.uk/data-and-information/publications/statistical/children-s-dental-health-survey/child-dental-health-survey-2013-england-wales-and-northern-ireland

Wadia R, Walter C, Chapple ILC *et al.* Periodontal diagnosis in the context of the 2017 classification system of periodontal diseases and conditions: presentation of a patient with periodontitis localized to the molar teeth. *British Dental Journal* 2019; **226**: 180–2.

Walter C, Chapple ILC, Ower P *et al.* Periodontal diagnosis in the context of the 2017 classification system of periodontal diseases and conditions: presentation of a pair of young siblings with periodontitis. *British Dental Journal* 2019; **226**: 23–6.

Chapter 42

Beck JD. Periodontal implications: older adults. *Annals of Periodontology* 1996; **1**: 322–57.

Billings M, Holtfreter B, Papapanou PN, Mitnik GL, Kocher T, Dye BA. Age-dependent distribution of periodontitis in two countries: findings from NHANES 2009 to 2014 and SHIP-TREND 2008 to 2012. *Journal of Clinical Periodontology* 2018; **45**(Suppl. 20): S130–S148.

Clark D, Kotronia E, Ramsay SE. Frailty, aging, and periodontal disease: basic biological considerations *Periodontology 2000* 2021; **87**(1): 143–156.

Fuller E, Steele J, Watt R, Nuttall N. 1: Oral health and function – a report from the Adult Dental Health Survey 2009. 2011. https://files.digital.nhs.uk/publicationimport/pub01xxx/pub01086/adul-dent-heal-surv-summ-them-the1-2009-rep3.pdf

Jones JA, Wehler CJ. The Elders' Oral Health Summit: introduction and recommendations. *Journal of Dental Education* 2005; **69**: 957–60.

Klinge B, Norlund A. A socio-economic perspective on periodontal diseases: a systematic review. *Journal of Clinical Periodontology* 2005; **32**(Suppl. 6): 314–25.

Lopez R, Smith PC, Gostemeyer G, Schwendicke F. Ageing, dental caries and periodontal diseases. *Journal of Clinical Periodontology* 2017; **44**(Suppl. 18): S145–S152.

Papapanou PN, Wennstrom JL, Sellen A, Hirooka H, Grondahl K, Johnsson T. Periodontal treatment needs assessed by the use of clinical and radiographic criteria. *Community Dentistry and Oral Epidemiology* 1990; **18**: 113–19.

Preshaw PM, Henne K, Taylor JJ, Valentine RA, Conrads G. Age-related changes in immune function (immune senescence) in caries and periodontal diseases: a systematic review. *Journal of Clinical Periodontology* 2017; **44**(Suppl. 18): S153–S177.

Wennstrom JL, Papapanou PN, Grondahl K. A model for decision making regarding periodontal treatment needs. *Journal of Clinical Periodontology* 1990; **17**: 217–22.

White D, Pitts N, Steele J, Sadler K, Chadwick B. 2: Disease and related disorders – a report from the Adult Dental Health Survey. 2011. https://files.digital.nhs.uk/publicationimport/pub01xxx/pub01086/adul-dent-heal-surv-summ-them-the2-2009-rep4.pdf

Chapter 43

British Society of Periodontology. Implementing the 2017 Classification of Periodontal Diseases. www.bsperio.org.uk/assets/downloads/111_153050_bsp-flowchart-implementing-the-2017-classification.pdf

Dental Defence Union. Probing deeper into periodontics claims, 2014. www.theddu.com

Dietrich T, Ower P, Tank M *et al.* Periodontal diagnosis in the context of the 2017 classification system of periodontal diseases and conditions – implementation in clinical practice. *British Dental Journal* 2019; **226**: 16–22.

NHS England. Commissioning Standard for Restorative Dentistry, 2019. www.england.nhs.uk/publication/commissioning-standard-for-restorative-dentistry/

Index

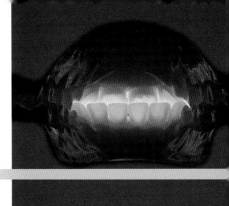

Periodontology at a Glance, Second Edition. Valerie Clerehugh, Aradhna Tugnait, Michael R. Milward, and Iain L. C. Chapple.
© 2024 John Wiley & Sons Ltd. Published 2024 by John Wiley & Sons Ltd.